REFLECTIONS ON THE LANGUAGE AND CULTURE OF DEAF AMERICANS

Louis L. Aymard, Jr.

Christine Winstanley

Anne Arundel Community College

Foreword by McCay Vernon

KENDALL/HUNT PUBLISHING COMPANY
2460 Kerper Boulevard P.O. Box 539 Dubuque, Iowa 52004-0539

We dedicate this book to

Kathy and Roger

whose love and constant encouragement made it possible.

A portion of the royalties from the sale of this book are being donated to the National Association of the Deaf.

List of Credit lines:

Table of Contents

Foreword ix

Preface xi

Acknowledgements xiii

Introduction. xv

Chapter 1: Understanding Hearing Loss
Confronting Deafness in an Unstilled World 3
Harold Orlans
Thought Before Language: A Deaf-mute's Recollections 15
William James
The Newly Deafened 25
Jean A. Mulrooney
Acquired Hearing Loss—Shifting Gears .29
Holly Elliott
Communication: Our Highest Priority 31
Roderick J. MacDonald
Two Views of Deafness 35
Chris Wixtrom

Chapter 2: Historical Foundations of American Sign Language
Notes For A Psycho-history of American Sign Language 39
Harlan Lane
The Value of the Sign Language to the Deaf 49
Edward M. Gallaudet
Thomas Hopkins Gallaudet on Language and Communication: A Reassessment . .55
James J. Fernandes
Laurent Clerc: America's Pioneer Deaf Teacher 63
Loy Golladay
Everyone Here Spoke Sign Language 69
Nora Groce
The Revolution of the Deaf 75
Oliver Sacks

Chapter 3: The Structure of American Sign Language
They Finally Listened 91
Bart Barnes

The Roots of Language in the Sign Talk of the Deaf 93
   Ursula Bellugi and Edward S. Klima
The Facial Behavior of Deaf Signers: Evidence of a Complex Language 99
   Charlotte Baker-Shenk
ASL: Adjective Before Noun or After Noun? 105
   M. J. Bienvenu
The Transparency of Meaning of Sign Language Gestures 109
   Harry W. Hoemann

Chapter 4: Sign Language Systems

Controversy Within Sign Language 119
   McCay Vernon
Signing Exact English 125
   Gerilee Gustason
Seeing Essential English: SEE 129
   David Anthony
An Historical Sketch of the Manual Alphabets 135
   Edward R. Abernathy
Cross-cultural Communication with Foreign Signers: Fact and Fancy 141
   Robbin Battison and I. King Jordan

Chapter 5: Deaf Culture

Inside the Deaf Community 153
   Barbara Kannapell
Name Signs as Identity Symbols in the Deaf Community 157
   Kathryn P. Meadow
Deaf Women: We Were There Too! 163
   Roslyn Rosen
Poetry Without Sound 169
   Edward S. Klima And Ursula Bellugi
Reflections of American Deaf Culture in Deaf Humor 181
   M. J. Bienvenu

Chapter 6: Family Life

The Jaech Family: From Dad with Love 187
   Timothy A. Jaech
Nothing Is Impossible: The Hughes Family 191
   Patty Hughes
Bilingual Experiences of a Deaf Child 195
   Judith Stein Williams
The Empty Crib 199
   Lou Ann Walker
The Deaf Child in Foster Care 205
   M. Teresa Arcari And Beth Gwinn Betman

Chapter 7: Sign Language Interpretation

Being Ignored Can be Bliss: How to Use a Sign Language Interpreter 213
Barbara Fink

You're a What? Interpreter for the Deaf 219
Gallaudet University Public Service Programs

On Guard! 221
Elaine Gardner

Code of Ethics: The Registry of Interpreters for the Deaf 229
The Registry of Interpreters for the Deaf, Inc.

Chapter 8: Resources 233

Organizations, Agencies and Educational Institutions 233

Professional Journals 235

General References on Deafness 236

Classic Titles 236

Current Books 236

Autobiographies, Biographies and Novels 237

Sign Language Books 237

Dictionaries of Signs 238

Texts of American Sign Language Grammar 239

Linguistic Analyses of American Sign Language 239

Books for Children 240

Additional Aids for Sign Language Students 240

Videotapes 240

Sign Language Flash Cards 241

Games 241

Computer Software 242

Telecommunication Devices for the Deaf (TDDs) 242

History And Explanation of the TDD 242

The Personal Computer as a TDD 243

Electronic Signaling Devices 243

Continuing the Study of American Sign Language 244

Chapter Summary 245

Glossary 247

References 251

Article Evaluation Sheet 253

FOREWORD

Authors Aymard and Winstanley's *Reflections on the Language and Culture of Deaf Americans* is a timely, highly readable book which meets what has previously been a huge vacuum in the literature on deafness. The authors have brought to the reader concise, interesting discussions and data on American Sign Language, the culture of deaf people, interpreting issues, and hearing loss. To this solid core of knowledge they add information about resources of value to deaf persons, their families and professionals in the field.

With objectivity and scholarship, the book confronts directly some of the more controversial linguistic and psychological issues in deafness. In doing this, the authors have brought to these concerns not only their own thinking, but that of other recognized scholars in the field.

McCay Vernon, Ph.D.
Professor Emeritus
Western Maryland College
Editor, American Annals of the Deaf,
1969-1990

PREFACE

American Sign Language (ASL), the language of Deaf Americans, is flourishing in a manner undreamed of just a quarter of a century ago. Some linguists estimate ASL is the third most frequently used language in America today. Hundreds of colleges and universities offer credit sign language courses, Sesame Street features it for their preschool viewers and many graduate schools accept fluency in ASL as fulfilling the modern language requirement for doctoral students. From preschool to doctoral levels, the language of Deaf Americans is being valued in significant ways.

Students in colleges and universities are responding to this trend in a heartening manner. They are turning out in record numbers to take sign language classes. At our college, enrollment in credit courses in American Sign Language has increased several hundred percent in the last five years.

Our experience as teachers of ASL and our constant search for better material with which to teach, led us to this project. We discovered many fine dictionaries of signs, but nowhere could we locate a text that gave students a sense of the richness of Deaf Culture, facts about hearing loss, a perspective on the history and structure of American Sign Language and comprehensive re-sources. We discovered numerous articles in the periodic and scientific literature covering a broad spectrum of issues in the field of deafness. After extensive research, we collected these articles into a database of references on the history, culture, and language of Deaf Americans. Secondly, we retrieved and carefully reviewed each article for content, readability, and inherent interest to students. The articles which met these criteria and dealt with the topics often addressed in college-level ASL courses were included in our reader.

This book was originally intended for sign language students only. However, midway through the project, we realized that this information would be valuable for students in speech pathology, linguistics, special education, audiology, social work and psychology. Deaf Americans can be found in nearly every walk of life. Each is linked to the larger society by family, work and friends. Deaf persons deserve to be respected and understood. It is our hope that reading and discussing these articles will enable students to achieve a greater appreciation of the American Deaf Community and their language.

Louis L. Aymard, Jr.
Christine Winstanley

ACKNOWLEDGEMENTS

The publication of a book is seldom the solitary effort of an author. This book emanated from the collective energies of several people who are special to us. We want to acknowledge them for their respective roles in making our publishing dream become a reality. Foremost, we thank our spouses, Kathy and Roger, and our children, Kristin, Marc, Annie and Jacob. They generously shared us on weekends and at other inopportune times when family fun was scheduled. Their love was the source from which we derived the strength to see this project through to completion.

We would also like to thank the students of Anne Arundel Community College for reviewing the manuscript and providing insightful suggestions, especially Sue Seighman who undertook the yeoman's service of collating the original database. A special debt of gratitude is due Robert Ringle for his dedication to the American Sign Language Program at Anne Arundel Community College. The competent, professional staff of the Andrew G. Truxal Library made the research phase of this project less burdensome. They were helpful to us in innumerable ways, particularly Janet Pumphrey who consulted with us about manuscript preparation and publication. Thanks also to our capable editors Joan Albert, Joan Doolittle, Rebecca Kajs and Carol Miller for their patience and incisive reviews of our work.

We were fortunate to work with Jerry Hart and Carol Lucas of Kendall/Hunt Publishing Company, who believed in us and this project from the start. Their wonderful support, assistance with permissions and editorial revisions were invaluable. We appreciate the encouragement we received from friends and colleagues to complete this book. It was a solace to us and the reason we prevailed in difficult times. Last, but by no means least, we are deeply grateful to the authors who graciously granted us permission to reprint the products of their labors. It is our hope that their work will be read widely by students and valued as an outstanding contribution to the field of deafness.

LLA
CW

INTRODUCTION

Reflections on the Language and Culture of Deaf Americans is a book of readings which is intended to supplement a sign language dictionary or text. It is organized around specific themes that relate to content areas as they are taught in sign language classes. This book contains articles, written by deaf and hearing individuals who are well respected in the field. The authors chosen for our book present their ideas and findings with particular skill and clarity.

Chapter 1 is entitled Understanding Hearing Loss. This chapter is an overview of the experience of deafness, contrasting such topics as adventitious and prelingual deafness, mild versus profound hearing loss and the impact of deafness on communication.

In Chapter 2, students are introduced to the writings of the earliest advocates of ASL, who saw this language as the cornerstone of the American Deaf Community. Also included are articles which trace the evolution of attitudes about ASL as a language.

Chapter 3 deals with the structure of American Sign Language. It contains technical articles on the grammar and syntax of ASL. Some of this contemporary research documents the importance of nonmanual features in communicating in sign language.

Summaries of the various systems of Manually Coded English and international sign language are found in Chapter 4. Several of the articles are written by the scholars who developed these systems. Also contained in this chapter is an article which summarizes the controversy surrounding the use of Manually Coded English.

Chapter 5, Deaf Culture, embraces those readings which explore the cultural legacy of deaf persons. This heritage is evidenced in the folklore, theater, dance, and poetry of the Deaf Community.

The articles in Chapter 6, examine deafness in the context of family life. How do members of the family communicate with one another, and how do they relate to the world around them?

Chapter 7 discusses Interpreters and Interpretation in American Sign Language. These articles provide a glimpse into a relatively new profession, and the problems and possibilities therein.

One of the unique features of this book is the resource chapter. Chapter 8 is filled with information regarding organizations and agencies for and by deaf persons and their families. There are also lists of books, journals and videotapes that may be of interest to sign language students. Also included is information on Telecommunication Devices for the Deaf (TDD) and other electronic signaling devices for deaf people.

Lastly, we have added a glossary which contains definitions and clarifications of terms commonly found in the field of sign language and deafness. It was developed to help students define some of the technical language found in the articles in this book.

Reflections on the Language and Culture of Deaf Americans presents the beginning sign language student with a broad spectrum of topics, and therefore will enhance students' general understanding of the richness and the complexity of the American Deaf Community and its language. It is our hope that this book will also fill a void in the market of available sign language texts.

Chapter 1

Understanding Hearing Loss

Deafness has been likened to a glass wall which separates people. It is an invisible handicap which has a significant impact upon human interaction. If we are denied the experience of expressing ourselves and understanding others, we become isolated cells in the society in which we live. Deafness affects more than a person's ability to hear, it influences human communication in a profound way.

The loss of hearing can occur at any stage in the course of human development. An auditory loss that is inherited or develops *in utero* is referred to as congenital deafness. When the hearing loss is so severe that the young child cannot process speech sounds, the development of oral language is significantly altered. Even with a hearing aid, these profoundly deaf infants will not acquire spoken language without specific and intensive training. They are, however, able to develop language naturally if it is presented visually. American Sign Language is the visual language used by most Deaf Americans.

Some infants who acquire deafness genetically often have deaf parents or other deaf family members who use American Sign Language. If all the members of the family use ASL, this language is passed on to the child visually, just as spoken language is transmitted through auditory means to the hearing child. Other deaf infants are born to parents who may not be skilled in the use of sign language. In these cases, the young child is often left with the task of acquiring language without the benefit of visual or manual cues.

Not all hearing loss occurs at birth. Adventitious deafness is the loss of hearing due to accident, illness or complications of an unknown etiology. When a hearing loss occurs later in life, usually the individual has already mastered a native language. The adventitiously deaf person must make many adjustments and face new frustrations when communicating with family and friends.

The degree and time of onset of a hearing loss are critical to the type of adjustment an individual makes. A person who experiences a sudden, severe hearing loss at age twenty or thirty will need to make comprehensive changes in the routine of daily life. A profound hearing loss in a young child of two or three will change that child's entire life and all those who are close to him or her. However, a mild hearing loss late in life may require only minor modifications of lifestyle.

The articles in this chapter are accounts of the authors' personal struggles with the loss of hearing. They provide a basis for understanding hearing loss and its pervasive impact upon interpersonal communication.

Confronting Deafness in an Unstilled World

Harold Orlans

"Man was born free, and he is everywhere in chains." With this call in *The Social Contract,* Rousseau may be said to have launched the Romantic, not to mention the French, Revolution. To Rousseau, society was the enemy: convention, ostentation, the clever chatter in the salons was false; society constrained the freedom of the individual to live and speak honestly and virtuously, just as chains then constrained the residents of mental institutions. The theme of society and the individual dominates the experience of deafened adults; but to most, society is paradise lost, the false friend who betrays and ejects them from their accustomed place. As their sense of exclusion grows, they may come to feel, like Rousseau, that society is indeed the enemy and that peace can be found only in solitude.

The adjustment of adults to progressive hearing loss can be viewed as a conflict between their drive for continued sociability and their need for the relief that solitude offers from the tensions and blows that sociability now brings. I shall review some of the common feelings about and adjustments to hearing losses of varied severity and age of onset reported by some 1,500 members of Self Help for Hard of Hearing People (SHHH), the large American voluntary organization of hearing-impaired persons. Their accounts were obtained by a four-page questionnaire inserted in the January-February 1984 issue of *Shhh,* the bimonthly magazine distributed to all SHHH members. I will try, in part, to summarize these comments and, in part, to depict and interpret the emotional and social dynamics of increasing deafness in formerly hearing persons, as reflected in this material. All unidentified quotations in this

article are drawn from these questionnaires, and each in a series of quoted passages represents a different individual.

Most quotations come from responses to five open-ended questions: "How has your hearing loss affected your personal life (e.g., family, social life, leisure activities)? How has your hearing loss affected your working life? Who and what has best helped you adjust to your hearing loss (e.g., spouse, friend, hearing aid)? What could be done to help you now? We welcome any other comments you wish to make about your hearing loss and any suggestions you have for SHHH activities or articles." Only one page was allotted to replies, but many members attached additional pages of comment; some even enclosed a copy of their audiogram.

The questionnaire was prepared jointly with Kathryn P. Meadow-Orlans, Research Scientist at Gallaudet University, in cooperation with SHHH President Rocky Stone and Vice President Patricia Clickener. Michael Karchmer, Susan King, and other staff of the Gallaudet Research Institute undertook the computer programming and statistical analyses; the project was authorized by Raymond Trybus, Dean of the Institute, and financed by Gallaudet.

Questionnaires were received from 1,670 persons, 28 percent of the 6,000 SHHH members. Seventy respondents (audiologists, teachers, counselors, and other professionals working with hearing-impaired persons or family members of a hearing-impaired person) had normal hearing. The number and quality of responses to specific questions varied: 1,518 persons replied to the question about the effects of hearing loss on their personal life, 1,415 to the question about its effects on their work, and 1,069 offered suggestions for SHHH activities. The average age of respondents was sixty-two; 30 percent were seventy or older and only 11 percent, under forty; 62 percent (and 70 percent of those under sixty) were women. In this preponderately elderly, female population, only 22 percent were employed full-time and another 9 percent, part-time; 48 percent were retired; 18 percent classified themselves as housewives and 5 percent, as unemployed.

Most respondents had a major hearing loss. The difficulty of assessing the severity of loss by a series of graduated questions (the Gallaudet Hearing Scale) was evident; nonetheless, as estimated by this method, which a good many respondents criticized, 53 percent had a loss of 56 decibels or more and another 34 percent, of 41-55 decibels, in their better ear. Nineteen percent said that they had lost some or all of their hearing by the age of nine or earlier; and from 11-14 percent, during each succeeding decade (their teens, their twenties, and so on, up to and including their sixties).

These SHHH members are heavy users of hearing aids: 89 percent owned one or, more often, two, and most wore one or both "all the time." The remaining 11 percent included some with a small loss and some who refused to wear an aid, but most were evidently too deaf to benefit from one and some could not endure the excruciating noise.

From all the evidence provided, Kathryn Meadow-Orlans and I attempted to assess the adjustment—the degree of personal acceptance and contentment or bitterness, anger, and dissatisfaction—of each respondent. Of the 1,388 persons we ventured to classify, we judged the adjustment of 33 percent to be "poor," 31 percent as "good," and 36 percent as intermediate or average. On a five-point scale, we classified the adjustment of 7 percent as "very poor"; 26 percent, "poor"; 36 percent, "average"; 23 percent, "good"; and 8 percent, "very good." The proportion classified as "poor" was higher among women, those with a severe loss, and those who were divorced or separated as compared with those who were either living with their spouse or widowed. Relatively fewer of the oldest respondents (those over seventy) were classified as poorly adjusted: old age brought a greater degree of either peace or weariness and a disinclination or inability to protest.

Undetected Loss

Hearing loss is not only invisible, a fact often lamented as adding the burden of disclosure to that of the condition. It may go undetected by those with the loss. Adults who suffer a sudden loss are, at least, inescapably aware of that traumatic event. If awareness is the first step in the long process of adjustment, that step is thrust upon them. It would follow, as some argue, that their adjustment is earlier or, at any rate, quicker than it is for the person with a gradual loss. Both the theoretical point and the empirical facts are debatable. One can also argue that a great deal of adjustment proceeds unconsciously and that the perfect marriage between consciousness and reality exists only in the minds of some intellectuals.

Certainly, some hearing loss can go undetected at all ages: in infants and children, because they have never experienced any other kind of hearing, and in adults, because their loss is so slight it can be misinterpreted. After all, to miss a word, especially in a noisy place, is entirely normal. Who can hear anything in a disco? Many people with a "good" ear live so completely in the hearing world that they are seldom considered, and do not consider themselves, "impaired."

If hearing impairment is the most prevalent disease [one respondent writes], I wonder why I meet so few who have it. I go to a spa, to classes, to clubs. Occasionally someone says he or she is hard of hearing, but there is either no hearing aid or a dainty behind-the-ear model and you don't even have to raise your voice. Where are all those people, in hiding?

The answer is that most have a loss that is functionally insignificant. If the line between an insignificant and a significant loss is drawn between "having difficulty only with faint speech" and "frequent difficulty with normal speech" (which the National Center for Health Statistics places between the 40 and 41 decibel levels), in 1981 roughly 3.1 million or 1.5 percent of the United States population had such "frequent difficulty," while over 11 million or 5 percent had a lesser loss in one or both ears. Thus, the population with some hearing loss fades into the hearing population much as the population with some loss of hair fades into the population with a full head of hair.

That is both the opportunity and the aggravation of adults who, as puzzling episodes, miscues, and misadventures mount, finally realize that something may be wrong with their hearing. "I couldn't figure out how the other kids heard what they did," a twenty-two-year-old girl, who evidently had some hearing loss since infancy, writes: "after high-school graduation, it 'clicked' in my mind." Similarly, a girl of twenty, also with an early loss, for many years "didn't realize how much I was missing." How can you know everything that you do not hear?

Passing and Bluffing

A loss not noticed by the person who has it can also be overlooked by friends and family, who may attribute the nonresponsiveness they observe to personality, not physiology. "During school years, before I *knew*, I had a hearing loss, my friends always complained that I was stuck up and thought I was better than anyone. They said I never answered them when they spoke to me!"

Passing, or being taken, for someone with normal hearing but not normal conduct— "unfriendly, uncooperative, stupid, no personality" —is common. Indeed, it is unavoidable in casual encounters in public places, crowds, and social gatherings; for, whether a hearing aid is worn or not, few people are as alert to the presence of hearing loss as the person who has it; and the opportunity to disclose it may not arise. Thus, be it vigilant or, as the years go by, dulled and weary, the deafened person's passage through the hearing world, oblivious to much that transpires, is characteristically guarded and uncertain, hoping to avoid but necessarily encountering pitfalls, surprises, misunderstanding, error, frustrations, irritation, embarrassment, pain, puzzlement, and a simple lack of comprehension. Surprise, irritation, and puzzlement can be experienced both by the person who hears and the one who does not.

A condition that is not anticipated, that can go undetected, and, if detected, cannot be quickly, precisely, and fully known, invites further disguise:

Have become an excellent bluffer.

I used every cover-up known! The only ones who suspected were my children.

I'm apt to laugh in response to [the movie] audience rather than what I've heard and comprehended.

I am one of the greatest hypocrites in pretending that I can hear or understand.

In most social situations I resided in my glass coffin, putting up an appearance. . . . I appeared pretty, neat, and smiling.

I wear two "faces" —one usually has a smile and has been described as vibrant—the other is bewildered.

Grin and act pleasant.

Smile a lot! Look pleasant!

The anthropologist Ruth Benedict, author of *Patterns of Culture*, often wore that smile, as if to ward off or soften the annoyance that might arise from her failure to reply to what she did not hear.

The difficulties and perplexities of not understanding what one is assumed to hear, may, it is said, be relieved by a public declaration of hearing loss. That is one function of the visible hearing aid, of signing, of the pin or other symbol which is often suggested and sometimes worn, and of the individual signs and notices that deaf or deafened persons sometimes use: one woman wears a "Deaf and Bright" button; another, a pin, "I READ LIPS."

A public declaration can relieve only the misconception that one hears well; it does not explain how a conversation should proceed thereafter and exactly what will and will not be grasped. To determine that requires familiarity, frankness, and close and patient attention. The normal pace of conversation must be slowed, which does not happen in a crowd; and if it does, in a smaller group or party, the deafened person can become the center of unwanted attention.

> I . . . often resisted even to attempt conversation because of the awful result when I lost the topic, and said something irrelevant because I misunderstood. When, worse yet, the group realized I wasn't hearing and several people at once attempted to tell me what was said, resulting in a loud jumble, and me still not understanding. At this point I would "freeze," pretend [to understand], and retreat as unobtrusively as possible, figuratively licking my wounds.

Noisy Groups

To deafened adults, noisy places—gatherings, parties, dances, playgrounds, stores, restaurants and bars, any busy unshielded place with a hubbub of voices, traffic, machines, or music—are a hostile setting for conversation. The quieter the place, the fewer the voices, the closer and clearer the speaker, the easier is it to converse by lipreading, partial hearing, and careful speech. The hearing aid, which magnifies background noise and nearby speech alike, can be a mixed blessing when ears register only distorted sound, recruitment (the intense magnification of sound) renders loud noise unendurable, and tinnitus (a noise in

the ears) adds its distressing accompaniment. Thus, the adult with a growing hearing loss tends increasingly to forsake group socializing and to see only a few people or one person at a time in a quiet location.

This tendency may be altered or delayed with a moderate loss well corrected by a hearing aid, good lipreading ability, a strong, confident personality adept at handling people, or simply persistence, a determination to continue social activity despite inescapable blunders and blows. The comments of three respondents, all relatively young women in their twenties to forties, illustrate this attitude:

> I have two choices . . . to continue going out and do normal things and to try extra hard to get along . . . or . . . to stay away from people. To me there is only one choice.

> My hearing aids help some, but mostly [it takes] sheer determination to not hide. Constantly reminding myself that I'm a person too and I have the right to work and enjoy life the same as anyone else.

> I try not to moan about my hearing loss or feel defeated. If someone isn't speaking loud enough, I say "Please speak up—I'm hearing impaired!" No apologies from me! . . . I am not going to withdraw from life because of feelings of embarrassment.

Straining to Socialize

Socializing imposes a physical and emotional strain. The concentration required to diagnose the meaning of distorted, half-heard speech, other sounds, lip movements, and facial expressions is tiring; requests to repeat or to face the listener can be made just so often and shy people may not make them at all; attempts to position oneself closer to speakers and to look at their lips may make them uncomfortable and disturb the conversation.

> I believe I am a source of annoyance to people who must repeat what they have said.

I am very intelligent and articulate but feel dumb when I ask to repeat and even then I don't understand what is said so I just let it pass.

If you ask people to speak up repeatedly and they don't, then you try and move your ear closer to their mouth; they draw away, as if you have a contagious disease, or else they are stymied by my staring at their lips.

Inappropriate remarks, talking too much or too little, too loudly or softly, a hearing aid that whistles or crackles or is often adjusted can upset the flow of conversation and reduce the pleasure of the occasion. When socializing is not relaxing but becomes an ordeal— "I'm terrified that someone will talk to me and terrified that no one will talk to me" —and the deafened person feels embarrassed or lost in the midst of the group, he or she may wonder if it is really worth the effort:

Seems like one can never relax when with others.

It is very stressful for me to mix with hearing people.

I have to look at people's faces and never know in what direction the next person's going to speak. I am exhausted after group meetings.

People become annoyed at having to repeat themselves, and I become embarrassed when I misunderstand what was said. . . . in such situations I often say something that had previously been stated. Many people find it amusing, and I usually laugh along with them even though I am feeling embarrassed or frustrated.

Miss "small talk" and jokes. Therefore feel left out. . . .

Discomfort, embarrassment, confusion, and loss of confidence are common. "Embarrassed times without number." "I don't always know how to handle it [misunderstanding]." "I have lost confidence and social comfort." It "has resulted in a lack of confidence, feelings of inadequacy and extreme sensitivity." "Confidence and

ease have been replaced with anxiety and apprehension."

Resentment and anger can grow. "I resent very much being deaf." "I get angry over the insensitivity of people who don't understand hearing loss." "I was very anxious, frustrated, angry, embarrassed and humiliated." A married woman of fifty-five, a secretary who is apparently well adjusted, acknowledges "a great sense of anger at my situation. Actually I function very well; most people are not aware that I wear an aid. . . . But I am still angry since my loss is not my fault, and I expect consideration for this."

Feelings and concomitant behavior may swing between a determination to persevere and overcome the obstacles to social activity; anxiety or frustration, the fear or experience of failure in that effort; and withdrawal to rest and recuperate.

I want to withdraw and have to push myself to attend social functions.

Sometimes I stay at home for a while and then get up enough courage to go out and face life again and try not to let it bother me.

I go between painfully shy and overcompensating aggressiveness.

How [do] people weigh whether doing something is worth the energy (of trying to hear) to participate[?] . . . some people pull back too soon and maybe others frustrate themselves by doing too much.

Selective Socializing

In ventures into society, the individual becomes more selective. Smaller groups with friends who "know" are preferred to large gatherings with strangers. Visiting may be undertaken only with one's spouse or a friend, who can repeat a remark, correct a mistake, or keep one abreast of the conversation. Small parties at home, where the number of guests, seating, and lighting can be controlled, may replace attendance at large gatherings. Conversation with strangers is avoided: "I am afraid of being asked something I won't hear so I avoid eye contact and people in general whenever I can. . . . My worst times are with casual 'How are you doing?' . . . I don't relax, joke, smile, and enjoy people."

Friends who recognize the hearing problem and show patience in dealing with it are retained, while others are dropped. "I pick friends . . . I can lipread well." "I avoid people who are irritated by requests to repeat a phrase." "I catch myself avoiding . . . people with soft light voices." ". . . selected a husband because of loud voice." "Those friends who understand my problem and I enjoy a good social life. I *refuse* to let my hearing loss make me an introvert." "When choosing friends, I'm very careful. . . . My best friends understand my hearing problems. In a way, I *don't* want too many friends."

Even a small group of understanding friends can present hazards. As they turn to talk to each other, the deafened individual is left out: "In a group, the interaction they have between one another causes them to forget or choose to ignore my hearing loss." "My friends have been good to me, but at times forget my hearing problem and get me into situations . . . where I cannot function properly."

As deafness grows, socializing may be reduced to one-on-one encounters, to life within the home and family, to dependence on the spouse, or, ultimately, to utter solitude. Some may seek the company of other deafened people, which is more easily done in urban than in rural areas. Some want to learn lipreading, fingerspelling, and/or signing, partly as a means of communication and partly to meet other people with similar problems. It may be difficult to find an instructor, to get enough people together to justify a class, and also to induce a spouse or relative to learn so that there is someone with whom to practice and communicate. Also, after a lifetime spent in hearing society, most have no wish to sign. They would rather remain isolated in the society they have known than enter a new one.

Prospects of Solitude

At each stage in this gradual removal from hearing society, the prospect of solitude emerges, either as a desolate state or as a condition which, if not as idyllic as Rousseau's in *Reveries of the Solitary Walker,* is at least relaxing and preferable to the constant pains of contending with people who think that you hear. Upon occasion, each feeling may prevail, as the individual struggles with himself, not knowing which course is best, perhaps not knowing the kind of person he or she has already become. As time goes by, the extrovert can become an introvert, the partygoer stays increasingly at home, and the socializer turns into a loner.

> When I had my hearing I was an outgoing person. I don't care to be with people any more.

> I have become more isolated, personality changes from a fun loving type to a more skeptical person, less willing to confront rejection.

> I avoid socializing and going out. It's too painful to sit there and be left out. . . . I'd rather stay home—alone!

> It's a *lonely* disease. My love of people, and being with them, diminishes daily.

> I tend to enjoy being with myself, because it is easier.

> I am least alone when I am alone. Most alone at a dinner or cocktail party.

The saddest condition portrayed in our responses is that of some very deafened elderly persons, usually but not always living alone. They desperately want some human contact but no longer know how to obtain it. Thus, a woman of seventy-three, a former public school teacher, widowed twice, now lives by herself in a city apartment. Her hearing loss began at age sixty-three; one ear is now "useless"; she wears an aid in the other but cannot make out words: "I cannot communicate with people—it takes so long—trying to comprehend, their point. . . . Learning *anything* is not easy at my age. I'm alone—no one to try to talk to, no one to say *'you are too loud!'* etc. I can't understand T.V., so I keep it on to feel that someone is with me." A man of sixty-five, recently retired from work as a draftsman, lives with a wife who is apparently considerate and understanding. His hearing loss began at twenty-eight; despite two aids, he can now barely hear loud noises: "I am very despondent and wonder if life is worth living. . . . I don't feel even a psychiatrist can help me. . . . I am ready and waiting for God to take me out of my miseries and know that when I get up to heaven I'll be able to hear." An eighty-nine-year-old woman, whose long, gradual loss started at eighteen, is now so profoundly deaf that she does not use her aid— "Too noisy. Sounds like an iron foundry." Never married, she lives alone:

> My greatest need is more companionship. There is an *awfulness* about silence. If someone would just drop in once in a while—smile—say Hi! and hand me a note "I'm on my way to the store—do you need anything? Postage stamps? Could I make a phone call for you?" etc. My only female neighbor said "I could visit you oftener but I haven't time to sit down and write." Understandable, isn't it? I am days at a time without speaking a word. It is affecting my voice and I fear for my mind. I can't hear the alarm clock, telephone ring, door bell, radio, television—or the human voice. . . . HAVE SOMEONE CROSS THE THRESHOLD OF THE SHUT-IN . . . EVERY DAY.

Family Accord and Discord

As the case of the despondent husband may suggest, even a good marriage and loving family give no immunity from the pains of deafness. Deafened people can find refuge and comfort at home, where family members are sympathetic, familiar with the condition—here, at least, they do not have to announce it—and can cater to special needs. Some adults whose families have an established history of hearing loss (with either an early or late onset) seem to be among our better

adjusted respondents. Living with hearing loss and expecting it themselves, members of such families may take it for granted, like poor eyesight, obesity, or other defects that "run in the family." "My hearing loss never affected my personal life because my mother taught me just what a hearing loss meant," a woman of sixty-seven, with an 80 decibel hearing level in her better ear, writes: "She was developing her hearing loss when I was born so I had no fear when I was hearing less at age twenty-five." A librarian with a moderate hearing loss, who hears fairly well with an aid, says, "five of my children have hearing loss so we all understand each other."

As other respondents attest, hearing loss in the family affords no assurance of a satisfactory adjustment. Obvious maladjustment and an inability to accept and cope with the loss can be shared by several family members and passed from parent to child. Far more information than is available would be needed to allocate responsibility for family discord. Some respondents accept primary responsibility; some blame their spouse or relatives; plainly, all parties can contribute. The same battles that are waged in public—for respect, understanding, accommodation, acceptance, and participation—can be fought at home. Familiarity can breed either sensitivity or contempt.

Respondents complain about family members' "mumbling," talking from another room or over background music, and their impatience or anger at not being understood and having to repeat what they said. Respondents acknowledge similar feelings of frustration, impatience, and anger.

> My own husband talks to me from another room or with his back to me. My own mother forgets that I am deaf.

> With my family it's a constant conflict between their desire to have background music and my desire to join in conversation.

> I felt he [her husband] mumbled and he felt I didn't pay attention when he was talking.

After 10 years, my wife cannot make allowance for my inability to hear her from another room.

My husband gets mad because I can't hear, and I get angry because he can't remember to look at me when talking to me.

On the humorous side: My husband will sometimes *yell*: "Are you deaf?" I yell back: "YES!"

Even a spouse who is usually patient and considerate, "an in-house saint," can at times be curt and impatient. Hearing as well as deafened persons can get weary of conversation that requires close attention and careful enunciation. When family members talk to one another, deafened people can feel as left out as if they were at someone else's party. In the family as in society, good conversation with them must be one-on-one or, at least, one at a time.

If only my family . . . would try a little harder to make me feel more comfortable—sitting one to one for instance, but they'd all rather sit around the living room and converse among themselves.

My worst problem is my husband's family—they all have very tiny soft voices—a nightmare! They don't seem to speak up no matter how often I remind them, so the past year I've been practicing "not caring" what they say unless they make a point to speak clearly and directly to me—it was (is) too frustrating to rush from one side of the room to the other trying to catch every word!

My family and long time friends are supportive, but it is inconvenient to include me in most communication. My pad and pencil slow them down.

My large family has a reunion at Thanksgiving. I feel like an outcast. They try so hard to include me but the quick repartee is impossible.

Reflective respondents recognize that adjustment in the family is an intricate, interactive process requiring accommodations on both sides of the sound barrier. "There has been more ad-justment needed for my family than me," observes a man who hears well with an aid. "They are the ones who must speak up to be heard." One woman complains that "My family always wanted me to wear my hearing aid for THEIR convenience" and another that "My parents treated me normal. I think *too* normal." It is evident that excessive sensitivity and moodiness—defining expected conduct too strictly and changing that definition too often—can be obstacles to successful adjustment in the family.

What Help Do Deafened Adults Want?

Responses to the question, "What could be done to help you now?" evoked comments such as "new ears," "a medical cure," "give me my hearing back," "Miracle!" "some miracle to stop the progression of loss!" "Outlaw mustaches and dark or mirror sunglasses and send hard to lipread people to Beirut!" "Nothing," "I don't really know," "a long walk on a short pier."

In a more serious vein, respondents hope for research, medical treatment, or surgery to prevent hearing loss, restore their hearing, or at least arrest further loss; and for effective relief from tinnitus. Some have had repeated operations and a few, cochlear implants; some have doctored themselves with medications, including niacin and zinc, vitamins, special diets, and dubious regimes to promote fitness, increase the flow of blood, and "clear the ears." The hearing aid receives much comment. It is "my lifesaver," "my dearest possession," "my crutch," "my friend and my enemy." "I sometimes fantasize about smashing them on the ground to relieve the frustrations they cause." The frustrations include amplified noise, distorted and "artificial" sound, feedback, the expense of purchase and maintenance, short-lived batteries, unreliable operation, and slow and unreliable repair service. Respondents would like cheaper, better, and directional aids that clarify speech, amplify only selective frequencies, and screen out background noise, loud sounds, and such noises as rustling clothing and paper; some want waterproof aids that can be worn while swimming. The volume control should work more simply, quickly, and inconspicuously. Ear molds should fit comfortably and not cause pain or tenderness, rashes, swelling, seepage, or perspiration.

Reimbursement for hearing aids under medicare and medical insurance, and the subsidization of—at least the removal of taxes on—aids, amplified telephones, and other assistive devices would help many deafened persons, especially those who are unemployed, retired, have high medical expenses, and live only on social security benefits. The better regulation of hearing-aid dealers and of audiologists who dispense only one manufacturer's products is also requested.

Most respondents use telephones with a loud ring and volume control, but some cannot obtain them or object to the added charges. The court-ordered breakup of the American Telephone and Telegraph Company has led to a proliferation of instruments, some of poor quality and not compatible with a hearing aid. Many respondents are poorly informed about such devices as the telephone switch on a hearing aid or the use of a tape recorder to play back messages or have them transcribed.

The provision and clear signposting of more amplified phones in offices, public facilities, and motel rooms is often requested. Those who cannot use a phone ask for message services or teletypewriters, especially at hospitals and police and fire stations. The increasing use of word processors and home computers that can be linked to telephone lines may soon provide broader communication, to those who can afford it, than that available with teletypewriters.

Respondents want more audio loops and infrared sound systems installed in theaters, churches, and meeting halls; visual signals and notices to augment loudspeaker announcements in airports, planes, buses, schools, and so on; more and better captioned films and television programs (and superscripts in theaters, such as those at Sydney opera house performances). The video cassette recorder offers a new way to view captioned films and educational programs.

Many hope for the elimination of noise and blaring commercials on television and the omnipresent background "music" in films, elevators, telephones, and restaurants; plainly, under a dictatorship of the deaf, juke boxes and Muzak would be extirpated. A suggestion many hearing people would welcome is the establishment of quiet sections, comparable to "no smoking" areas, in restaurants, bars, and other public places.

Half of our respondents had some assistive device besides an aid and amplified telephone: the most common were captioned television, a teletypewriter, a signal light on the doorbell or alarm clock, a vibrator alarm, and television or radio earphones. Few had an audio loop or broadcasting system. Many knew little about these and other devices, but would like to learn and to try them out. Even some severely deafened faculty at Gallaudet University, with its many special provisions for assisting the communication of deafened persons, have been surprised at how much better they can hear with a loudspeaker and loop. A service displaying a range of hearing aids, telephones, and other instruments; providing information about their quality, cost, benefits, and limitations; enabling the equipment to be examined and tried out; and helping to install and maintain it would be of significant help to deafened persons.

Stricter enforcement of laws barring employment discrimination against handicapped persons is mentioned by relatively few respondents (only a minority were working); evidently still fewer consider it likely or practicable. Although many jobs can be reorganized so that a deafened person can perform them well without having to use the telephone or talk with clients, respondents evidently feel that, because the cooperation of their employer and workmates is required, this is best done voluntarily.

Requests are made for help in finding: good, secure jobs; good audiologists, surgeons, and hearing aid dealers; instruction in lip reading, signing, and cued speech; penpals; "singles" services to locate friends and companions of the opposite sex; and tour groups and clubs for hearing-impaired persons.

Discovering SHHH and reading its bimonthly magazine have given many people comfort and help, a sense of dignity, and a feeling that they are, at last, understood and not alone. Often the magazine is also read by family members and friends, and the information in an article (for example, on how to talk to a deafened person) may be photocopied and distributed to others. Our questionnaires abound in comments such as "I can not state often enough the help your organization has been to me in adjusting to my handicap." "The SHHH organization and journals have given me much joy and encouragement, as well as information." "SHHH is a real inspiration and help." "Just knowing there are so many other people going through what I am gives me the courage to carry on with hope." Members also benefit from joining local SHHH chapters and meeting others with similar hearing problems.

Their comments also indicate that it is difficult for a single organization of volunteers, with low dues and very modest resources, to serve the needs of all hearing-impaired persons, whose conditions, circumstances, age, education, income, and interests differ so greatly. Young persons want to meet other young people; some members are, and others are not, sophisticated about technical and policy issues; some are affluent and others, poor; some do, and others do not, hear fairly well with an audio loop. A few sign but most do not and, in some chapters, conflict has developed between the two groups. Sadly, some persons go to a SHHH meeting and come away having heard, lip-read, and understood very little.

Educating the Public

Everyone, it seems, wants to inform and educate the public, their family, their friends. They want them to know how to talk to them; to understand that a hearing aid does not enable the wearer to hear normally; to realize that they are not stupid, that only their hearing, not intelligence, is impaired and that otherwise they are ordinary, normal people who, with patience, consideration, and some practical help, can function well at work and at home. Even doctors, audiologists, psychologists, the staff of retirement and nursing homes, and teachers of the deaf, some respondents say, have much to learn about dealing with hearing-impaired persons.

> Everyone talks too fast. Tell the whole world to talk slower and more distinct.

> Public servants, clerks, waitresses, etc., think that just because you have a hearing aid you can hear.

> Educate all of the people with whom I have contact—family, friends, other social groups—about the aspects of deafness that I call psychological, physiological. Most audiologists, and all doctors, that I have had need this education.

It would be splendid if everyone could be thus educated, but most unlikely. The hectic pace, the appalling noise and clatter of urban life will not stop and few people will change their normal style of conversation because three in two hundred have "frequent difficulty" hearing and one in a thousand may say so. The public will not and cannot learn everything that every sect and party, every organization and interest group, would like them to, anymore than they can buy everything that advertisers would like them to.

Help and Self-Help

Abstract knowledge is not enough for incorporating hearing-impaired persons—or those who want to be incorporated—into hearing society. Social scientists tend to make too much of abstract knowledge, the "laws" and generalizations they formulate. Personal experience, rapport, perceptiveness, patience, and sympathy are vital. Can we teach a busy, selfish, insensitive person—hearing well or poorly—to be patient, sympathetic, and sensitive? One woman writes, "My husband will never understand my loss," and another, "My husband is unbelievably understanding—he doesn't even notice when he has to repeat something three times!" Can we teach understanding and affection?

To the question, "Who and what has helped you to adjust to your hearing loss?" too many people reply, "I don't think we ever really adjust," "I shall *never* completely adjust," "I am still . . . trying to adjust." A twenty-two-year-old woman says, "God, mostly. I never have to ask Him to speak up."

In recounting the responses of SHHH members to their hearing loss, I do not mean to suggest that all deafened persons follow the same path from sociability to an unhappy or contented soli-

tude. Certainly, many do; some—either with a mild, well-corrected loss or with a severe loss and remarkable lipreading ability and character—remain socially active; and some oscillate between the poles of sociability and solitude. One-to-one conversation is the fulcrum on which the deafened adult's adjustment hinges and a spouse or relative often serves as the indispensable partner in that adjustment.

If the spouse's commitment can be critical to a successful adjustment, so is the deafened person's resolve. "Who . . . has helped you to adjust?" A common reply is *"me!"* "myself," "my willpower," "The Lord and myself," "what there has been has been by myself" "I feel that I myself have been the best help, because no one could do that for me." Nothing can be added to that simple truth.

Thought Before Language: A Deaf-Mute's Recollections

William James

On page 266 of the first volume of my work *The Principles of Psychology*, I quoted an account of a certain deaf-mute's thoughts before he had the use of any signs for verbal language. The deaf-mute in question is Mr. Melville Ballard, of the Institution for the Deaf and Dumb at Washington; and his narrative shows him to have had a very extensive command of abstract, even of metaphysical conceptions, when as yet his only language was pantomime confined to practical home affairs. Professor von Gizycki of Berlin, whose nominalistic prepossessions were apparently startled by Mr. Ballard's account, wrote to me to ask if I had made sure of his being trustworthy. This led me to make inquiry amongst those who knew Mr. Ballard intimately, and the result was to show that they all regarded him as an exceptionally good witness.[1] Mr. Fay (the gist of whose statement about Mr. Ballard I print below) was kind enough to refer me to another printed account of a deaf-mute's cosmological ideas before the acquisition of language; and this led me to correspond with its author, Mr. Theophilus H. d'Estrella, instructor in drawing (I understand) at the California Institution for the Deaf and Dumb, and the Blind. The final result is that I have Mr. D'Estrella's permission to lay before the readers of the PHILOSOPHICAL REVIEW a new document which, whilst it fully tends to corroborate Mr. Ballard's narrative, is much more interesting by its intrinsic content.[2]

---

1   Professor Samuel Porter (who first published Mr. Ballard's statement in the Princeton Review for January, 1881) says: "I regard him as a person quite remarkable for the clearness and accuracy of his recollection of matters of fact, especially such as have occurred under his own observation or in his own experience, and as scrupulously honest and truthful. Indeed his traits of character, both intellectual and moral, are such that I cannot conceive of a case in which testimony of the kind in question could be less open to suspicion and objection."—Mr. Edward Allen Fay writes: "Mr. Ballard is an exceptionally conscientious person in making statements. There is nobody whose testimony with respect to any facts of which he might have knowledge I should more readily accept than his. I place implicit confidence in his honesty as a witness. Is it possible that he is himself deceived, and that, as Prof. V.G. suggests, he 'verlegt sein jetziges gebildetes Denken in die Seele jenes Kindes zurück?' I suppose it is possible, but it does not seem to me probable. His recollection of those early years is so distinct, he recalls so vividly other circumstances which are directly associated with the train of thought described, and about which there could be no mistake, that I am compelled to accept his statement as 'unconditionally trustworthy'"—Mr. J.C. Gordon says: "Mr. B. is peculiarly qualified to relate incidents interesting to him in the order in which they originally occurred, and with extreme accuracy. His perceptions are acute, and his power of recollection of facts within the range of his experience I consider quite extraordinary. He is not a great student of books, and probably has no idea of the bearing of his statements on metaphysical speculations."

2   Mr. W. Wilkinson, Superintendent of the Institution, writes to me of Mr. d'Estrella that "he is a man of the highest character and intellectual honesty. He was the first pupil that ever entered this Institution, and when I took charge of the school in 1865 he was about fourteen years old. It was at that time that I became specially interested in his account of his explanations of the various physical phenomena as they presented themselves to his untutored mind. At that time I wrote

The printed account just referred to appeared in the *Weekly News* (a paper published at the Institution at Berkeley, California, and printed by the pupils) for April 27, 1889. Although expressed in the third person, Mr. d'Estrella informs me that it was prepared by himself. I give it here as it stands, in the form of a note to a paper by Mr. J. Scott Hutton on the notions of deaf-mutes before instruction:

This interesting extract reminds Mr. d'Estrella of his similar notions. Nothing stimulated his curiosity like the moon. He was afraid of the moon, but he always loved to watch her. He noticed the shadowy face in the full moon. Then he supposed that she was a living being. So he tried to prove whether the moon was alive or not. It was accordingly done in four different ways. First, he shook his head in a zig-zag direction, with his eyes fixed on the moon. She appeared to follow the motions of his head, now rising and then lowering, turning forward and backward. He also thought that the lights were alive too, because he repeated similar experiments. Secondly, while walking out, he watched if the moon would follow him. The orb seemed to follow him everywhere. Thirdly, he wondered why the moon appeared regularly. So he thought that she must have come out to see him alone. Then he talked to her in gestures, and fancied that he saw her smile or frown. Fourthly, he found out that he had been whipped oftener when the moon was visible. It was as though she were watching him and telling his guardian (he being an orphan boy) all about his bad capers. He often asked himself who she could be. At last he became sure that she was his mother, because, while his mother lived, he had never seen the moon. Afterwards, every now and then, he

saw the moon and behaved well towards his friends. The little boy had some other notions. He believed that the earth was flat and the sun was a ball of fire. At first he thought that there were many suns, one for each day. He could not make out how they could rise and set. One night he happened to see some boys throwing and catching burning oil-soaked balls of yarn. He turned his mind to the sun, and thought that it must have been thrown up and caught just the same—but by what force? So he supposed that there was a great and strong man, somehow hiding himself behind the hills (San Francisco being a hilly city). The sun was his ball of fire as a toy, and he amused himself in throwing it very high in the sky every morning and catching it every evening.

After he began to convince himself about the possible existence of such a mighty god, he went on with his speculations. He supposed that the god lit the stars for his own use as we do the gas-lights in the street. When there was wind, he supposed that it was the indication of his passions. A cold gale bespoke his anger, and a cool breeze his happy temper. Why? Because he had sometimes felt the breath bursting out from the mouth of angry people in the act of quarrelling or scolding. When there were clouds, he supposed that they came from the big pipe of the god. Because he had often seen, with childish wonder, how the smoke curled from lighted pipes or cigars. He was often awed by the fantastic shapes of the floating clouds. What strong lungs the god had! Where there was a fog, the boy supposed that it was his breath in the cold morning. Why? Because he had often seen his own breath in such weather. When there was rain, he did not doubt that the god took in much water, and spewed it from his big mouth in the form of a shower. Why? Because he had several

---

out many pages of his story, but this account, with a good deal of other material, was destroyed in our great fire of 1875. It very often occurs that deaf-mutes are not able to distinguish between the concepts obtained before and after education. By the time they have obtained education enough to express themselves clearly, the memory of things happening before education has become dim and untrustworthy; but Mr. d'Estrella was, and is, unusually bright and of a very inquiring turn of mind, so that before coming to school he endeavored to explain to his own satisfaction the reason of many things, and it is quite surprising how similar his explanations were to the explanations which are found in the childhood of many races. Mr. d'Estrella is imaginative, but quite as much so before education as since, and the early age at which he gave me the account of himself forbids the notion that he could have been influenced by mythologies, and the nearness of time, taken with his honesty, is sufficient assurance of the accuracy of his statement. You may trust Mr. d'Estrella perfectly for any statement he may make.

times watched how cleverly the heathen Chinese spewed the water from his mouth over the washed clothes. The boy did not suppose that the people grew. He seldom saw a baby, but when he did, he hated it, and thought it a horrid-looking thing. He had contempt for girls. He was never bad on Sundays. In fair whether he would always go to church and Sunday-school. Why? Because he fancied that the moon wanted him to go, as he had been in the habit of going to the Catholic church with his mother. He was in rags sometimes, but the church-people and Sunday-school children were generally kind to the homeless little boy. He had some faint idea of death. He saw a dead baby in a little coffin. He was told that it could not eat, drink, or speak, and so it would go into the ground and never, never come back home. Again, he was told that he would get sick and go down into the ground. He got angry. He said that he would go up to the sky where his moon-mother wanted him.

Mr. d'Estrella's autobiographic letter to me runs as follows:

The history of my parents is very little known. I never saw my father. He was a French-Swiss. My mother—a native of Mexico—died when I was five years old. Then I had no other living relative known to me. It is about seven years ago when I first learned that I had one aunt and two cousins yet living. I am now forty years old.

I was born quite deaf. However, I have been able to hear a little in the left ear only. About eight years ago my ears were examined, and it was said that the external ear and the drum as well as the nerves going to the brain were perfect, but the trouble was the inner ear or the mechanism of the internal ear. Suppose, if I were not born deaf, it must then be that I became deaf somehow in my infancy. My two friends who saw me in my infancy said that I was not born deaf. They remembered that everybody would speak to me, and I should immediately turn towards the. The doctors attributed my deafness to a fall or fright. I cannot see that either the fall or the fright had anything to do with my deafness. It is said that those who are born deaf never hear in their dreams. I am strongly subjected to dreams, but I never heard any sound in my dreams until once in 1880. Since then I had not heard again till 1890. Later, since, I have heard three times—making up five times in all my life hitherto.

However I do not believe that fact, because I know that a good many deaf mutes who lost their hearing at five or six years have never heard in their dreams.

The first recollection is that I cried. I think I was four years old then. One morning my mother left me alone for the first time in a room and locked the door. I was afraid because I had never remained alone in a closed room. So I cried. She came back in soon and ran laughing to me. She comforted and caressed me with kisses of love. This only is all what I can think instinctively of a mother's love. Probably the next recollection is one of the few I have cherished through years of memory. I remember it as though this had occurred yesterday. While walking one sunny Sunday morning with my mother to a Catholic convent, it took me by surprise when I heard the bell tolling. Rapture seized me at once. I cried joyfully. Then I felt a dreamy, wandering sensation amid the bustle of the people. Even after the good bell ceased tolling, the vibrations continued ringing in my over-excited brain for a while. Often do I think of this undying recollection—sometimes with awe, sometimes with delight. When I think of it, I feel as though I were *actually* hearing the bell toll—tolls slowly and sweetly. Even, while writing this part, I feel apparently paralyzed in my senses as if my soul were giving way to the mesmeric spell of the very recollection.

I have several other early recollections, more or less perfect. I remember that I saw a priest burning a number of Bibles; that I attended a Catholic spelling-school (I often wonder if I learned to say "papa" there. I can say "papa" as plainly as any one can—this is the only word I have ever lisped); that I saw much excitement in moving the furnitures and other household articles in a hurried and confused manner, because there was an earthquake (with I afterwards learned in the Annals of S.F.—I was born in S.F.); that I saw a great red comet; that my mother told me that we all should be knocked down if the comet struck the ground; that I watched the comet every night until it disappeared; that I saw a man lassoing another, both on horseback at full speed through the street; that I saw two fires near my home; that my mother took me to church on Sundays and on other days oftener early in the morning. If I was restless during the service, she would give me something to eat. (Although I am not a Catholic, yet now and then I go to the Catholic church, and enjoy my meditation mainly to keep the memory of my mother.) While my mother was alive, I did not know that I was deaf. I did not see the sun and stars figuratively. I remember that I had never observed the moon but once with a sort of wonder,—the moon was new. I seldom went out by myself and played with the children. I was then passively quiet and good, almost an intellectual blank.

I know almost nothing about my mother's death. While she was sick, she gave me some marmalade and kissed me, for the last time. I was then put away. I do not remember if I saw her corpse or attended her funeral, nor how I felt about her death. Only that my friends said that she had gone to the sky to rest.

What then became of me after my mother's death? I remember at best that I was taken to the house of my god-mother. Since she was my mother's best friend, I did not miss my mother consciously at all. A short time afterwards, a French consul (I believe, my father's brother) took me to the house of a Mexican woman and left me there, with a box of Noah's animals, in her charge. I did not feel homesick. She continued as my guardian until I was taken to school (I was the first pupil then, in the California institution). I remained about four years with her. She, I learned when in school, was my mother's bitter enemy out of jealousy in love affairs.

Hitherto till this time I had but a little, if ever possible, of instinctive language. I could hardly make intelligible signs; but my mother might understand my gestures, that is, such as were moved by feelings for what I should either wish or deny. For example, the idea of food was aroused in my mind by the feeling of hunger. This simply constitutes the Logic of Feeling; bear in mind that it is different from the Logic of Signs. I could neither think nor reason at all, yet I could recognize the persons either with delight or with dislike. Still, nearly all the human emotions were absent, and even the faculty of conscience was wanting. Everything seemed to appear blank around me except the momentary pleasures of perception. What happened at home had not come back within my memory until I went to school. The state of my mental

isolation, I believe, is wholly due to my confinement at home. I was then five years old, though.

But no sooner had I been left in charge of my guardian than the knowledge of good and evil was opened to me slowly but surely. As Minerva the goddess of wisdom was said to have leaped forth out of the brain of her father Jupiter, full grown and full armed for the business of life, so was my new life formed apparently mature and complete. The unwomanly treatment of my guardian was, in truth, the direct cause of the evolution of my instinctive—or better speaking—latent feelings for the higher. Not only could I think in pictures, but almost spontaneously I was also able to learn how to think and reason. Thinking in pictures or images is prevalent among most of the congenitally deaf children at different degrees in proportion to the different powers of perception. That faculty predominates in this class, and consequently compensates for the loss of hearing, no matter even if they do not think at all. I learned to know that there was a difference between right and wrong, and to understand that there was a relation between cause and effect. This proves that my conscience must have been in the act of developing. My mental condition was favorable elaborated and properly reduced to the Logic of Signs.

How were the essential signs acquired? My mother must have known my wants beforehand, without any forced attempt on my part. But my guardian was a stranger to me, and could not understand my desires. It was necessary that she or I would seek something rational or conventional to make us understand each other. So we made signs, one after another. Imitation constitutes the foundation of the sign language. We traced as intelligibly as possible the shapes and peculiarities of the objects and the actions of the bodily movements. The language thus acquired was greatly augmented by the expression and play of the features to emphasize the meanings of the signs. She soon made herself a good sign-maker. The Mexicans, as well as the people of the Romance races, are expert in pantomimic gestures which they are in the habit of using while speaking to one another. How natural all the imitative signs are! When I came to school, I had no difficulty in understanding the true deaf and dumb language of signs—the conventional language. The sign language is the universal one. (I do not pretend to say that I am about the best sign-maker in this institution. This must be attributed to the early training of the mind during my ante-speech days.)

My guardian let me go about in the rear yard. There I learned to love hens, ducks, turkeys, parrots, canary-birds, dogs, cats. Quite a bustle of life. A novelty of observation.

The woman often went out shopping. I sometimes accompanied her. As I had learned to remember the places she frequented—within a radius of two or three blocks—she sent me to the grocery to get something, such as bread, milk, potatoes, etc. I enjoyed it, because she would not let me go otherwise. While out on errand, I now and then might make acquaintances with boys and play with them for a little time. One morning I was carrying a pitcher of milk. A boy accidentally broke it and let the milk spill. I cried and went home with the broken vessel. I told the woman honestly about it. She would not listen, but she got angry and whipped me. I believe that this was the first whipping I had every got from any person. Because I thought that it was not good, my blood rose in protest. She whipped me harder, and I yielded reluctantly.

I now began to notice the gambols of the boys out on streets. So new and keen was my instinct for sport that I envied their play. Then I slipped stealthily out of the yard to the gate and looked at their pranks with delight. At last I went out to play. The woman caught and whipped me. I played again. She whipped me again. Well, I then began to think why. I thought and thought. She could not make me understand that I was a bad boy. Playing seemed to be *good*. I soon learned to hate her. If she had scolded me gently and gave me decently to understand her command, it might have been all right. But it was too late. I made up my mind that I would have my own way, regardless of consequences. I did not want to be whipped so often. I all at once hated whipping. It would make me anything but good. I played out whenever I liked. She whipped me nearly every time. It did me no good. It hardened my body as well as my heart. She desired some other way of punishment by taking off my hat. It failed. She then took off my shoes. It met the same fate. She took off my jacket. I still played only with pants and a shirt

on. It availed nothing. I had already determined that she would be revenged. She found it useless to break down my obstinacy. Now and then she would whip me very long and hard when I was out too long. I saw it rationally, but I delighted in following the boys on the alert far from home—say, ten blocks. One day I was playing with two larger boys. There was a large miry pond across the alley. We wanted to cross it. They succeeded, but I was unfortunate. While I was walking along the picket fence, one of the pickets gave way and I lost my balance, falling flat into the mire. I, from head to foot, was covered with the mud. I waddled and cried until I got out of the pond. By chance, my guardian, who had made a call, saw and took me. It was quite a far way off. The children out at recess stared at me and laughed "wickedly" like the imps. What a funny picture it must be! As soon as we got home, she made me strip off my clothes and wash them. I was then completely naked—still worse, I was made to do the washing out in the yard. It meant punishment. Several of the boys peeped over the yard and made faces at me. I rebelled, but the woman was the more determined, and the boys were the most delighted. I had to remain so in this uncomfortable place for hours until the clothes got dry enough.

A good many of the neighbors knew from the hearsay of the children and by hearing my cries that I must have been cruelly treated. They were kind to me, and would let me come in and have something nice to eat. Several of them dared to see the bad woman, and tell her not to be so hard on me. But she had her own way.

Her new husband was an American captain and owned some barges. The woman sometimes took me with her to his office at the wharf where she usually got meat. Afterwards she sent me alone to the wharf and bring the meat. What a long journey it would take for a small boy to cross a dozen of blocks—alone! However, what a splendid tramp it was! How much I loved to go to the bay! The sea was a wonder to me—nay, a wonder of wonders, since even a boat was a marvel. What a variety of life along the wharves! Such a life with such a variety awakened in me a vague feeling of mystery—sadness(?)—loneliness(?). At my request, the woman would let me go to the wharf early in the morning to get the meat. As soon as I brought it home, I made haste to the bay, and spent many long hours to view the cosmopolitan sights. I made acquaintance with the rough-looking though good-natured sailors. They taught me many good and bad ways. I was quick to see and understand. I learned from them how to draw a picture of a ship. I made very good pictures, indeed, for a boy of my age. I sometimes doubt if I can draw a ship with her details so good now as I did that time, because I used to notice all the parts of the whole ship. (I am now an amateur artist and photographer. I teach drawing at school.)

I loved money. I liked best to have dimes and half-dimes. The love of money led me to steal some little money. I was an adept in theft. I could steal some small thing easily, most without being detected. Yet my friends or some other person know from hearing my steps that I had taken something, usually eatables. But I never confessed it, even by threats, nay, by ready force. That habit was mainly owing to the condition of hunger; this was an excusable necessity, I say. I was often ill-fed at home. It meant punishment for staying away too long. This stung me dearly towards stubbornness, and I became worse and worse. It shows plainly that there is no greater fallacy than "the child's will must be broken!" Will forms the production of character. Without strength of will there will be no strength of purpose.

I began to find a new kind of pleasure in being out at night, because I could see more vicissitudes of evil amid the din of dissipation peculiar to the early days of California, then before the sixties. I was as a moth midst the dazzling lights of the night revels. I became quite a nocturnal being. In this way I contracted many bad things during my abandoned youth,—a period of four years. The influence of this evil has still retained some fascinating but unhealthy influence over my imagination. On this account I sometimes ask myself, with a certain sense of mystery and gratitude, if I had left school twenty years ago, and gone somewhere for a living, what might have become of me? I have been connected with this school thirty-one years. My long, home-like stay prevents me from ever returning to that pernicious life too soon.

More about stealing. Often did I go out at night with an empty stomach. I had to find something to satiate my hunger. Sometimes I returned home at midnight without a morsel, and entered the kitchen quietly. I took bread or meat, or what else I could hold, and slipped away. Sometimes it was done at the different houses of my friends. They would be good glad to give me some food, but I was too proud or ashamed to beg. Sometimes I took a loaf of fresh bread off the doorsteps where the baker put it. Sometimes, while passing close to the fruit-stand, I slipped one apple or two into my pockets or shirt. I had no intuitive conscience at all. There might possibly be a mote of it when I thought of the moon (you have already known my cosmology). Of course, hunger was stronger than conscience. Yet that faculty seemed to be more or less active. I shall say how I was cured of stealing. I frequented a meat-shop. The good-natured butcher let me go about at large. I happened to see some money in a box under the counter behind. I thought of getting some little money there. So I went back and crept slowly to the box and took a dime. I feasted on its worth of candy. Fond of sweets I was. I stole another dime in a few days. I wanted more money, so I stole a quarter of a dollar. My conscience worked up as though saying that it was too much. I knew that it cost two dimes and one half dime together. As long as I had it with me I felt peculiarly unhappy. I turned around to see if it was all right. I spent all of it, and saw how much more good time I could have with one of greater value. I did not come back to the shop so soon for the money. A good while later I stole the other quarter, and so on about weekly I took the quarters, piece after piece. That never-forgotten morning I wanted a quarter. While behind under the counter, I was about to put my hand into the box. The man opened it. I was quite frightened, but remained still. I would not leave, but I waited and slipped my hand into the box. So nervous was I that I took whatever piece I could touch first. I took one, and thought from the size of the piece that it was a quarter. I made haste to the nearest grocery-store and asked for candy. I put the money on the counter. It was gold!—ten dollars!! I felt as though I were a fish out of the water, with my eyes shooting out. At once I took it back and ran out. I could see nothing but gold everywhere. My heart beat. Did I know that I was guilty? If so, how could I know? Simply by seeing that I had stolen *too much*. Although I did not know the relative value of gold, yet I knew that gold cost more than silver. Because it was heavy, bright, and could be had only by the rich. I felt that it was too much for me. I never saw gold among the poorer people, and always noticed it in the hands of the more respectable ones. How could I get rid of the gold? I ran and ran with the gold tight in my hand until I returned to the senses. Then I went to the confectionery and bought much candy, regardless of the consequences about the change. The man looked surprised, buy yet, knowing that I was deaf, he might not suspect anything ill with me. He gave me the change all in silver, many halves. I was quite bewildered, but I tried well to be still. The silver was not too heavy for me to carry along as easily. The conscience came, saw, and conquered. I went some way with caution, and hid all the money under a saloon. I felt free. I thought of going to the minstrels in the evening. When the time came I went back for the money. I found it all gone. I was momentarily disappointed, but in fact I felt happier than sorry for conscience's sake. Strange to say, anybody, even the butcher, never gave me to understand that I had been suspected of theft. Still more strange, I have never stolen money again. Besides, I did not steal as many other things, particularly food, as I used to. My conscience must have become keen enough. It began developing more and more, mainly owing to the influence of the moon. (Then the moon was full, when I found the money gone.) Therefore my cosmological speculations came out, as those already given in the Annals.

Let me add as to the origin of the ocean. One day I went with some boys to the ocean. They went bathing. I first went into the ocean, not knowing how it tasted and how strong the waves rolled. So I was knocked around, with my eyes and mouth open. I came near being drowned. I could not swim. I went to the bottom and instinctively crawled up on the sand. I spit the salt water out of my mouth, and wondered why the water was so salty. I thought that it was the urine of that mighty god.

I hated girls with contempt. I never played with them. I would not visit my friends who had girls at home. Why? Because from my accidental observation I found out the difference between the girls and boys,—not in dress, but in sex. This led me to despise female animals. When I was hungry, I might occasionally go to the women for foods, but I could not stay long with them. While at school, I retained this dislike three years before I could like a girl.

I cannot remember if I ever knew that I was deaf. I knew that I could not talk, but I never asked myself why, not because I was satisfied with my condition, but because I was too wide awake to think of my own self. I often wondered how others could speak, particularly while they were quarrelling. I believed that the people could never grow. I had never wanted to be a man, because I could do enough what I liked to. I seldom saw a baby. I hated it and thought it a dirty thing. I have still retained the dislike for babies. (I am single.)

This is all what I can say for the present. Mr. Wilkinson, when he was my teacher, used to make me write about what I did before I came to school. It helped me much thus to repeat the memory. Ever since my recollections have been the same, though the words have changed now and then to get better style and more definite meanings in language.

It shows that I thought in pictures and signs before I came to school. The pictures were not exact in details, but were general. They were momentary and fleeting in my mind's eye. The signs were not extensive but somewhat conventional after the Mexican fashion—not at all like the symbols of the deaf and dumb language. I used to tell my friends about some of my cosmology. Several of them encouraged me.

One always took so much interest in me that he attempted to teach me. But he knew almost nothing, only he could say yes or no with more or less emphasis in gestures, when I said in pantomimic what I did or what I saw, or what I thought. He was the means of sending me to school as soon as he learned that the school started. He was an Italian. Some of the signs I used were beard for *man*, breast for *woman*, moustache with spelling papa for *papa*, the hand moving over the face and one finger of each hand meeting parallel (alike, meaning that someone looked like me) for *mother*, the hand down over the shoulder moving like a bell for *Sunday*, two hands open before the eyes for *book* or *paper*, one hand stretching sideways for *going*, the hand moving backwards for *coming*, the hand moving slant for *whipping*, the fingers whirling for *stealing*, the rubbing of the thumb and one of the fingers for *money*, two hands turned opposite for *breaking*, one finger stretching from the eye for *seeing*, one finger stretching from the mouth for *speaking*, one finger stretching from the forehead for *understanding*, one finger rapping lightly on the forehead for *knowing*, ditto with negation for *not knowing*, one finger resting on the forehead with the eyes shut for *thinking*, one finger now resting on the forehead and then stretching with emphasis for *understanding*, etc., etc. The signs for meat, bread, milk, water, chocolate, horse, cow, were as natural as the Mexicans make nowadays. The Mexicans generally ask with facial gestures, "What do you do?" "How do you do?" "What is the matter?" "What is the news?" It is natural. I could then understand these questions.

The reader will have noticed that many of the signs which Mr. d'Estrella reports himself to have used are regular conventional gestures of the deaf-mute sign language. Some of these may be used habitually by the Mexicans, others the poor boy probably captured out of the social atmosphere, so to speak, in the way in which needy creatures so generally find a way to the object which can satisfy their want. It will be observed, however, that his cosmological and ethical reflections were the outbirth of his solitary thought; and although he tried to communicate the cosmology to others, it is evident, since the most receptive of his friends could only say "yes" or "no" to him in return, that the communion must have been very incomplete. He surely had no conventional gestures for the causal and logical relations involved in his inductions about the moon, for example. So far as it goes, then, his narrative tends to discountenance the notion that no abstract thought is possible without words. Abstract thought of a decidedly subtle kind, both scientific and moral, went on here in advance of the means of expressing it to others. To a great extent it does so in all of us to-day, for nothing is commoner than to have a thought, and then to seek for the proper words in which to clothe its most important features. The only way to defend the doctrine of the absolute dependence of thought on language is so to enlarge the sphere of this latter word as to make it cover every possible sort of mental imagery, whether communicable to others or not. Of course no man can think without some kind of

mind—stuff to think in. Our general meanings and abstract conceptions must always have for their vehicle images more or less concrete, and "fringes" of tendency and relation which we feel between them. To a solitary untaught individual (could such a one exist) such unverbalized images would be rationally significant, and a train of them might be called a monologue. But such a monologue is not what any one naturally means by speech; and it is far better to drop the language—doctrine altogether than to evaporate its meaning into triviality like this.

Mr. d'Estrella's reminiscences also help to settle the question of whether moral propositions are "intuitive" or not. He begins life as a thief, with, as he says, "no intuitive conscience at all," and yet with a knowledge that what he does is an outward social offence, since he must needs do it secretly. At last he is converted to honesty—by what? Not by the teachings of others, not by detection and punishment, but by the very magnitude of his own crimes. He steals so much that the burden becomes too heavy to bear. It sobers him; and a success which would have turned a non-moral or an immoral boy into a confirmed criminal, produces in him a reaction towards honesty. This would seem to be a common experience. A youth tries dissipation, or indulges himself in tyranny or meanness, till at last an experience supervenes which tastes too strong, even for him, the agent. He didn't intend quite *that!* It casts a "lurid light" on all the rest of the performances, so he cries "halt" and "turns over a new leaf." Now I take it that the doctrine of an innate conscience in morals, as opposed to the pure associationist doctrine of nursery-teaching *plus* prudential calculation, means no more than this, that bad deeds will end by *tasting* bad, even to the agent who does them successfully, if you let him experience them concretely enough, with all the circumstances that they comport. They will, in short, beget an intrinsic disgust; the need of stealthiness in our tread, the satiety which our orgies leave, the looks and cries of our victims lingering obstinately behind, spoil the fun for us and end by undermining it altogether. For the poor deaf and dumb boy the fun of thieving stopped as soon as the ill-gotten gold-piece saddled him with so important a responsibility that even his moon-mother in the sky grew mixed up with the affair.

Few documents, it seems to me, cast more light on our unsophisticated intellectual and moral instincts than the sincere and unpretending narrative which Mr. d'Estrella has allowed me to print.

The Newly Deafened

Jean Mulrooney

The experience of the newly deafened is one meant to be shared. I share this experience with you from two perspectives, my own personal experience of sudden profound hearing loss and that of a psychologist using the best tools available to help another through a similar situation.

In November of 1961, I was a Registered Nurse employed in a medical division of a large suburban hospital. Prior to that time, I had worked two years as a psychiatric nurse and was familiar with both the dynamics of human behavior and the need for, function, and sheer beauty of interpersonal communication.

While driving to work early one fall morning, I was involved in an auto accident and sustained bilateral basal skull fractures that destroyed the functioning of both acoustic nerves and caused damage to the inner ear mechanism. I was comatose and near death for days.

Let me share with you my immediate memories before the accident and a few glimpses I had in the fleeting seconds of consciousness the first few days following this trauma.

I remember entering the intersection near a library I frequented. The light was green. I drove into the intersection and then ...

A strangeness, something was wrong. "Why is the library sign so close?" And I was cold all of a sudden, a chilling, pervading cold. Things were blurred and my head felt enormous, weighted, as if it would drop off. My groping hand told me it was still there. But my hand was moist, filled with a strange sort of wetness. I was falling somehow, falling, and falling. I remember seeing blue, a deep blue, with silver glinting on it and then nothing, nothing more.

Like hope, from out of nothingness a face appeared. A face of concern, competence and compassion. A face familiar to me. It was that of the head nurse in the Emergency Room of my home hospital. For that is where the silver-badged ambulance team had brought me as I hemorrhaged from the ears and head. A fleeting glimpse of reassurance and then once again, the dark, silent void.

Much later I woke to a world of effort. Effort to breathe, to think, to focus my eyes, to stay alive. I saw a yellow paper I knew had to be a head chart. That confirmed that I was in Intensive Care and dangerously ill. I knew I had left for work on Tuesday and that the first 48 hours are crucial in a head injury and thought, "If I can just make it until Thursday, I'll be all right." Then the effort overwhelmed me and I fell into a deep, troubled sleep.

It did not last long. It was broken by tidal waves of nausea and viselike throbbing in my head. I knew it was the night shift because one of my classmates was on duty. I thought, "It must be Wednesday," and then for awhile, I thought no more.

There was daylight, a presence. A figure in white by my bed. It was my sister who is also a nurse. It is strange how we ask of another what we cannot ask ourselves. "Am I going to die?" I said, for I wanted to know. She shook her head negatively quite strongly.

I was aware that the day's routine was in progress. I saw nurses preparing medications and physicians making rounds. I remember the few minutes my parents visited. I saw their concern and wanted to tell them it was all right, but I was uncertain.

It was afternoon. My sister was back with the hospital chaplain. I asked again, "Am I going to die?" They shook their heads in the negative, and Father said, "I wouldn't lie to you." I wanted to ask why they looked so gloomy then, but I didn't speak at all.

The day faded to early evening. My sister was back with a resident physician I knew. I was fighting nausea, exhaustion and pain. I wanted to sleep but there was something to ask. "Tom?" I said. He smiled and shook his head yes. He was talking to me, but I didn't know what he was saying. I said it very calmly, "I can't hear you." And then I realized that I was deaf.

The realization was the beginning of a long journey through the paths leading to a new identity as a deafened individual. It was not a simple trip. It involved learning and relearning, unbelievable isolation, barely controlled rage, the depths of depression, personal devaluation, acute sustained anxiety, frustration of the most basic human needs, and continual feelings of conflict in interpersonal relations.

But I was lucky. It also involved a few people, those precious few, who although I am sure they did not fully fathom the implications or dynamics involved in such a profound hearing loss, were willing to walk with me part of the way. Willing to try and understand what was happening to me, to share what I was experiencing, to accept my negative feelings as a fact without moral judgment, to listen with me to the strange, new, overwhelmingly confusing, cacophonous song that was then my life.

Before going on to discuss a fruitful approach to helping others with a similar loss, three more things should be said. First, there was nothing in my experience that contradicted the psychological teachings about anxiety, frustration, conflict, depression, what have you. On the contrary, my experience substantiated them all! I did find knowledge of these principles helpful in identifying what I was experiencing and getting a per-

spective on what it would lead to and how it should be handled.

Secondly, there were some things unique to profound hearing loss I think should be briefly noted. One is the feeling that "nothing seems real" coupled with the full conscious awareness that it was real and the fact that I was responding appropriately. This should not be confused with withdrawal or denial. It seems to be simply the result of profound auditory sensory deprivation and not a behavioral dynamic to be assessed for motivation.

The other point may seem obvious. It is that the usual method of obtaining help in handling a disability through counseling was greatly compounded by the disability itself. All efforts to communicate with a helping person involved tension, exhaustion, ambiguity and frustration, no doubt for *both* of us.

Third, although nothing in my experience contradicted what I knew of adjustment mechanisms, I always had the feeling, "Yes, that's right, but it doesn't adequately convey what I am experiencing. There is something more I do not have words or theories for." That something more is the process of grief. Grief is the human reaction to loss. It is a growth-like process and not a state. It can be delineated into stages and recognized by its symptoms. An extensive discussion of this can be found in books, such as Collin Murray Parkes' *Bereavement: Studies of Grief in Adult Life*.

Those helping a newly deafened individual are faced with a difficult task. You are being asked to share a painful experience and one in which the usual approaches do not seem adequate.

The crux of scientific investigation is learning to ask the right questions. I am raising questions about the adjustment of a newly deafened person in the framework of the grief process. Those working with such a person in a helping relationship will need much more than the information given here. It is my hope, however, that by phrasing the questions in this manner you will include aspects of the person's experience that are often neglected and may not even be in the individuals' conscious awareness.

The first question often asked about a newly deafened individual is "How is he taking it?" or "Is he depressed?" That question implies there is an alternative to depression or perhaps that the experience will not bother him at all. Let me repeat, the human reaction to loss is grief. A more helpful question then is "What state of grief is he in, and how can he be helped to work through it constructively."

The newly deafened individual will need help in identifying just what was lost. He will need time to experience what the hearing loss means in various situations and relationships. He will experience both the *loss* of hearing that will cause him to search for what was lost and also the *deprivation* caused by the absence of hearing. He must be helped in this search and in handling the feelings of deprivation.

A second frequently asked question about the newly deafened is, "Has he adapted to his deafness?" This implies that the problem is in accepting or rejecting a single characteristic of the self. Actually, it involves much more extensive restructuring. A more inclusive question is, "Has he found or is he finding a new identity as a deafened person?" This involves a long, painful process of giving up the old self that may never be complete. The new identity is found neither in denying one's past life nor acting like a congenitally deaf person, but in the altered life situations of everyday experience.

The third question is, "Is he refusing to accept his deafness?" A better approach is to ask, "Is he showing evidence of an atypical grief reaction, and if so what help is needed?" Symptoms of excessive separation anxiety, delayed grief response, or unsuccessful attempts to avoid grieving may be indications of atypical grief. Atypical grief reactions require competent professional help. An important sub-question under atypical grief is, "Is the person's behavior or feelings evidence of an atypical grief reaction or simply the growing awareness of the pervasiveness of the effects of his hearing loss?" As the person continues to face altered life situations, he continually becomes more aware of just what abilities, experiences, identities were lost, in addition to the physical capacity to hear. Each new loss that is identified may precipitate additional grief.

The fourth question often asked is,"Is he preventing himself from getting the necessary help?" Loneliness knows not its own cure. A better question is, "How can I help reduce the loneliness and isolation and thereby help him tolerate the pain of grief better?" Well then, if he's not preventing himself from getting the necessary help, "Is he feeling sorry for himself?" What should be asked is "Is he using the loss for secondary gain?" This is an extremely rare occurrence and a less than satisfactory explanation for the person's behavior. It is more likely that his behavior is a reflection of the intensity of feeling that was bound up with what was lost rather than any indication of self-pity.

The last question frequently asked is this: "Is he 'over' the hearing loss yet?" This implies not a process of grief but a mythical obstacle to be overcome before returning to normal. A more honest question is, "Is he still encountering further awareness of the loss as the self knowledge of his new identity progresses?" and "How can it be helped?"

Learning to ask the right questions together is a beginning—the beginning of knowledge, of understanding, of sharing, of adjustment, of finding a new identity as a deafened person. It is also the beginning of victory, a victory over adult hearing loss in which you can share.

Acquired Hearing Loss—Shifting Gears

Holly Elliott

Not long ago a deaf man said to me: "I'm better off than you are. You lost something, I didn't." "Maybe I'm better off," I replied. "I had something, you didn't."

Even more recently, I was talking with a deaf man who is doing research on the attitudes of deaf people about hearing people in the general context of mainstreaming. "You may be hearing impaired," he said, "but inside you really feel like a hearing person."

True. I suspect that is the way it is with those of us who have lost our hearing after years of normal hearing. We can't deny what we were then any more than we can deny what we are now. You and I know that the transition from then to now was a rough road. We all have our own story of what we experienced when the realization finally hit: "I have a hearing impairment."

My problem began when I was nineteen and a music major in college. An otologist told me I had a severe hearing loss; it would probably get worse, a hearing aid would not help me, and I would have to learn to live with it. My response was rage and denial and I spent the next 30 years of progressive deafness trying to prove to myself that I could do anything I wanted to. I never allowed myself to experience grief and I paid dearly for those repressed feelings. I was forty-eight years old with a profound hearing loss, before I finally faced this issue, went back to college, learned sign language and found a new identity. It took me thirty years to shift gears.

One of the most important things I have learned in the last eighteen years is the difference between grief and depression. Hearing impairment supposes a frightening loss and grief is a natural response to loss, an active process that must be experienced to be resolved. Depression is a giving-up process, a long term withdrawal. The feeling of being "left out" —and not doing anything about it—is a feeling of depression. I have a hunch that depression interferes with communication more than hearing loss. The combination of impairment and depression makes communication very difficult. Hearing loss is not the handicap; the inability to communicate is the handicap. If I can overcome my depression, I will find a way to communicate: by writing, by signing, by lipreading, by helping the other person find a way that is comfortable for us both, or by a combination of these approaches.

I have also learned that sudden—and even progressive—deafness means an identity crisis. Even now I find myself wondering from time to time who I really am. Hearing people often think I am hearing because my speech is good; deaf people often think I am hearing because my signs are bad. Identity crisis. Hearing people have their culture based on spoken language and some deaf people have their culture based on sign and we are caught between incomprehensible speech on the one hand and incomprehensible signs on the other. If only those hearies would talk more clearly! If only those deafies would sign more slowly! Who's taking care of us?

I like Erik Erikson's definition of identity crisis: A crisis is a necessary turning point, a critical moment when development must move one way or another, gathering resources of growth and recovery, to prepare for further differentiation. Identity crisis means shifting gears. Have you read the book *Shifting Gears* by the

O'Neills? I recommend it. The O'Neills tell us that shifting gears is a process by which we choose change. Now that may seem crazy because we sure didn't "choose" hearing loss. But we can choose how we manage it. Life strategy consists of an approach to life that makes such change possible.

Some examples: see a rehab counselor; go back to school; use notetakers if you don't know sign language; learn sign language; find a commitment larger than yourself; find some creative solutions to problems.

From my own experience: I was frustrated when I could no longer use the phone. Now I have a TDD. Call me sometime! I grieved when I could no longer play the piano. Now I can be creative on the typewriter keyboard. Letter writing is my hobby. Write me a letter! I'm an old has-been church choir director and I miss church music. My sign language choir gives Christmas and Spring concerts every year. Last year we did the Hallelujah Chorus in sign language. Come and hear/see my sign language choir!

Make a list of your own creative solutions to big and little problems and invent a few more. It boosts the morale. We need these plusses, because loss of hearing can be very frustrating, and whatever the feeling—frustration, rage, fear—it must be experienced before it can be resolved. How do you experience the feeling? Do you have a punching bag? Do you jog? Do you let it out to a therapist?

Two of the most damaging words in the English language are: "if only." I'd like to take these two words, tear them up and throw them away. I'd like to replace them with: "That's the way it is. Now, where do we go from here?"

Shifting gears isn't easy. The road is full of bumps and detours and dangerous curves. We need a support system where we can get tuned up now and then. We sometimes need to shift into compound low before we can get going again.

May the road rise with you and the wind be always at your back.

Communication: Our Highest Priority

Roderick J. MacDonald

When we speak of a language, we usually refer to a group of words which, when put together in various ways, enable us to communicate with, to share ideas with, and to express needs in a manner readily understood by others. All formal languages, whether vocal or visual, have structure, syntax and "rules" for expressive communication. All major formal languages, vocal or visual, normally depend upon the sense of hearing or sight for effective reception.

In the case of a blind person, the lack of sight does not in any way diminish the ability to communicate effectively through the use of vocal languages. Similarly, a deaf person's ability to follow a visual language is in no way impaired by the loss of hearing. For the purpose of communicating with others through language, the substitution of sight for hearing, or hearing for sight, is a relatively simple transition.

However, for individuals who are both deaf and blind, the situation is entirely different. Deaf-blind people do not have a formal language of their own, for there is no language specifically designed for the sense of touch. A deaf-blind person must learn to communicate by adapting methods that normally would require the use of sight or hearing as, for example, following Sign Language tactually, or by following speech through the application of the Tadoma method.

It is readily apparent that deaf-blind persons face difficulties in the search for effective communication, yet they need that communication every bit as much as any other person.

A wide variety of methods and techniques are used by deaf-blind individuals in their quest for effective, meaningful communication. For example, a person who was born deaf, grew up as a deaf person and later became blind, might find Sign Language the most comfortable means of communication, and attempt to follow signs tactually when no longer able to follow it visually.

In such a case, the deaf-blind person employs an alternate technique in following a communication method employed by deaf people. Similarly, a person who became blind early in life, grew up as a blind person and later became deaf, might well prefer to continue to employ the English language as his or her primary mode of communication, and employ fingerspelling or print on palm, as the most comfortable way of following this method. This has been the case with me.

Communicating in English via fingerspelling presents some obvious problems. For one thing, it is not possible to fingerspell faster than about 60 words per minute, a communication rate far slower than normal speaking or signing. A great deal of pressure can be placed on the interpreter in such situations, and the physical and emotional strain can be very taxing.

I remember well the time I was making a formal presentation at work with my wife interpreting for me. I was very anxious to learn the reaction to what I had said, and my wife was aware of this. The first person to speak was my boss, who exclaimed, "Good!" However, in her haste to communicate this to me as quickly as possible, my wife got her letters a little mixed up and instead spelled out "Goof!" for my benefit. This is the type of mechanical dysfunction that I try to be careful about.

Sometimes the pressure of interpreting via fingerspelling can lead to rather humorous slips. I was once attending a meeting at which the subject of training interpreters to work with the so-called "low-verbal" deaf individual was being discussed. The speaker was talking quite rapidly, and my interpreter was having problems in keeping up. When she informed me that the subject was "Training Low-Verbal Interpreters," I began laughing so hard I had to leave the room.

One of the most common problems faced by deaf-blind people, as well as other handicapped individuals, is that many people feel it is necessary to protect the deaf-blind individual from the hard knocks of this cruel world. Parents, for example, often feel that a deaf-blind child should not grow up with daily contact with non-handicapped children. The argument is often that children can be very cruel in their teasing, and a deaf-blind child has enough to bear without that. I feel very strongly that deaf-blind people can learn from the School of Hard Knocks just as other people can, and it is a vital part of their education to do so. There are exceptions, but by and large allowing deaf-blind people to experience "real life" situations is very important to their development. The deaf-blind individual must learn how to cope with these situations just like others must learn to do.

When I first started working for the Federal government, there was a young man in the office who loved to tease me about my "sex life." During the 1950's, it was referred to as one's "social life," and in the 1960's, it was called one's "love life." But this was in the early 1970's, and it was referred to as a "sex life." Every time he asked me, I became very embarrassed and did not know what to say. Well, one day he asked me the inevitable question at a farewell luncheon we were having for a coworker. He wrote me the note and, at the same time, spoke his question for the benefit of the others. Everyone became very quiet to hear what I would say. As usual, I was very embarrassed and did not know what to say. Without thinking, I blurted out that "My sex life is all

screwed up!" My friend never teased me again. It was a learning experience for me—and for him, too, I think.

The question of what to do, and what not to do, in interpreting situations with deaf-blind persons has long been a topic of discussion in the college-level communication class I teach. For example, I am a teacher and have responsibility for maintaining order in the classroom. I normally have the assistance of an interpreter in my classroom, who fingerspells for me and signs for the benefit of deaf students in the class when I speak.

Now suppose a deaf student in the class is "goofing off"—does the interpreter tell me about it? If the interpreter's primary role is seen to be working with deaf students in the classroom, the interpreter should not speak about the student's behavior. Yet, as an interpreter for a deaf-blind teacher, the interpreter should give the visual information which the teacher misses by virtue of being blind.

Here we have an interpreter with a dual role, a difficult assignment. The consensus of opinion is that the teacher should explain to the students that the interpreter will be giving the teacher visual information. But this question is one which illustrates the type of ethical difficulty an interpreter can face when working with a deaf-blind person. There is no formal code of ethics or guidelines especially established for this type of situation. Knowing what to do, how to do it, and when is often a matter of learn-as-you-go.

Knowing what information to provide can also involve what information not to provide. For example, consider the situation of an interpreter who is assisting with the communication at a meeting between a teacher, a counselor and a deaf-blind student. Let us suppose that the counselor arrives late, and greets the teacher but not the deaf-blind student. Does the interpreter tell the student that the counselor did not greet him or her?

A little thought will no doubt suffice to show that the interpreter should not convey this information, for it is calling upon the interpreter's judgement in deciding upon what happened. The interpreter should simply convey the information that the counselor greeted the teacher. With sufficient experience and confidence, the deaf-blind individual will learn to evaluate the situation from the facts given, and will know not only what happened, but what did *not* happen as well. This can be very important because if the interpreter specifically calls the omission to the attention of the deaf-blind person, it tends to imply fault on the part of the counselor, which an interpreter should never do.

The question might well be asked here just how an interpreter can be expected to make appropriate judgements about conduct when there have never been any guidelines established for correct behavior, as there have been in the case of interpreting with deaf persons. My only suggestion would be for the interpreter to ask himself or herself the question: "Why am I here?"

The answer is that the interpreter is there to provide auditory information which the deaf-blind person misses because he or she cannot hear; and also to provide visual information which the deaf-blind person misses by virtue of being blind. The interpreter can bring the question down to this: "Is this information needed by the deaf-blind person because of deafness or blindness?" If the answer is yes, the interpreter should go ahead and provide the information. If the answer is no, the information should not be conveyed.

I have been asked by interpreters what they should do when they are asked to stop interpreting because what is said is not intended for the deaf-blind person's benefit. The answer I give is always the same: "Interpret it." If the speaker does not wish the conversation "overheard," it is quite appropriate to leave the room, just as it is appropriate to do this when a hearing person is involved. To ask an interpreter not to communicate is equivalent to asking a hearing person not to listen—if one does not want a hearing person to listen, one gets out of earshot.

Interpreting effectively with a deaf-blind person is a difficult assignment, yet it can be done and, when it is, it can fill the deaf-blind person with a feeling of self-worth, a deep-down feeling that he or she can do things just like everyone else, and do them well. A deaf-blind person can stop worrying about whether or not information will be provided, and instead concentrate on how it will be used. A good example of how this can work out can be seen from the following story.

Not long ago, I had an appointment with IBM, and went to my appointment with my interpreter. As we entered the lobby of the building we were met by a security guard. I said, "Good morning! We would like to see so-and-so." The man called upstairs on the telephone and was informed that the person we wished to see was out, but was expected back shortly. He then turned to us and explained. My interpreter fingerspelled the information into my palm, and I turned to the guard and said, "That's fine, could we see someone else?" Well, he looked at us for a moment and then called back upstairs on the telephone.

This time he tried to muffle his voice so that we could not hear him. He said, "I have a girl here who can't speak, but has a gentleman with her who does all the talking. They want to see somebody else." He then turned back to us but, instead of speaking, this time he wrote a note and held it up for my interpreter to read. She, in turn, fingerspelled it for me, and I again spoke. We carried on a conversation in this manner for 15 minutes, and all the while the guard thought he was dealing with a young woman without speech, and that I was her interpreter. Eventually we took care of our business and had a good laugh over this on our way down in the elevator. At my suggestion, my interpreter waved to the guard as we left and said, "Bye! Thanks very much!" He was still staring after us as we walked down the street.

What is important here is that a deaf-blind person, with the assistance of an interpreter, was able to get "Out there" and conduct normal, everyday business effectively, without the other person even suspecting that he was both deaf and blind. I was not in any sense pretending I could see or hear—sight and hearing were just not important in this situation, because I was provided with the information I needed to conduct my business. But I can tell you there certainly was an inner feeling of excitement, even of pride, that I could do this, and it was because of the assistance of my interpreter that it was possible.

Communication is a challenge for all of us. For some it is more difficult, which makes it more of a challenge. It is also a challenge for those who try to help us in our search for communication. Communication is the key to participation in the mainstream of life, and in this regard it can be said that communication is the highest priority.

Two Views of Deafness

Chris Wixtrom

1st View: Deafness as Pathology

With this perspective, a person might:

Define deafness as a *pathological condition* (a defect, or a handicap) which distinguishes *abnormal* deaf persons from normal hearing persons.

Deny, downplay or hide evidence of deafness.

Seek a "cure" for deafness; focus on ameliorating the effects of the "auditory disability" or "impairment."

Give much attention to the use of hearing aids and other devices that enhance auditory perception and/or focus on speech. Examples: Amplifiers, tactile and computer-aided speech devices, cue systems. . . .

Place much emphasis on speech and speechreading ("oral" skills); avoid sign and other communication methods which are deemed "inferior."

Promote the use of auditory-based communication modes; frown upon the use of modes which are primarily visual.

Describe sign language as inferior to spoken language.

View spoken language as the most natural language for all persons, including the deaf.

Make mastery of spoken language a central educational aim.

Support socialization of deaf persons with hearing persons. Frown upon deaf/deaf interaction and deaf/deaf marriages.

Regard "the normal hearing person" as the best role model.

Regard professional involvement with the deaf as "helping the deaf" to "overcome their handicap" and to "live in the hearing world."

Neither accept nor support a separate "deaf culture."

2nd View: Deafness as a Difference

With this perspective, a person might:

Define deafness as merely a *difference,* a *characteristic* which distinguishes *normal* deaf persons from normal hearing persons. Recognize that deaf people are a linguistic and cultural minority.

Openly acknowledge deafness.

Emphasize the abilities of deaf persons.

Give much attention to issues of communication access for deaf persons through visual devices and services. Examples: telecommunication devices, captioning devices, light signal devices, interpreters. . . .

Encourage the development of all communication modes, including—but not limited to—speech.

Strongly emphasize the use of vision as a positive, efficient alternative to the auditory channel.

View sign language as equal to spoken language.

View sign language as the most natural language for people who are born deaf.

In education, focus on subject matter, rather than on a method of communication. Work to expand all communication skills.

Support socialization within the deaf community as well as within the larger community.

Regard successful deaf adults as positive role models for deaf children.

Regard professional involvement with the deaf as "working with the deaf" to "provide access to the same rights and privileges that hearing people enjoy."

Respect, value and support the language and culture of deaf people.

Chapter 2

Historical Foundations of American Sign Language

This chapter begins with the ideas, teachings, and writings of several scholars who profoundly influenced the course of Deaf History. These pioneers were primarily educators. They saw sign language as an essential tool for teaching deaf children. One of these trailblazers, Thomas Hopkins Gallaudet, founded the first school for deaf students in America. He believed in the " . . . indispensable necessity of the use of natural signs in the education of the deaf" (Gallaudet, 1887, p. 144). Gallaudet's fervent feelings about sign language helped nurture its development in the United States. Thomas Hopkins Gallaudet, Laurent Clerc, and Edward Miner Gallaudet insisted upon the value of sign language in teaching and communicating with deaf children. Their innovative ideas were not always accepted by their contemporaries. Proponents of the oral philosophy advocated the exclusion of sign language from the curriculum. "Oralism" teaches deaf children speech, lipreading, and the use of residual hearing. From these historic roots, a controversy known as the oral-manual debate arose and continues to the present.

Articles by Harlan Lane, James Fernandes, and Loy Golloday describe the development of sign language in Colonial America. The common theme among these articles is that the hearing majority suppressed the language of Deaf Americans. Nevertheless, deaf persons and sign language showed an extraordinary resiliency.

In contrast to the general suppression of American Sign Language was the complete acceptance of deaf people and their language on Martha's Vineyard in the 1700s. The hearing citizens on Martha's Vineyard learned sign language to communicate with their deaf friends, neighbors and relatives. Deafness was not seen as a handicap and deaf citizens were included in all facets of island life, such as town meetings and political decisions. Deaf and hearing settlers lived in harmony.

In modern times, deaf people have not always been permitted to have a say in shaping their own future. As recently as 1988, the students at Gallaudet University protested the administrations insensitivity to their call for a deaf president. The ensuing strike gathered enough momentum to change the minds of the trustees. Oliver Sachs chronicles the students' strike and reports on their attitudes and feelings. In this "revolution," the Deaf Community asserted itself and let the world know they were ready and able to make their own decisions. Their efforts helped elect Dr. I. K. Jordan as the first deaf president of Gallaudet University. Dr. Jordan now takes his place as a contemporary leader in the Deaf Community.

The history of American Sign Language and the Deaf Community in the United States from humble, obscure beginnings to front page, prime-time news is an interesting and often controversial story. The articles in this chapter convey the richness of this history.

Notes For A Psycho-History of American Sign Language

Harlan Lane

Part I: Two deaf sisters and the Abbe de l'Epee

The setting: The French Enlightenment, a time of enormous intellectual excitement. Painting, theater, music and literature were flourishing. Rousseau had advanced his theories of social contract and of education. Condillac had published his treatises on grammar, on sensation, and on the origins of human knowledge. The glittering salons of Madame Récamier, Madame de Staël, and others were the rendezvous of the intellectual and social elite. Science was thriving. Pinel had just written the first book on psychiatric diagnosis and had ordered the insane unchained. Jenner discovered that people could be protected against disease by giving them a benign form of the disease itself; no one knew why. The first anthropological society was formed and data were pouring in on the flora, fauna and tribes of Africa, Indonesia and the New World. The seemingly unlimited possibilities of the new social order were on everyone's mind.

The problem: Until the middle of the 18th Century, it was generally believed that the deaf were inherently uneducable and, consequently, properly denied their rights as citizens, among those rights the opportunity to attend public school, to vote, to serve in public office and so on. There were, of course, a few deaf individuals who, by their accomplishments, called this image of the deaf into question. They were usually the children of extremely wealthy nobility who, through the painstaking labors of a dedicated instructor, could achieve a certain measure of

skill in lipreading and pronunciation. Then, along came a priest by the name of Charles Michel, the Abbé de l'Epée.

According to the official version of the story, the abbot was wandering about Paris one day and decided to pay a courtesy call on a woman of his acquaintance. She was not at home but one of her two daughters ushered him to a seat, indicating that he might await her return. As he waited there, it struck him as odd, even allowing for the dignity of his office and the girls' modesty, that they would not address a single word to him for hours on end. Finally, the mother returned from her errands and explained that, alas, her daughters were deaf. To make matters worse, the neighborhood priest who had begun to teach them some notion of salvation with the aid of engravings had recently gone to his own salvation, leaving that of her daughters in some doubt. She appealed to the abbot as a friend and priest to consider her daughters' cause and he put his mind to this problem. What can you do to educate people who have neither speech nor hearing? How do you give them an idea of the Trinity, the heavenly hosts, their guardian angels or the cherubim and seraphim?

The solution: Epée remembered something from his own education, something taken no doubt from John Lockes' book, *An essay on human understanding*, which had been published in French at about that time, that is, the 1740's. Locke said:

It was necessary that man should find some external signs whereof his invisible ideas might be made known to others. For this purpose man adopted a variety of sounds he was able to use. Men came to make use of words as the signs of their ideas. Not by any natural connection, for if one existed, all the languages of the world would be the same, but rather by a voluntary imposition whereby a particular word is arbitrarily made the mark of a particular idea.

On reading this, Epée had an amazing idea, an unimagined solution to his problem. Perhaps it is obvious to this audience, but to the eighteenth-century European it was not at all evident. It is deeply ingrained in human character, I think, to give one's own language, whatever it may be, a special status in the scheme of things; to imagine that if you wake a foreigner in the night he would cry out "What's the matter?" in your language, not his; to feel that words we know are connected in a compelling and necessary way to the things to which they refer. We can observe that tendency openly among us in the taboo on saying certain words—like the name of God in the Hebrew religion. Words still contain a lot of magic for us all and the arbitrariness of their linkage to their referents was not an obvious fact. But Epée grasped it. If the connection between words and their referents is arbitrary, he reasoned, then the gestures of the deaf can serve equally well. "The natural language of the deaf," he wrote, "is the language of sign. Nature and their different wants are their only tutors in it. And they have no other language as long as they have no other instructors." The problem: how to educate a deaf person. The solution: to realize the arbitrariness of speech, to employ signs instead.

The myth: The Abbé de l'Epée then proceeded to make up sign language and to educate the deaf. The reality is, of course, that the Abbé de l'Epée did not invent the sign language of the deaf, he adopted their signs, the signs of the deaf people that he gathered together in Paris. We have his disciple's word on it. The Abbé Sicard wrote: "The Abbé de l'Epée saw that the deaf-mute expressed his physical needs without instruction, that one could with the same signs communicate to him the expression of the same needs, and

could indicate the things that one wanted to designate. And these were the first words of a new language which this great man has enriched to the astonishment of all Europe." And Europe was indeed astonished. Epée's accomplishment was on everyone's lips; laymen, physicians, royalty, philosophers—what would now be called psychologists and linguists and anthropologists, and many more came to his public demonstrations year after year.

To the core group of signs that he got from the deaf, Epée did add something of his own. Something foolish, something that obstructed the progress of the education of the deaf. He added what he called "methodical signs." It is important to understand what Epée thought he could and could not accomplish. He thought he could succeed in teaching deaf children to render written French into sign and sign into written French, so that with two deaf children, one signing a text and the other transcribing the signs, a perfect replica of the original text could be obtained. To train copyists in this way, he needed a sign language that not only had signs for most French words but also could represent the grammatical apparatus of French: the article *a,* in French *un* (or *une* in the case of a feminine noun); the suffixes of French words like *-able* and *-ment,* and so on. For *un,* a "masculine" article, he chose the sign for a man's hat. And for the "feminine" article, *une,* he chose a bonnet. Well, the result, and I have this from a first-hand observer, was that when his students referred to a bench, *un blanc,* they would sign a hat and a bench, and when they wanted to sign a table *une table,* then they would sign a bonnet on the table. You can imagine that putting hats and bonnets on everything did not speed up the progress of conversation or enhance the education of the deaf.

As a result of this effort to build a kind of bastard language, something that was signed but French, Epée was able to train some extremely skilled copyists. But nothing more.

Sicard writes, "All the words of the French language had their counterpart in that of the deaf by the time Epée was through. Nothing was easier than to get words and signs committed to memory, engraved there; all that was required was ordinary attention, since each gesture accompanied the invariable combination of letters that form the corresponding word. Entire pages of the most abstract books were copied from simple dictation by sign."

As an example of expressing abstract words in sign, Epée's books on the instruction of deaf-mutes recounts how he taught them to sign the French *inintelligibilite*, that is, unintelligibility. He says, "I needed only five signs, performed in an instant. The first announced an internal activity; the second represented the activity of someone who reads internally, that is who understands what is said to him; the third declared that this arrangement was possible; does that not give *intelligible*? But with the fourth sign I transformed this adjective into an abstract quality.

Isn't *intelligibilite* the result? Finally, by a fifth sign I added negation. And then do we not have the entire word, *inintelligibilite?*"

The reality: If Epée did not invent sign language, if indeed the methodical signs he did invent were what one of his successors called "an elaborate and cumbersome scaffolding on the language of the deaf," then why do we revere him? Epée did not devote his life to the education of the deaf. He took it up, *faute de mieux,* for lack of something better, at the age of sixty, having failed to rise higher than the deaconhood because of his disputes with the church hierarchy, having failed to complete the legal studies that he began as a result of those disputes. Why do we revere him? Because he did two things that are terribly important: first, because he was a priest, and because he was concerned with the poor, he saw that he would have to bring the deaf together to educate them. It was impossible for a poor deaf child to have a private, live-in tutor. Instead, because Epée was a priest, he said, "I must bring the poor deaf together. I must make this training available to them." And as a by-product, he created a deaf community. He created the essential

circumstances in which a language could develop. Not because he understood this necessity, but for an adventitious reason. Here is what Jean-Marc Itard, physician to the institution for deaf mutes and teacher of the Wild Boy of Aveyron, had to say about Epée's school four decades later.

> A large and seasoned institution of deaf-mutes, bringing together individuals of diverse ages and degrees of education, represents a genuine society with its own language, a language endowed with its own acquired ideas and traditions, and which is capable, like spoken language, of communicating directly or indirectly all its intended meanings. In fact, the deaf-mute raised in the midst of such a gesturing society sees not only the signs that are made to communicate with him but also those that are exchanged in conversations among the deaf that are within his view. [The impact of this indirect communication] explains how these children who have only been taught the names of objects, after several months in a large institution, can conduct sustained animated little conversations with their peers that require a knowledge of [how to sign] adjectives, verbs, and tenses.

If Epée's first accomplishment was the formation of a deaf community, his second was to call attention to that community. I fear we have little reason to believe he did so because of his deep commitment to the deaf. He did so because, like so many others of his time (and ours), he enjoyed glory. And he did get a lot of glory. He held public demonstrations in which the deaf transcribed the signs that he dictated into French, Italian, Spanish and, of course, Latin, the language of the church. These demonstrations brought about a tremendous flurry of efforts in behalf of the deaf. This was a time when mental retardation was believed untreatable; when deafness and the ignorance of the deaf were considered similarly invincible; and here was a man who taught the deaf to converse in the tongues of the world, or so it would appear to the casual observer. The casual observer included kings and princes and emissaries from throughout the world.

As a result of his proselytizing, schools for the deaf were opened throughout Europe and, following the French Revolution, the newly-elected National Assembly declared that the deaf shall be members of the new fraternity of man. They further declared that Epée's school shall become a national school, the National Institution for Deaf Children, which has shaped the lives of untold deaf children down to the present day.

Part II: Jean Massieu and the Abbé Sicard

The setting: When Epée died in 1789, the French government found a brilliant way to choose his successor. The French have always been great enthusiasts for *concours,* competitions. They still are. "We'll have a competition," they reasoned, "and we'll pick the director by choosing the best deaf student." What a brilliant idea! I wish we chose our educational leaders nowadays by evaluating their students. The various teachers entered their best students in this competition; the winner was one Jean Massieu. And so they said, "You're a knowledgeable young fellow, Massieu. You must have a wonderful teacher, let's have him as our director." And that was the Abbé Sicard of Bordeaux.

The problem: How to make the deaf more than just copyists. Sicard believed, even while he was studying with Epée, that it was necessary to progress beyond Epée's methods. And Epée criticized him for this conviction. There's a wonderful passage in a letter he wrote to him: "Sicard, what are you up to? You insist on training writers but my method can only produce copyists. Content yourself modestly with the share of glory that you see me enjoying. Teach your children the declensions and the conjugations. Teach them the signs from my dictionary of verbs. Teach them to do the parts of the sentence following my diagrams." (That, of course, was French grammar.) "Do not delude yourself that your students are going to express themselves in French, any more than I can express myself in Italian although I can translate that language." Sicard said, "The Abbé de l'Epée thought his work was through when he invented all these signs. He was giving the deaf only signs and not meanings. He failed to see that nothing was easier than to make them write words for signs, but they knew nothing of the former and little of the latter, he led them from the unknown to the unknown. He succeeded in making them copy whole pages of abstract books, but they conveyed no meaning since words can only be conventional signs and there must be some language mutually understood."

The solution: What did Sicard do to make French meaningful for Massieu? He tells us in a book he published describing his method of instruction. He prepared some twenty sketches of familiar objects and, in the first lesson, Massieu learned to fetch the object given the sketch, and vice-versa. For the second lesson, Sicard had lettered the names of the objects above their corresponding sketches on a blackboard. When the outlines were erased, Massieu was unable to fetch the various objects, with only the names as a guide. Sicard then redrew the objects with the letters on, not above, them; the letters extended between the borders so that the printed name had roughly the conformation of the object. Next the outlines were erased carefully between the letters, and an observer was used as a model to fetch the objects according to their printed names. Massieu was puzzled.

Sicard repeated the procedure but had Massieu copy the names of the iconographs, lettering each one just below the corresponding letter-design, which was then erased. The observer then fetched the various objects guided only by the names Massieu had written. Massieu was overjoyed, we are told, at his newfound ability to communicate and learned to fetch all that he had transcribed. Quite soon the intermediate steps of sketching and copying could be dropped. Massieu pointed to all manner of things around him, wanting to know their names.

The myth: Sicard, a brilliant grammarian, professor at the newly opened national teacher's college, head of the school for the deaf, taught the deaf sign language and through it French and, through French, a knowledge of the world. His most famous pupil was Jean Massieu, whom he raised up from an ignorant shepherd to be a great spokesman for the deaf.

The reality: Sicard did not teach Massieu sign language, Massieu taught Sicard sign language. Sicard says so himself. He says, and I quote, "There wasn't a day in which by this method Massieu didn't learn more than fifty names. Never a day in which I didn't learn from him the signs of as many objects . . . Thus by a happy exchange, when I taught him the written signs of our language, Massieu taught me the signs of his. "Thus," writes Sicard, "neither I nor my illustrious teacher is the inventor of sign language (it must be said) and, as a foreigner cannot teach a Frenchman the French language, so a man who speaks should not get involved in inventing signs."

Now just in case you like Sicard too much for all of that, I must tell you that he was an awful man. An utterly crafty, cunning man of low principles. Let me tell you a true story that Lou Fant first called to my attention: how Massieu saved Sicard's life. The story is not only interesting in itself, but tells us something about who is in debt to whom, and about the social and linguistic skills that Massieu was able to achieve. We may well ask ourselves how much more progress we have made in the education of the deaf, how much further our pupils can go than did Massieu. Toward the end of the 1700's, at the time of the French Revolution, there was a great deal of bloodshed as you know. One day some sixty armed citizens stormed into the Celestine Cloister where the Institution for the Deaf was temporarily located. They seized Sicard as he was preparing his lecture. The Revolutionary Commune had ordered his arrest along with that of many other priests because he, like Epée years before him, had refused to take the oath of civil allegiance. And thus he began an incredible week of flirtation with death during which he was swept into the bloody vortex of the September Massacre. He was led at saber point through the streets to the City Hall. He was brought before the *Comité*

d'Exécution, he was stripped of his personal effects, including his breviary. He was minutely searched for counterrevolutionary propaganda. And he was locked up. The following morning Massieu arrived. "I've written a petition to the National Assembly. Surely they will step in. What do you think of this?" And he handed Sicard a petition he had composed.

> Mr. President, The deaf and dumb have had their instructor, their guardian angel, and their father taken from them. He has been locked in prison like a thief, a criminal, but he has killed no one, he has stolen nothing. He is not a bad citizen. His whole time is spent in instructing us, in teaching us to love virtue and our country. He is good, just, and pure. We ask for his freedom. Restore him to his children for we are his. He loves us like a father. He has taught us all we know. Without him we would be like animals. Since he has been taken away we are sad and distressed. Return him to us and you will make us happy.

Massieu, the former shepherd boy, went to the National Assembly. The secretary read his petition and the assembly rose and applauded at the miracle of a deaf person petitioning that body. They ordered Sicard's immediate release. But the days passed and the order was ignored. The prosecuter of the Revolutionary Commune arrived and told the prisoners that if they could prove they belonged to the clergy, they would be spared. Sicard hastened to point out that he did indeed belong to the clergy. He decided that he would open an institute for the deaf somewhere else and offered to leave the country at once if they would release him. Most of the clergy were herded off as promised but, for some reason, Sicard was left behind in prison. A day or two later, some more prisoners arrived and the visitors reported that the priests who had been herded off were actually not being deported, but were being sent to the Abbey of Saint Germain de Prés for execution. The Minister of the Interior instructed the mayor of Paris to show cause why Sicard had been arrested, and why he should not be released immediately as ordered by the National Assembly; he replied that it was not his province but that of the *Comité d'Exécution*. The committee replied that since Sicard's papers had been seized for prosecution their contents could not be revealed, and hence they could not answer the minister's questions. On September 2, 1792, the signal for the bloodbath was given: with the third firing of the cannons, the people were to slaughter the enemies of the state. And slaughter they did. Soldiers entered the prison and led Sicard and others to the Abbey. The prisoners pleaded for carriages to protect them against the mobs, and the soldiers finally agreed but left the carriage doors open. As this pitiful caravan made its way through the streets, people attacked the riders in the carriages, hauling them out and killing them right on the street.

When they arrived at the Abbey, one of Sicard's group leapt out, made a dash for shelter, and was grabbed by the crowd and his throat cut. A second tried to slip out and disappear in the tumult, and the cutthroats fell on him. A third was seized and swallowed up by the mob as the carriage approached the main door. The fourth was struck by a sword as he entered the building. Somehow Sicard, cowering in the back of the carriage, was overlooked. And the crowd moved on to the second wagon. Sicard slipped into the Abbey where an administrative meeting was in progress. He begged for their protection. While he was making his entreaty, there was thunderous knocking on the door. Sicard gave his watch to one of the people there and said, "My life is over, but tomorrow a young deaf boy will come here asking after me and I want you to give him this watch." That of course was Massieu who had a passion for watches. Sicard knelt, he prayed, the doors were thrown open and the crowd rushed in and screamed, "There are the bastards we're after! Let's get them!" One of them said, "Why, it's the Abbé Sicard. The father of the deaf." The crowd hesitated for just a moment and Sicard leapt up on a ledge and he said, "Yes, that's me. Look, there are many deaf people in France and they're all poor. I belong to them, and hence, I

belong to you." And the voice cried, "We must spare Sicard. He's too useful to kill. Anyway, he doesn't have the time to be a conspirator." "Spare Sicard, spare Sicard!" the crowd chanted. The cutthroats rushed forward and embraced him. They offered to lead him home in triumph, but Sicard preferred to wait for an official release. In that, he made a grave error, because in the morning a messenger arrived to tell him that he would be executed at 4:00. "How can that be? I was to be spared." He quickly wrote a note to a deputy at the National Assembly, "Stop this. Come wearing the tricolors, and lead me away from this carnage." The messenger hastened to the assembly, but it was no longer in session. He found the deputy, however, and the deputy found the president and the president of the assembly went before the Committee on Public Instruction which sent an officer to the Abbey to give Sicard safe escort. He led him back to the National Assembly, meantime reconvened, which rose to applaud the father of the deaf. Within hours Massieu was back in his arms and the deaf were united with their benefactor.

A few years later Sicard was in trouble again, this time for publishing a religious political newspaper. He narrowly missed deportation and was forced into a sort of exile in the outskirts of the city for over a year. Finally he published a remarkable avowal which will help you to understand why I called him earlier a person of few principles: "For me, all authority exercized by the powers that be is by that very fact, legitimate. Thus, by the same faith that I was a royalist in '89, '90, '91, and '92, I am, since the Proclamation of the Republic, a zealous Republican. The monarchy is, as far as I am concerned, as if it had never existed." When Napoleon was exiled and the Bourbon monarchy restored, Sicard changed his tune again, and when Napoleon threatened to return, Sicard fled with Massieu to London, where he met Gallaudet.

So the myth is replaced by the reality. Massieu taught Sicard sign language. Massieu saved Sicard's life, and not the other way around. I thought you might like to hear a little bit of Massieu's story, in his own words.

> I was born at Semens in the department of La Gironde. My father died in 1791. My mother is still live. There were six deaf-mutes in my family: three boys and three girls. Until the age of 13 years 9 months, I stayed in my region without receiving any sort of instruction. I was in the dark. I expressed my ideas through manual signs and by gestures, which I employed to communicate with my parents and brothers and sisters. These signs were quite different from those of educated deaf people. Strangers did not understand me when I expressed myself in this way, but neighbors understood me well enough. I saw cattle, horses, mules, pigs, dogs, cats, vegetables, houses, fields . . .

Do you know why he's going through this list? Because at that time it was reasoned that you could not have thought without language, and since the deaf had no language, they presumably could not think about things and could not remember their perceptions.

> Having considered these objects I remembered them well. Before my education, when I was a child, I did not know how to read and write. I wanted to read and write. I often saw young boys and girls going to school. I wanted to follow them and I was very jealous of them. I asked my father with tears in my eyes for permission to go to school. And my father refused, signing to me that I could never learn anything because I was a deaf-mute. And then I cried. Despairing, I put my fingers in my ears and I asked my father impatiently to unstop them! He answered that there was no remedy. One day, I left my father's house and went to school without telling him. I went up to the teacher and with gesture I asked, "Teach me to read and write." He refused and sent me away. I was twelve . . . When I was a child, my father made me pray in the morning and evening with gestures . . . I knew how to count, my fingers taught me. I didn't know the numbers. I counted on my fingers and when the number passed 10 I made notches on a piece of wood . . . One day, a man who passed while I was tending my flock took a liking to me and invited me to his house to eat and drink. The man, when he went to Bordeaux, spoke about me to the Abbé Sicard, who agreed to take charge of my education . . . In a period of three months I knew how to write several words and in six months I knew how to write several sentences. In one year's time, I wrote fairly well. In a year and some months, I wrote better. And I responded well to questions. I was with the Abbé Sicard three and a half years when I left with him for Paris. In four years, I became like people who can hear and speak.

The reality then is that the credit for this collaboration goes primarily to Massieu. But Sicard, like Epée, helped to perpetuate the signing society and thus the sign language, which continued to evolve. Jean-Marc Itard gives us a very interesting description of the difference, as a result of this evolution, between Massieu and his successor Laurent Clerc, both of whom Itard knew intimately.

> Comparing our current deaf-mutes with those first pupils trained in the same institute, by the same method under the same director, we are led to recognize their superiority which can only be due to their having come later, at a more advanced stage of the signing society. There they found two sources of instruction that could not exist in its earliest days: the [signed] lessons given by the teachers, and their conversations with pupils already educated. Thus it is that instruction is easier and more widely effective than it was twenty years ago. At that time, Massieu was a dazzling phenomenon in the midst of his unfortunate companions, who remained well behind him, still at the first stages of their education; nowadays, he is nothing more than a highly distinguished student. Instruction, powerfully assisted by tradition, has more rapidly developed and civilized his companions; one among them has equaled him, and several have come close and would have surpassed him had they not so promptly left the institute . . .
>
> Let us contrast Massieu . . . with [Laurent] Clerc, this student whom I said was his equal in instruction but who, having come quite recently to the institute, ought to have profited by all the advantages that a more advanced civilization can offer. Massieu, a profound thinker, gifted with a genius for observation and a prodigious memory, favored by the particular attention of

his celebrated teacher, benefiting from an extensive education, seems nevertheless to have developed incompletely: his ways, habits, and expressions have a certain strangeness that leaves a considerable gap between him and society. Uninterested in all that motivates that society, inept at conducting its affairs, he lives alone, without desires and ambition. When he writes, we can judge even better what is lacking in his mentality: his style fits him to a tee, it is choppy, unconventional, disorderly, without transition but swarming with apt thought and flashes of brilliance.

Clerc with a less encompassing and towering intelligence, trained as much by the institute as by any teacher, presents a picture of much more uniform development. Clerc is entirely a man of the world. He likes social life, and often seeks it out, and he is singled out for his polite manners and his perfect understanding of social custom and interests. He likes to be well-groomed, appreciates luxury and all our contrived needs, and is not insensitive to the goads of ambition. It is ambition that snatched him from the Paris institute, where he had a worthy and comfortable existence [as a teacher], and led him across the seas to seek his fortune.

Part III: Laurent Clerc and the Reverend Gallaudet

The setting: Hartford, Connecticut. The year is 1805. Thomas Gallaudet was graduated from Yale that year and, like Epée, took up studies for the ministry. Like him, he encountered a young deaf woman, or rather a girl, Alice Cogswell. He tried to teach her to say a few words and had some success.

The Problem: To begin the education of the deaf in the United States. The clergymen's association of Connecticut reported that there were some 89 deaf people at the time in the State. By extrapolation, that meant that there might be perhaps 2,000 in the United States. There was no institution for the deaf here.

The solution: Alice's father, Dr. Mason Cogswell, persuaded Gallaudet to go to Europe to learn methods for educating the deaf and to return to Hartford and open a school.

The myth: Gallaudet heard about sign language through Cogswell's collection of books by the Abbé Sicard. He went to France to learn the sign language and returned to the United States to introduce it to the deaf and thereby to educate them.

The reality: He didn't want to go to France. He didn't speak French. He was a confirmed oralist, to start with. In the end, he was forced to study with the Abbé Sicard. Gallaudet went first to London as part of his plan to learn how to educate the deaf. He knew that the Braidwood School, which originated in Edinburgh, had a monopoly on the education of the deaf in the United Kingdom. He hoped to learn the Braidwood method, which was reportedly so successful in teaching lipreading and pronunciation. He went to London to a school run by a relative of Thomas Braidwood. The instructor told him, "I'm very sorry, but I can't teach you the method because I'm under a thousand pound bond never to reveal the Braidwood art of instruction." Gallaudet was dismayed. He went to another school outside of London, which was part of the same monopoly and received the same answer. Then he learned that the Abbé Sicard was in London with Massieu and Clerc demonstrating his method before the Pariliament. Gallaudet went to the performance and was very impressed. He asked for an introduction to Sicard, and got it. Sicard said to him, "If you'd ever like to come to Paris and learn our method, learn our language, you'd be most welcome." Gallaudet said "Thank you, no. That's very nice of you." He set out for the Birmingham school, where he was turned away. Then he went on to Edinburgh, where Thomas Braidwood's grandson said, "I can't reveal the method to you, but my brother John will open the school with you in America." Gallaudet didn't have that in mind, the more so as John was a drifter and alcoholic. But he wanted to learn the oral method. Braidwood offered to train him. "If you commit yourself to spend six months—at most a year—here as one of our students, then we'll accept you." But he said, "No, I don't have six months, or a year."

So Gallaudet went to Paris. He took the Abbé Sicard up on his offer. When Gallaudet arrived, Sicard said, "Let's get to work. We'll teach you sign language. In the morning Jean Massieu will give you private lessons. In the afternoon you'll attend a class taught by Clerc. And you and I will meet once a week to talk over the whole thing, the metaphysical principles on which my system is based."

Two months went by and our hero became impatient. He wasn't making that much progress in the language. He was anxious to get back to Hartford; so he went to Clerc and asked, "Will you come back with me?" Imagine! Clerc was, first of all, a man terribly attached to France and to Paris. It was his land, he was fluent in French. He was a bit of a boulevardier, a man about town. He liked the bistros, he liked a little white wine, he liked his croissant in the morning, he liked the art galleries, he liked French clothing. And here was a man who proposed that he go live with the Indians somewhere across the ocean. If today the French think that Americans are primitive, just imagine what they thought of us then. And Clerc said, according to his diary, "You know, I don't want to go, but I think I must." He went home to see his mother to say good bye. And she said, "I've just gotten a letter from the Abbé Sicard and he pleads with me to stop you." And Clerc said, "Mother, I must."

And, as you know, he left.

During the voyage, Clerc continued to instruct Gallaudet in sign language. He wrote and eventually published his diary. By the way, the Hartford School printed it, and it's available today. He taught Gallaudet sign and Gallaudet taught Clerc his second foreign language, English.

After arriving in Hartford they went about New England raising funds. They opened a school, the American Asylum for the Deaf, now the American School. It was from this nucleus that the sign language Clerc imported from France spread throughout the United States.

Clerc taught the hearing people who went on to become the directors of the New York School, the Kentucky Institution, the Virginia School, the Pennsylvania School, the Ohio School, the School in Quebec, as well as others. These people went out then and taught "the sign language" as it was called in those days. And of course, Clerc taught the deaf, first and foremost, Alice Cogswell, and then others, who studied this language and, integrating it with the gestural communication they already employed, made it their own.

Nowadays there are over two hundred schools for the deaf in the U.S. and perhaps half a million children and adults who communicate in American Sign Language.

Part IV: Pupils Deaf and Hearing

Epée, Sicard, Gallaudet: these are not the real heroes of our story. I should say, of your story. I suggest that leafing through documents in the National Library and Institution for Deaf Children in France, in the American School in Harford and in other institutions, will convince you, as it has me, that the real heroes of this story are the deaf. I would like to say a word as a teacher to other teachers here. Society puts us in a false role. We are presented as the purveyors of wisdom. But that was not the contribution of Epée, that was not the contribution of Sicard, nor of Gallaudet. The genius of these men was to have the sensitivity, the openness to observe their pupils. I think that's what makes a great teacher: a willingness to be the pupil oneself. Gallaudet was ready to be Clerc's pupil. Sicard was ready to be Massieu's pupil. Epée was ready to learn from the handful of children at his school. The willingness of the deaf to collaborate with them was also required for these teachers to become successful pupils. Without Clerc, Gallaudet would have returned from Europe emptyhanded; ignorant of both oral and manual methods of educating the deaf, without a highly educated deaf person to show what could be achieved, he might have gone to serve some parish anonymously in one or another New England town. Without Massieu, Sicard would have died amid the misdirected passions of the Revolution, if indeed he ever made it to Paris from the provinces. No Clerc, no Gallaudet; no Massieu, no Sicard; and, without the six anonymous young deaf children to whom we owe the greatest debt, no Abbé de l'Epée.

The milestones in the education of the deaf were placed there jointly by hearing teachers with the humility to become pupils and by deaf pupils who cared enough to teach them. Thank you for teaching me. Long live the collaboration.

The Value of the Sign-Language to the Deaf[1]

Edward M. Gallaudet

A few isolated instances are recorded, previous to the last century, of deaf persons who, under favorable conditions, have developed for their own use a measurably complete language of signs. But it was only toward the middle of the eighteenth century that this language was used by considerable numbers of deaf-mutes. Before describing this general use, however, it is important to consider, somewhat carefully, the limitations as to means of communication which absolute deafness imposes on those who suffer from it.

The means of expression possible to creatures of intelligence, by which information as to thought and feeling may be given and received, are five in number, corresponding to the senses. All expression, *i.e.*, all communication from one intelligent being to another, must, therefore, be either audible, visible, tactile, odorice, or palatal. The senses of taste and smell are addressed so rarely and with such difficulty, for the purpose of communicating thought, that they may be left out of view. The same may be said of the sense of touch, except that, in the case of persons both blind and deaf, it becomes the main channel of communication, and may be made useful under certain conditions with such as are only deaf; as, for example, in the dark, or when it is desirable to address the deaf without diverting the eye from some object—such as a landscape, a passing pageant or spectacle. George Dalgarno, in his curious and interesting work "Didascalocophus," or "The Deaf and Dumb Man's Tutor," published in Ox-

ford in 1680, presents an alphabet arranged upon the palm of the hand, certain letters being associated with certain joints and other parts of the hand, by the use of which one may communicate with a deaf person without demanding the attention of his eyes, his hand being touched by the fingers of the speaker so that words are rapidly spelt. The Morse telegraph alphabet may also be made use of in communicating through the sense of touch, by giving taps or pressures of varying length as to time, the hand of one resting lightly on the arm of the other.

Visible expression employs a great variety of forms in the accomplishment of its purpose, but these forms may be grouped in two perfectly distinct classes; the *gestural*, which produce their effects only from moment to moment, having no enduring quality, and the *graphic*, which are more or less permanent.

Audible expression, almost infinite as it is in variety, is susceptible also of division into two great classes, *articulate* and *inarticulate*, the former comprising all forms of word utterance, and the latter including cries, moans, sighs, music, percussions and explosions.

Among all these possible means of transmitting intelligence from one to another, it will readily be seen that the three principal means of communicating thought and feeling made use of by man are: 1, *articulate speech* addressed to the sense of hearing; 2, *gestural;* and 3, *graphic expression* presented to the sense of sight.

---

1   Extracted, by permission, from an article in Buck's "Reference Handbook of the Medical Sciences" (William Wood and Company, New York, 1886), entitled "The Language of Signs and the Combined Method of Instructing Deaf Mutes."

which are not in any manner recorded or made permanent.

Graphic expression will then include all forms of writing and printing, all productions in the fine arts, all marks, of whatever character, that are in any degree permanent, and are designed to communicate information or to express thought and feeling. And the range of this form of expression is wide enough to embrace at one extreme the Duomo of Milan, or Milton's noblest poem, and at the other the cattle brand of a Texan cow-boy, or the blaze of a backwoodsman's axe in the primeval forest.

In determining the value of gestural expression to the deaf, it is necessary to keep constantly before the mind the fact that, where hearing does not exist, no mental impressions can be received through the means of articulate speech. In other words, that he who would communicate with the deaf is limited to gestural and graphic means. Even in cases where a deaf person retains the power of speech, or is taught to speak and to understand the speech of others by watching the motion of the lips, such motions are to him nothing other than a certain form of gestural expression. The peculiar element of sound, the perception and understanding of which enables a hearing person to comprehend speech *without* seeing the vocal organs of the speaker, is wholly wanting to the deaf. And so essential is the possession of hearing to the free use and enjoyment of articulate speech as a means of communication from man to man, that to the deaf this can be no more, at its very best, than what an artificial leg is to one who would walk, or run, or dance. Serviceable, no doubt; far better than no leg at all; but never an equivalent for the missing member.

Have the deaf, then, no means of expression that can be as free and as perfect as speech is to their more favored brethren?

A distinguished scientist and philanthropist, justly honored and respected in the city of his adoption (Washington, D.C.), who has long been interested in the education of deaf-mutes, but who has had little experience in teaching them,

said recently, in a paper read before one of the learned societies of Washington:

> "Nature has been kind to the deaf child; man, cruel. Nature has inflicted upon the deaf child but one defect, imperfect hearing; man's neglect has made him dumb, and forced him to invent a language which has separated him from the hearing world." "Let us then," says the learned writer, "remove the afflictions that we ourselves have caused." And, after some eminently reasonable suggestions, he adds: "And last, but not least, let us banish the sign-language from our schools."

Nature has indeed been kind to the deaf child, in that she has left him capable of using as freely as his hearing brother the gestural and the graphic means of communicating thought; in that she has made it natural and easy for him to employ a method of expression, in the use of which he is at no disadvantage as compared with his hearing brother, and which is, beyond all dispute, the *only* means of communication which can be to the deaf what speech is to the hearing as a vehicle of thought. And this "language of action," which philologists agree is the foundation of all human intercommunication, which is the acknowledged vernacular of the deaf, the distinguished theorist, and not a few others with him, would "banish from our schools." Of such an act of "kindness" proposed by certain teachers of the deaf on both sides of the Atlantic, one of the most eminent and successful oral teachers of deaf-mutes in Germany says: "If this system were put into execution, the moral life, the intellectual development of the deaf and dumb would be inhumanly hampered."

The founder of deaf-mute instruction in America, who is to be ranked among the most successful teachers of the deaf in the world, says, in an article on "The Natural Language of Signs," written some years after he had completed his work for the deaf, and when he had had time to review his methods with calmness:

> My object is to show the intrinsic value and, indeed, indispensable necessity of the use of

natural signs in the education of the deaf and dumb. * * * In attempting this, I wish I had time to go somewhat at length into the genius of this natural language of signs; to compare it with merely oral language, and to show, as I think I could, its decided superiority over the latter, so far as respects its peculiar adaptation to the mind of childhood and early youth.

In what relates to the expression of passion and emotion, and of all the finer and stronger sentiments of the heart, this language is eminently appropriate and copious.

So far as objects, motions, or actions addressed to the senses are concerned, this language, in its improved states, is superior in its accuracy and force of delineation to that in which words spelt on the fingers, spoken, written, or printed are employed.

This claim of the superior accuracy and precision of the sign-language, as compared with words, may perhaps excite surprise at first thought. But it is believed that its reasonableness will appear when it is remembered that the meanings attached to words are almost wholly arbitrary, very few giving the slightest hint of their signification in their shape or sound; while nearly every gesture used in the sign-language carries with it a plain suggestion of its meaning, and in very many instances gives a vivid and easily recognized portrayal of the idea to be conveyed.

The signs for such objects, for example, as *salt, pepper, milk, coffee*, would be at once understood by one unaccustomed to the use of gestures, were they made at the table. In a school-room the most ignorant child would catch the meaning at once of signs for such objects as *slate, pen, book*, and, indeed, of a host of familiar things.

But slight explanation is needed to make clear to one uninstructed in gesture-language the meaning of the signs in common use for such emotions as *love, hatred, fear, pain, anger*.

That children often learn, repeat, and sometimes even make use of words the meaning of which they comprehend very imperfectly, is a familiar fact to parents and teachers. An incident in the childhood's experience of a lady belonging to one of the most cultivated families of New England well illustrates this point. The pastor of the church to which her family belonged was in the habit of teaching the children of his charge the Assembly's Shorter Catechism *viva voce;* and the children committed it to memory thus, without making use of any book. Mrs. T——— said that, when nearly grown, she came across a copy of the book, and was much surprised to find that the first question was not "What is man's chefand?" which she had always supposed it to be.

Since experience has proved that the sign-language is natural to the deaf, that it is acquired and made use of by them more easily than speech is by the hearing, that it furnishes a full and adequate means for communicating thought and feeling, often surpassing speech in vividness and exactness, it is not strange that teachers of the largest experience and broadest view unite in approving its use in the education of the deaf.

Nor is it surprising that those who would "banish signs from the school room" are, for the most part, persons who have never learned to use them, and have, therefore, no experimental appreciation of their value in teaching. And these persons are utterly incapable of giving the deaf, either in school or after they have passed into adult years, the great comfort and benefit of public addresses. For it is through the use of the sign-language alone that the deaf can enjoy lectures, sermons, or debates.

At this point the question will naturally arise in many minds: "Does the sign-language give the deaf in these respects *all* that speech affords to the hearing?"

The experience and observation of the writer lead him to answer the question with a decided affirmative. On many occasions it has been his privilege to interpret, through signs to the deaf, addresses given in speech; he has addressed assemblages of deaf persons many times, using signs for the original expression of though; he has seen hundreds of lectures and public debates given originally in signs; he has seen conventions of deaf-mutes in which no word was spoken, and yet all the forms of parliamentary proceeding were observed, and the most excited and earnest discussions carried on; he has seen the ordinances of religion administered, and the full services of the church carried on in signs; and all this with the assurance growing out of his own complete understanding of the language, a knowledge of which dates back to his earliest childhood, that for all the purposes above enumerated, gestural expression is in no respect inferior, and is in many respect superior, to articulate speech as a means of communicating ideas.

But the greatest value of the sign-language to the deaf, when the whole period of their lives is taken into account, is to be found in the facility it affords for free and unconstrained social intercourse. And in this, as in the matter of public addresses, nothing has been discovered that *can* fully take its place. It may even be asserted that so long as the deaf remain without hearing, nothing else can give them what speech affords their more favored brethren. They may have much pleasant intercourse with others by the employment of writing-tablets, they may even enjoy conversation under many limitations with single individuals through articulation and lip-reading; with the aid of the manual alphabet they may have a still wider and more enjoyable range for the interchange of thought; but it is only by employing signs that they can gain the pleasure and profit that comes from conversation in the social circle, that they can enjoy such freedom of intercommunication as shall make it possible for them to forget they are deaf.

Graduates of oral schools from which the attempt has been made to "banish signs," have repeatedly testified that they could in no way attain to such pleasure in social intercourse as through the use of the sign-language, ability to employ which they readily acquire by mingling with those more favored deaf-mutes who have become familiar with it earlier in life.

"But," say those who urge that the use of signs is an injury to the deaf, "they can use that language only with their fellow-unfortunates, or with the very few others who learn it for their sake, and their use of signs tends to make them clannish, thus narrowing the sphere of their lives and leading them to employ in excess a language other than the vernacular of their country."

It is admitted that, in the education of the deaf, injudicious teachers may allow, or even encourage, too free a use of the sign-language in the schools—that such teachers may suffer their pupils to go out from under their influence without being impressed with the importance of making special and persistent efforts to overcome the *tendency* to clannishness which is natural to the deaf, no matter what method of instruction is employed.

It is not disputed that in teaching the deaf, signs may be so employed as to affect unfavorably the acquisition by the pupil of verbal language, whether in its written or spoken forms.

But nothing is more certain, as proved by the experience of nearly three-fourths of a century in this country, than that the unfavorable results, which some have charged upon the use of the sign-language, are attributable in all cases to its *abuse* by injudicious, incompetent, or inexperienced teachers. Since 1817, when the first school for deaf mutes in this country was established, more than twenty-three thousand children have been educated in forty-nine schools now in successful operation, in all of which the sign-language has been made use of. A majority of these persons are living to-day, and may be found in every city, probably in every county of the land.

Among these, thousands could be named who, while associating freely with their fellow deaf-mutes, and deriving both profit and pleasure from such association, mingle readily with persons who hear; who are not clannish to any degree that would subject them to just criticism; who use the vernacular of the country with freedom and reasonable accuracy; who maintain themselves reputable and comfortably by their own labor;

who are, in short, good and intelligent citizens, adding strength, wealth, and character to the communities in which they reside.

And could the history of these persons be fully known to one competent to attach due weight to all the elements that had combined to give them what they have enjoyed, it would certainly be discovered that no one factor had contributed more to the sum of their happiness than the free and intelligent use of that form of communication which a beneficent Providence has made easiest and most natural to them—the language of signs.

Thomas Hopkins Gallaudet on Language and Communication: A Reassessment

James J. Fernandes

Though he is best known for his innovations in deaf education, T. H. Gallaudet also contributed insights and ideas to the study of language and communication. An investigation of his writing in this field indicates that some of his ideas about sign language have been misunderstood or overlooked and that in several instances he anticipated the work of 20th-century linguists, anthropologists, and rhetoricians.

Thomas Hopkins Gallaudet is revered and rembered as the founder of American education of the deaf and the man who, with Laurent Clerc, helped promote the use of sign language as an instructional method in the United States. Yet many misconceptions are commonly held about why and how Gallaudet became a staunch supporter of sign language, and one of his major arguments—that hearing people could greatly benefit from the study of sign language—has long been forgotten. Based on a reexamination of Gallaudet's correspondence and published works on the topic of sign language, this paper intends to clarify some misunderstandings about the origins of sign language instruction in the U.S. and to point out the relevance of Gallaudet's innovative ideas to educational practices and the study of communication today.

Misconceptions

Why Gallaudet Adopted the Manual Approach

When students are taught the history of deaf education, they are usually told that T. H. Gallaudet went to Europe in 1815 with the goal of learning the British (oral) system of instruction and that, frustrated by the secrecy and lack of cooperation of British educators, he turned to the French for help and thus adopted the manual approach. At best, this explanation is oversimplified, and it may be inaccurate as well. It is true that Gallaudet wanted to learn about the educational methods employed in England, but there is evidence that from the start he intended to investigate both the French and English systems with the aim of combining them. In the first place, he was familiar with the French system of instruction before visiting Europe. An early biographer writes that in Gallaudet's first informal attempts to teach his young deaf neighbor, Alice Cogswell, he was guided by "a publication of the Abbe Sicard which Dr. Cogswell had procured from Paris" (Barnard, 1859, p. 13). Apparently the book by Sicard, who was the head of the school for the deaf in Paris, enabled Gallaudet and others to learn the manual alphabet and some sign language. While Gallaudet was abroad, Alice was "mainstreamed" in a school run by the poetess Lydia Huntley Sigourney, who described how Alice was taught, revealing that Alice and her fellow students were already familiar with signing:

Words or historical facts thus explained by signs, were alphabetically arranged in a small manuscript book for her to recapitulate and familiarize. Great was her delight when called forth to take her part. Descriptions in animated gesture she was fond of intermingling with a few articulate sounds. Fragments from the annals of all nations, with the signification of a multitude of words, had been taught little by little, until her lexicon had become comprehensive; and as her companions, from love, had possessed themselves of the manual alphabet and much of the sign-language, they affectionately proposed that the examination should be of themselves, and that she might be permitted to conduct it. (Sigourney, 1866, p. 221)

Further evidence that Gallaudet's original intention in traveling to Europe was to synthesize the French and English modes of instruction comes from a letter he wrote to Mason Cogswell (Alice's father) from England on August 15, 1815. In the letter, Gallaudet described the difficulty he was having with gaining access to the trade secrets of the Braidwood schools, but said he would keep trying, for "I should wish, and yet hope, to combine the peculiar advantages of both the French and English modes of instruction" (T. H. and E. M. Gallaudet papers).

Finally, Gallaudet's decision to abandon the British teaching method was not merely the result of the Braidwoods' unwillingness to cooperate. A major influence on this decision was Dugald Stewart, a Scottish philosopher whom Gallaudet met while in Edinburgh and came to view as an esteemed mentor. As a "philosopher of the mind," Stewart studied what we would today call psychology. His understanding of sensory perception and language acquisition led him to believe that a purely oral approach was an unsatisfactory way to teach language to deaf children. Stewart helped convince Gallaudet that the French system of teaching the deaf was superior to the English system.

Another influence on Gallaudet's decision about instructional methods was his own observation. Despite the reluctance of the Braidwood family to reveal their teaching methods to him, Gallaudet was able to visit their schools in England and Scotland several times. In Scotland he attended a public examination of deaf students and concluded, in an entry to his journal on August 27, 1815: "The definitions were good, the composition quite interesting and ingenious, the communication by signs very partial and imper-

fect, and the articulation not of such a kind as to lead me to form any very favorable idea of this branch of the instruction of the deaf" (T. H. and E. M. Gallaudet papers).

A final, and most significant, influence on Gallaudet's decision to opt for the French mode of teaching stemmed from his own motives in becoming a pioneer of deaf education. He was a Protestant minister, an evangelist committed to the spread of Christianity, and he saw sign language as an efficient tool for teaching the deaf about God and as a means for deaf people to conduct their worship and prayer. It seemed to Gallaudet that the British system, with its emphasis on the slow and tedious process of teaching articulation, was not suited to the urgent need to provide religious education to deaf people.

Speech Training in America

A second misconception about the early education of the deaf in the United States is that no training in speech was provided at the American School in its first years. This view is fostered in part by Gallaudet's own published writing, but a careful examination of the historical evidence shows that it may be incorrect.

In 1818-1819 a lively debate about the better method for teaching the deaf (oral versus manual) was carried out in the pages of the *Christian Observer*, a British monthly, between Gallaudet and an anonymous correspondent. In his letters to the *Observer*, Gallaudet cited Dugald Stewart's remarks on the inexpedience of teaching articulation and complained that time spent on such teaching "prevents the instructor from devoting his time to more pupils, and to a more important part of education—the actual communication of knowledge, and the unfolding of the powers of the human mind" (Gallaudet, August 1818, p. 515). He went on to illustrate how the use of signs and pantomime to convey the significance of words was prerequisite to the acquisition of spoken or written language and presented a further argument in favor of sign language: that it could be used for religious instruction:

As this language of signs is capable of becoming a vehicle of all important religious truth, and as this truth can thus be communicated to the deaf and dumb long before they are able to read and write the English language correctly; another powerful reason is thus furnished for its cultivation and use. (Gallaudet, October 1819, p. 649)

Gallaudet questioned the utility of teaching articulation as an aid to languge acquisition. Since the significance of spoken words must be conveyed by referring to objects and pictures or through the use of sign language, he argued:

Why then perplex (the pupil's) mind with two arbitrary modes of communication during the progress of his education, when one is so easy and natural to him, and the other so difficult and constrained? Much time is lost, much embarrassment produced, and a great waste of labour takes place. (Gallaudet, December 1819, p. 786)

Because students stayed an average of only 3 years at the Hartford school, Gallaudet saw the teaching of speech as a laborious and time-consuming distraction from the more pressing needs of providing religious instruction, general education, and the acquisition of written language. Furthermore, the early pupils at the American School tended to be young people who were born deaf or deafened at an early age. Gallaudet's observations and experience convinced him that sign language was the most direct and expeditious method of imparting knowledge to such people.

However, there is some evidence that he was more open to instruction in articulation, even at the American School, than his letters to the *Christian Observer* would indicate. On February 1, 1818, he wrote to Connecticut Congressman Nathaniel Terry Washington and asked him to seek information on John Kirkpatrick, who, with the ill-fated John Braidwood, had briefly operated a small school for the deaf in Virginia (T. H. and E. M. Gallaudet papers). Gallaudet conjectured that if he were worthy, Kirkpatrick might be hired to teach at the American School. Since Gallaudet knew that Kirkpatrick's method of in-

struction would be the British one taught him by Braidwood, the letter to Terry was in effect an admission of Gallaudet's interest in offering oral training at the Hartford school. However, Kirkpatrick never did become affiliated with that school.

A final bit of testimony supports the contention that some type of instruction in oral communication skills has been given to select students at the Hartford school since its founding. In his history of the American Asylum, Job Williams declared:

Articulation has always had a place in the instruction given in this school. From the beginning the semi-mute and semi-deaf have had their speech kept up and improved by special attention. (Williams, 1893)

The safest conclusion to draw from the existing evidence, then, is that although Gallaudet favored the use of sign language as the most expedient means of conveying knowledge (especially about Christianity) to deaf students, he was not averse to training in oral communication for specific students. He reasoned that the visual language of signs was the most effective way of conveying knowledge to and establishing rapport and moral influence with students who could not hear. Noting that deaf people themselves were the originators of the language, he held that, in the conduct of education, "it is the part of wisdom to find the path which nature points out, and to follow it" (Gallaudet, 1847, p. 87). But his mind was apparently open to the utility of oral training for appropriate individuals and under appropriate circumstances. In fact, a posthumously published manuscript by Gallaudet, originally written in 1807, tells of his encounter with a man who, though deaf for 14 years, had laboriously learned to lipread and maintain clear speech in order to converse with family and friends. Gallaudet concluded: "This recital will not be altogether useless should it but prove the means of encouraging any who are deaf to attempt the acquisition of an art, which can restore to them one of the sweetest enjoyments of life" (Gallaudet, 1858, p. 249).

Innovative Ideas

Gallaudet's ideas about language acquisition and communication are surprisingly current and worthy of reconsideration, not only for the above-mentioned reasons but also as a rough gauge of educational progress (or lack of it) along the lines he suggested some 150 years ago. Gallaudet's thoughts in this regard appear in two essays published in three parts in the *Christian Observer* in 1826 and in an article appearing some 20 years later in the first volume of the *American Annal of the Deaf* (1847).

Language and Meaning

Gallaudet's first essay in the *Christian Observer* was devoted to consideration of "some of the elementary principles of language in general" (Gallaudet, August 1826, p. 465). The essay encompassed an analysis of meaning and the process by which meaning is learned and, in so doing, presaged some of the main tenets of 20th-century rhetorical theorists such as I. A. Richards. Richards is regarded as a major contributor to contemporary rhetorical (communication) theory (Johannesen, 1971), defining it as the "study of misunderstanding and its remedies" (Richards, 1965, p. 3) and focusing on language, the process of eliciting meaning, and the relationships among meaning, thinking, and human relationships (Golden, Berquist & Coleman, 1976, pp. 159-160).

Richards's definition of language is remarkably similar to Gallaudet's. According to Richards, a "language transaction" is defined as "a use of symbols in such a way that acts of reference occur in a hearer which are similar in all relevant respects to those which are symbolized by them in the speaker" (Ogden & Richards, 1936, pp. 205-206). Compare this with Gallaudet's definition of language, written a century earlier: "the expression, by visible, audible, or tangible signs,

of the thoughts, feelings, or state of one mind, in order to excite the conception of them in another" (Gallaudet, 1826, p. 465). Both definitions make the point that the true locus of meaning is in the mind of the communicator and that language is a tool or medium used to elicit "acts of reference" or "excite the conception."

Richards is recognized by communication scholars for unveiling what he termed the "Proper Meaning Superstition," i.e., the mistaken belief "that a word has a meaning of its own (ideally, only one) independent of and controlling its use and the purpose for which it should be uttered" (Richards, 1965, p. 11). Meaning is not contained in words; meanings are interpretations learned from paired encounters with words and their referents. According to Richards, "Our interpretation of any sign is our psychological reaction to it, as determined by our past experience in similar situations, and by our present experience" (Ogden & Richards, 1936, pp. 244-245). In this century Richards was acclaimed for these innovative observations on the nature of meaning, yet in 1826 Gallaudet had called attention to the same mistaken beliefs about the acquisition of meaning:

> It is a great mistake to suppose that language, in itself considered, ever conveys any emotions, or purposes; but the elements which compose these combinations must have been previously known, either by actual observation of external objects through the medium of the senses, or by the actual consciousness of the internal operations, emotions, and affections of the soul. . . .
>
> We are apt to attribute a sort of magical power to speech, as if the articulate sounds of the human voice were in themselves sufficient to convey the import of the language which is uttered. (Gallaudet, August 1826, p. 468)

Language Education

Not only did Gallaudet's sensitivity to and understanding of the nature of language and meaning anticipate contemporary communication scholars, he called for the same type of educational reform that is popular today. As he wrote in the continuation of his essay in the *Christian Observer:*

> When we consider the importance of language, with regard to the education of youth . . . and that this mighty instrument derives all its force from a few simple principles which are developed in the first stages of our being,—who cannot but lament, that so little has yet been done to carry these principles into correct and successful operation, and that children are left to acquire the elements of their mother tongue almost to chance; or, if entrusted to the care of a teacher, that it is deemed quite sufficient if he can lead them to pronounce, and spell, and read correctly. (Gallaudet, September 1826, p. 530)

Among the reasons Gallaudet cited for the "neglect of the early education of children in the import and use of language" was "the popular objection" to formal instruction in this area, it being commonly held "that children will take their own way in learning the elements of speech." Another reason for "the prevalent low state of improvement in the early education of children," according to Gallaudet, was inadequate fundings for schools, and a final reason was the failure of teachers to be child-centered in their approach to language instruction (Gallaudet, September 1826).

Interestingly, 150 years later, educators are calling for the same kind of reform and noting the same problems to which Gallaudet was sensitive. Ward (1971), for example, states that many parents today see no reason for language instruction. As Ward notes, "After all, the child will learn to talk—all children within (the mother's) experience have. She is more concerned about overt behavior, not his speaking ability" (p. 55). In response to this neglect, Allen and Brown (1976, pp. 241-251) propose that educators should have as a major concern "the development of the child as a message strategist"; that instruction in language "rules, norms, and conventions . . . may not be ignored or relegated to a small corner of the curriculum"; that "communication behaviors of children can be modified by training and by edu-

cation"; and that "communication educators should be child centered in their educational perspectives."

Thus, Gallaudet's ideas on language instruction are still being advocated today. The current concern with communication skills as part of a "back-to-basics" movement in education would no doubt have pleased Gallaudet. Larson, Backlund, Redmond, & Barbour (1978, p. 37) echo Gallaudet's words in this regard when they state their concern with developing communication skills in children and contend "that the focus of language-development education should emphasize not only correct or 'standard' language performance but also the use of language in various communication situations." In calling for this type of curriculum 150 years earlier, Gallaudet was clearly a man ahead of his time.

Recognition of Sign Language

Another area in which Gallaudet anticipated 20th-century scholarship relates to the nature and utility of sign language and visual-gestural communication. In his October 1826 essay in the *Christian Observer,* Gallaudet proposed sign language as a kind of *lingua franca* to be employed by missionaries in communicating with people in foreign lands. He argued that the universal intelligibility or transparency of mime and gesture, coupled with the iconicity of many signs, would make visual-gestural language appropriate as an international medium of communication. Citing the facility with which sign language makes communication possible between deaf and hearing people, Gallaudet suggested that it could similarly provide a channel of communication between people who spoke different languages. In effect, he proposed sign language as a second language to be used by foreign missionaries and others who might contact speakers of other languages.

Though Gallaudet called for an "experiment" in which sign language would be used to communicate with natives from other countries as a means of learning their languages and teaching them English, the idea never caught on. Thus it was that, in 1975, no less an authority on culture and pidgin languages than Margaret Mead proposed a "new" idea: that sign language be adopted as an international *linqua franca* just as Latin had been in the Middle Ages.

Gallaudet also foresaw the conclusions of 20th-century linguists by recognizing the viability of American Sign Language as a language. Gallaudet's definition of language, cited above, which noted that the symbols making up a language may be "visible, audible or tangible," indicates that he recognized that an essential feature of language is the use of symbols rather than the use of one particular mode (i.e., speech). While scientific investigation of the structure and syntax of American Sign Language had to await the latter half of this century, Gallaudet had attempted to prove much earlier, through the use of examples or "illustrations," that sign language included such grammatical niceties as adjectives, pronouns, and verb tenses and moods. His conclusion was "that the language of the countenance, signs, and gestures, is an accurate, significant, and copious medium of thought" (October 1826, pp. 595-596). Gallaudet frequently avowed in print that the signs of the deaf comprised a true language, but the preceding statement is significant for its recognition that sign language is not simply manual but rather a visual-gestural language, including not only signs but body movement and facial expression. Thus his understanding of sign language is in easy agreement with the conclusions of contemporary linguists (Baker & Cokely, 1980).

Nonverbal Communication

Gallaudet's awareness of the visual-gestural nature of sign language aroused in him an interest in nonverbal communication. As a New Englander, he looked with dismay on the lack of nonverbal skills of his fellow citizens:

It is greatly to be regretted that much more of this visual language does not accompany the

oral, in the domestic circle, and, indeed, in all our social discourse. Our public speakers often show the want of it, in their unimpassioned looks, frigid, often monotonous attitude, and quiescent limbs, even though they are uttering the most eloquent and soul-stirring thoughts. Would they but *look out* and *act out* these thoughts, as well as speak them, how much greater power their eloquence would have. Why has the Creator furnished us with such an elaborate and wonderful apparatus of nerves and muscles, to subserve the purposes of this visual language; with such an eye and countenance, as variable in their expressions as are all the internal workings of the soul and graphically indicative of them; and with such a versatility of attitude and gesture susceptible of being "known and read of all men," —thus to supply the deficiencies of our oral intercourse, and to perfect the communion of one soul to another, if we are to make no more use of these things than if we were so many colorless and motionless statues! (Gallaudet, 1848, p. 80)

In order to make better use of this God-given potential, Gallaudet advised that nonverbal skills be cultivated in children during early education in the family and school. If this were done, he predicted:

We should find its happy results . . . on all occasions when the persuasions of eloquence are employed, and in the higher zest which would be given to the enjoyments of social life. As a people, especially in New England, we ought to be sensible of our deficiency in this respect and labor to remove it. Let us begin in our discourse with children and youth, and lead them, by our example, to have the soul speak out freely in their looks and movements. (Gallaudet, 1848, pp. 80-81)

Gallaudet was not unique in calling attention to nonverbal communication. Indeed, 19th-century British and American elocutionists had popularized the study of gesture, movement, facial expression, and vocal control for public speakers. Gallaudet's friend, Chauncey Allen Goodrich, included delivery or nonverbal communication skills in his lectures on rhetoric and public speaking at Yale, though he apparently focused on the use of voice rather than on the visual aspects of nonverbal communication (Hoshor, 1965). However, Gallaudet's innovativeness came, not only with his emphasis on the visual aspects (i.e., facial expression and gesture) of nonverbal communication, but with his suggestion that these skills be taught to young children. He even proposed that teachers in "infant schools" might use sign language with their hearing students as a means of encouraging the development of visual-gestural communication skills. If this were done, Gallaudet declared, "I have no doubt the delight which . . . little pupils would take in this language, and the livelier attention and interest which it would excite in them in pursuing their studies" (August 1826, p. 465). Oddly enough, his advice seems only recently to have been accepted, with the appearance of sign language vignettes on such educational television programs as "Sesame Street" and the advent of new courses on the visual-gestural bases of sign language, designed for both hearing and deaf people, as a means of developing skills to improve both signing and nonverbal expressiveness.

Summary and Conclusions

In reinvestigating the writings of Thomas Hopkins Gallaudet on the subject of sign language and communication, this essay has revealed that some of his ideas regarding the use of sign language in teaching deaf students may have been partially misunderstood. It seems likely that his original intention was to combine the use of sign language with the British method of speech training. His decision to adopt sign language at the American School was not really the result of difficulties in gaining access to the methods used in the Braidwood Schools but was heavily influenced by the advice of a prominent philosopher-psychologist, Gallaudet's own observation, and his fervent wish to expedite the religious instruction of deaf people in the most direct manner possible. Despite his opting for the use of sign language as an instructional mode, Gallaudet apparently did favor the use of speech training for some students.

In addition, this analysis of some of Gallaudet's published work on language and communication leads to the inevitable conclusion that he was a man well ahead of his time. Many of his ideas and assertions are today being suggested anew or corroborated by recent research findings. For example, his analysis of the function of language and the creation of meaning is remarkably similar to the major premises of the rhetorical theory of the 20th-century scholar, I. A. Richards. In the same way, Gallaudet's suggestions about the teaching of language and communication skills are akin to the proposals of modern educators who assess curricula in American schools. Some 150 years ago, Gallaudet anticipated linguists' findings that American Sign Language is indeed a language in its own right, as well as the suggestion of a prominent anthropologist that signing might form the basis of an international *lingua franca*. Finally, his ideas on education and nonverbal communication skills are another innovation that only now is beginning to be put into effect.

Though Gallaudet is remembered chiefly as one who helped educate deaf people, this look at his work suggests that he was equally successful as a student of deaf people and their means of communication. His ability to learn about communication from his work with deaf people and to apply that learning to better understand the communication process in general is another noteworthy achievement.

References

Allen, R., & Brown, K. L. *Developing communication competence in children*, Skokie, Ill.: National Textbook Company, 1976.

Baker, C., & Cokely, D. *American Sign Language: A teacher's resource text on grammar and culture*, Silver Spring, Md.: T. J. Publishers, 1980.

Barnard, H. Tribute to Gallaudet. A discourse in commemoration of the life, character, and services of the Rev. Thomas H. Gallaudet, LL.D., delivered before the citizens of Hartford, Jan. 7, 1852 (2nd ed.). New York: F. C. Brownell, 1859.

Gallaudet, T. H. Expediency of teaching the deaf and dumb to articulate. *Christian Observer*, 1818, 17, 514-517.

Gallaudet, T. H. On teaching the deaf and dumb. *Christian Observer*, 1819, *18*, 646-650; 784-787.

Gallaudet, T. H. On oral language and the language of signs. *Christian Observer*, 1826, *26*, 465-470; 525-533.

Gallaudet, T. H. The language of signs auxiliary to the christian missionary. *Christian Observer*, 1826, *26*, 592-599.

Gallaudet, T. H. The value and uses of the natural language of signs. *American Annals of the Deaf and Dumb*, 1847, 1848, *1*, 55-66; 79-93.

Gallaudet, T. H. Reading on the lips. *American Annals Deaf and Dumb*, 1858, *10*, 249.

Golden, J. L., Berquist, G., & Coleman, W. (Eds.). *The rhetoric of Western thought*. Dubuque, Ia.: Kendall/Hunt, 1978.

Hosher, J. P. Lectures on rhetoric and public speaking by Chauncey Allen Goodrich. In L. G. Crocker & P. A. Carmack (Eds.), *Readings in rhetoric*, Springfield, Ill.: Charles C. Thomas, 1965.

Johannesen, R. L. (Ed.). *Contemporary theories of rhetoric: Selected readings*, New York: Harper & Row, 1971.

Larson, C., Backlund, P., Redmond, M., & Barbour, A. *Assessing functional communication*, Urbana, Ill.: ERIC Clearinghouse on Reading and Communication Skills, 1978.

Mead, M. Commencement address. Gallaudet College, Washington, D. C., May 19, 1975.

Ogden, C. K., & Richards, I. A. *The meaning of meaning* (4th ed.). New York: Harcourt, Brace & Company, 1936.

Richards, I. A. *The Philosophy of rhetoric* (Reprint ed.). New York: Oxford University Press, 1965.

Sigourney, L. H. *Letters of life*, New York: D. Appleton, 1866.

Thomas Hopkins Gallaudet and Edward Miner Gallaudet Papers. Library of Congress. Manuscript Division.

Ward, M. C. *Them children*, New York: Holt, Rinehart & Winston, 1971.

Williams, J. A brief history of the American Asylum, at Hartford, for the education and instruction of the deaf and dumb. In E. A. Fay (Ed.), *Histories of schools for the deaf*, Washington, D.C.: Volta Bureau, 1893.

Laurent Clerc: America's Pioneer Deaf Teacher

Loy Golladay

Since 1817, the hearing impaired in this country have had many outstanding leaders and teachers who were themselves deaf. With the 100th anniversary of the NAD coming up, deaf Americans have new reason to be interested in their heritage. And it is about time for a reappraisal of the role of one of the most influential persons in the history of the American deaf—Laurent Clerc.

Thomas Hopkins Gallaudet brought Clerc from France in 1816 to help start America's first permanent school for the deaf, in Hartford, Connecticut. This is rather well-known, but not many people—deaf or hearing—know how much Clerc did, directly or indirectly, to interest the United States Congress, various state legislatures and hearing people in general in making this first effort successful.

When the American School for the Deaf opened April 15, 1817, Clerc was Gallaudet's guide and teacher. He organized the courses, tested and placed the new students. Over the years he gave lessons to many others in how to teach the deaf.

Perhaps most important of all, he brought us our sign language, which today thousands of hearing people are learning, because it's a beautiful, expressive and fascinating way to communicate.

A year after opening, the new school was overcrowded with poor and uneducated deaf students. These ranged from 10 or 12 years of age to as old as 51 years. Very few could pay their way and the future looked dark. Classroom and living space, food and teachers' salaries had to be paid for somehow.

Clerc had already solved the problem of how to teach and communicate with the deaf. The problem of support was now at a crisis. Laurent Clerc was the most influential person in getting this support so that the school did not have to close.

But let us start at the beginning of this fascinating story.

* * *

The home of the mayor of LaBalme, France, was made joyful by the arrival of a baby son on December 26, 1785. LaBalme is 26 miles east of Lyons, in southeastern France, not far from the Swiss border. Mayor Joseph Francis Clerc and his good wife named the new baby Laurent, in honor of a favorite uncle. He also had a long string of other names, but we will not bother with them here.

The Clerc family was of some importance, for the eldest sons for 300 years had held the office of *tubelion,* or king's commissary. Clerc's mother's father was also a magistrate in a nearby community.

No doubt a great deal was expected of the new son. In those days in France, few common people learned to read or write, but the Clercs not only could do that, but knew common law.

When little Laurent was about a year old, somehow he fell into the kitchen fireplace and was severely burned on his right cheek. Clerc's name-sign comes from the resulting scar—the first two fingers of the right hand brushed down the right cheek near the mouth.

When Clerc recovered from the fever which followed, it was discovered that he was deaf and had lost the sense of smell. It seemed Laurent could never expect to follow his father in office, or learn to read or write! For most deaf children in those days were unable to get any education.

While Laurent Clerc was growing up, there was much confusion and political unrest in France. The people rebelled against unfair rulers and poor living conditions. Many noblemen lost their lives or had to escape to other countries. The king and queen were beheaded. Later, Napoleon's wars and final exile to a lonely island in the South Atlantic were to affect Clerc's life, too.

When Clerc was 12 years old in 1797, his uncle Laurent took him to Paris, to the Royal Institution for the Deaf. This school had been founded by the Abbe Charles Michel de l'Epee about 1760. It was then headed by the Abbe Roche-Ambroise Sicard. Clerc's first teacher was Jean Massieu—a brilliant deaf man who would become Clerc's lifelong friend.

When Clerc arrived at the school, the Abbe Sicard was in prison. It was expected that he would be put to death, because he was a priest, and most priests supported the king. Led by Jean Massieu, the deaf pupils of the school took a letter to the court, begging that their teacher be freed to teach them. This saved Sicard's life. Another time, Sicard also had a narrow escape from death at the hands of a mob.

Clerc proved to be a hard-working student. Besides his school subjects, he learned drawing and the printing trade. After only eight years as a pupil, Clerc was chosen to be a teacher. When Gallaudet arrived in France in 1816, Clerc was teaching the highest class in the school and was Sicard's chief assistant.

During this time, things were happening in America that would change Clerc's life. The poor deaf French village boy would become the key person to open the minds of thousands and thousands of deaf Americans who were not yet born.

In Hartford, Connecticut, Alice Cogswell, aged two, became deaf from a fever. Her father, Dr. Mason Fitch Cogswell, was a pioneer in operating on blind people for cataracts. He knew that no doctor could give Alice back her hearing. Instead, he began to think of how to start a school for Alice and others like her.

A young neighbor, Thomas Hopkins Gallaudet, was home from theological seminary and expecting to accept a job as minister to a church in New Hampshire. One day he succeeded in teaching Alice the word "HAT." More words followed, because Alice suddenly realized that things have names. Dr. Cogswell and eight other Hartford friends collected enough money to send Gallaudet to Europe. He was to learn to teach the deaf there and come back to start a school for the deaf.

Before that a few wealthy deaf children went to England or France for an education. But the only class in America, in Goochland County, Virginia, did not last long. It was started by a Colonel Bolling for his deaf children. Thomas Jefferson refused to support the idea of a school for the deaf in connection with the University of Virginia. (Ironically, Jefferson's great-grandson, Thomas Jefferson Trist, was born deaf and became a teacher of the deaf, but that was much later.)

When Gallaudet left for Europe, he wrote that he hoped to include the best parts of both the English (oral) method of communication and the French (manual) method which included speech training for some students. This is the first known mention of a "combined" system for America. Teachers may be interested in this fact.

It happened that the Abbe Sicard was in England when Gallaudet arrived in London, July 5, 1815. This was again because Sicard was a royalist, or supporter of the king. Napoleon had escaped from exile in Elba. He was gathering his old soldiers to overthrow Louis XIII. Sicard thought it wise to be absent in England for a while. He took with him his two star pupils and teachers, Massieu and Clerc. They supported themselves by giving demonstrations twice a week on how to teach the deaf. Many important

English people attended these programs. The War of 1812 against England had ended just six months before Gallaudet arrived in London, a lone American. He happened to read a notice in a newspaper about the demonstrations. On July 8, Gallaudet went to meet the three Frenchmen and on July 10 he attended one of their lectures and saw how the two deaf men could give replies to the many questions that people asked them. Gallaudet was very much impressed with their answers. They invited him to visit their Paris school when the political situation should be better. Soon after meeting Gallaudet, they returned to Paris.

* * *

In the following months Gallaudet was frustrated in his hope to learn to teach the deaf in England. The Braidwood family which started the first schools there, kept their methods secret. They made their teachers sign a contract to keep it secret for at least seven years. They wanted Gallaudet to stay for three years, and then sign a contract to keep methods secret. This was impossible for Gallaudet to accept. Finally, with time and money running short, Gallaudet went to Paris. He was welcomed warmly and soon began studying their methods. In March 1816, he was moving from class to class in the Paris school and taking lessons from Sicard, Massieu and Clerc. Clerc also gave him private lessons in his spare time.

Gallaudet heard that Clerc had once been considered to help start a school for the deaf in Russia—but he was passed over because he was deaf. Russia's loss was America's gain.

Gallaudet soon realized that he could not learn enough about teaching the deaf in the time he had left. We do not know for sure who first suggested that Clerc return with Gallaudet to America. Clerc wrote that Gallaudet suggested it. Gallaudet wrote that Clerc volunteered! On May 20, Clerc agreed to come to America for three years, to help organize the new school, to be its first

experienced teacher and to teach others how to teach the deaf.

The Abbe Sicard was then a very old man. He did not want to give up Clerc, but he finally was persuaded. On June 18, 1816, Gallaudet and Clerc sailed for America on the ship, *Mary Augusta.* During the 52-day voyage, Gallaudet taught Clerc the English language, and Clerc taught Gallaudet signs and teaching methods. Clerc kept an interesting diary of the trip, and very soon he was able to write important speeches in almost perfect English, to be given before meetings of several state legislatures and citizens' groups. This was necessary, because they found no money ready for the school when they arrived in Connecticut.

* * *

The year 1816 is sometimes called "eighteen-hundred and froze to death." A volcano in the Dutch East Indies near Java exploded and filled the air all around the world with dust. The sunlight was cut off and the weather was cold for many months. There was really no summer, for crops froze in the fields. A sheep froze to death in Maine and people kept their fireplaces going all summer. December was the warmest month, according to newspaper stories. Clerc got a rather "cold" reception in America as far as weather is concerned—but his diary does not mention this.

* * *

Clerc's education, culture and seriousness of purpose quickly won the interest of people at the meetings they held to raise money in several cities in the eastern states. Without clear proof in the person of Clerc, that deaf people could be educated, and educated well, the project to raise money for the school might almost surely have failed. People must see to believe about things like that. By giving speeches and demonstrations over about eight months, Gallaudet and Clerc raised about $5,000. The Connecticut General

Assembly voted another $5,000. This was the first appropriation in history for the education of the handicapped.

On April 15, 1817, the school opened in rented rooms in Hartford. Clerc examined and grouped the students. Soon he had things moving smoothly in spite of interruptions from curious people who wished to see the new enterprise. Before the year was over, it became clear that a regular source of money was necessary if the school was to survive. It was not supported by state or Federal government, and families of the pupils could not raise enough money to pay. Gallaudet and others had been preparing the way for a request for help from the United States government. But again the key man to unlock this source of support was none other than Laurent Clerc.

On January 15, 1818, Clerc left by stagecoach for Washington, D.C., to ask Congress for help. He was accompanied by a board member of the school, Henry Hudson. The House of Representatives voted a half-hour recess to hear the visitors. The Speaker of the House, Henry Clay, invited Clerc to sit beside him. He and other congressmen conversed with Clerc in both the French and English languages.

To Clerc's surprise, Clay said that he had seen him before in France! While on a diplomatic mission, Clay had seen him and another deaf gentleman (probably Massieu) talking in sign language at the cafe where Clay often lunched.

The next day Clerc met the French ambassador, M. Hyde de Neuville. He was taken to meet President James Monroe. Imagine how Clerc felt when the President wrote that he, too, had seen Clerc—in London, where Monroe attended one of Sicard's demonstrations with Clerc and Massieu. Incidentally, Monroe had helped arrange for a deaf student from Virginia to attend the Paris school, but we do not know for sure if he actually visited the school while Clerc was teaching there.

So it came about that in the 1819-20 session of Congress, Clay helped the congressmen from Connecticut to sponsor a bill that granted a township (23,000 acres) of government land in Alabama to the school. The name "American" came from this U.S. support. President Monroe signed the act, which is now in the American School's historical museum, along with many other mementoes of Gallaudet and Clerc. From the $300,000 or so that was obtained from sale of the land, the new school was able to put up a set of buildings and start a small endowment for income. Several state legislatures also paid for pupils from their areas.

Besides teaching and other duties, for many years Laurent Clerc trained other people in ways of teaching the deaf. Some school heads whom he taught included Abraham Stansbury (New York); The Rev. A. B. Hutton (Pennsylvania); H. N. Hubbell (Ohio); Roland MacDonald (Quebec, Canada); Joseph Dennis Tyler (Virginia); John Adamson Jacobs (Kentucky); J. S. Brown (Indiana); and Isaac Lewis Peet (also New York). As the United States spread westward, several of Clerc's deaf students also started new schools. Many of them became teachers, like Clerc. One of them, Edmund Booth, was the first chairman when the NAD was founded in 1880 in Cincinnati. (An article on Mr. Booth is being prepared for *The Deaf American* by this writer.)

On May 3, 1818, Laurent Clerc was married to Miss Eliza Boardman of Whiteborough, New York. She had been one of the very early pupils of the school. She lost her hearing at about the age of three, but had some speech. Attractive, vivacious, intelligent and of graceful manners, Mrs. Clerc was a good reason for her husband to spend the rest of his life in America.

The Clercs had six children, all with normal hearing. One, the Rev. Francis Joseph Clerc, D.D., became a noted Episcopal minister. Guy B. Holt, a great-great-grandson of Laurent Clerc, was president of the American School's Board of Directors many years, until his death in the spring of 1975. A high school boys dormitory at the American School is named for Mr. Holt, and a high school girls dormitory is named for Clerc.

* * *

Other schools began to spring up. Clerc was asked to become acting principal of the Pennsylvania Institution in August 1821. For over six months he organized classes and curriculum, trained the teachers and made plans for the future to give to the Board of Directors. While in Pennsylvania, Clerc, his wife and baby daughter were painted by the famous American artist, Charles Willson Peale. These oil portraits now belong to the American School, given by a Clerc descendant.

Clerc had agreed in 1816 to stay in America only three years, but he made only three visits to France during the rest of his life. These were in 1820, 1835 and 1846. The latter times he took along one of his sons, first Francis, then Charles, to improve their ability to speak the French language.

Schools for the deaf had been established in many states by 1850. That year the graduates of these schools decided to honor their first two teachers. They organized a special meeting in Hartford. Gallaudet had given up teaching the deaf in 1831 after 14 years, but he kept up his interest. He was a board member of the school until his death. At that time, 1850, Clerc had been teaching for over 43 years—about 10 in France, and 33 in America. The deaf presented each of them with an engraved, coin-silver pitcher and tray, specially designed. The Gallaudet silver is still owned by members of the family in Michigan.

Several very flattering speeches were made about Gallaudet and Clerc by their former pupils. It is interesting to read the modest and self-effacing Clerc's answer to these speeches. He had always given credit to Gallaudet and to God for blessing the new school. Now he also gave credit to Hartford citizens who gave money to send Gallaudet to Europe; to the Board of Directors; to the governors and legislatures of the New England states who gave support; and to the government of the United States for the important land

grant. In short, he gave the credit to everyone except himself. But Gallaudet made sure to name Clerc as the man that they could not have succeeded without.

In 1858, when Clerc was 73 years old, he was retired with a pension after teaching 50 years. In June 1864, then aged 79, he made the long and tiring train trip to Washington to speak at the inauguration of the National Deaf-Mute College, now Gallaudet College. Although Clerc had never had the chance to attend a college, he received honorary degrees from several New England colleges for his work with the deaf.

Clerc's last years were spent peacefully. He enjoyed visiting the library and reading rooms of Hartford, meeting his friends and keeping an interest in the school. He passed away July 18, 1869, at the age of 84 and is buried in Hartford.

* * *

Besides the two Charles Willson Peale oil portraits, John Carlin, a noted deaf painter and friend of Clerc, painted at least two excellent pictures of Clerc. One is at the Kentucky School for the Deaf, and the other belongs to the Episcopal Mission to the deaf in Philadelphia.

Clerc was a leading member of a committee for a monument to his old friend, Gallaudet, who died in 1851. In 1874, five years after Clerc's own death, his friends dedicated a beautiful memorial to him in Hartford. It is a bronze head-and-shoulders bust set on top of a polished black granite base. On the bottom is the name "Clerc" spelled out with bronze hands in the manual alphabet. The wording on the granite base calls him "The Apostle to the Deaf-Mutes of the New World" . . . "who left his native land to uplift (them) with his teaching and encourage them by his example."

Several organizations such as literary societies are named for Clerc. Besides the girls dormitory at the American School, there is an older one at the Kentucky School named for him—and, of course, the high-rise Clerc Dorm at Gallaudet College.

The best monuments of Clerc are not in brick, or stone or even statues. They are in the deaf people of America since 1817 who have followed Clerc's teaching: To stand on their own feet, to solve their problems in a realistic manner, and never to feel sorry for themselves. Thus the life of a little deaf boy, born in an obscure French village, has made a difference.

"Everyone Here Spoke Sign Language"

Nora Groce

The fifth of April, 1715, had not been a good day for Judge Samuel Sewell of Boston. On his way to the island of Martha's Vineyard there had been trouble finding a boat to cross Nantucket Sound. The vessel then lay for hours without wind, and once it was across, the horses had to be pushed overboard to swim for shore on their own. Sewell and his company reached shore at dusk—cold, hungry, and in bad humor. Finding a group of local fishermen nearby, the judge engaged one of them to guide him to Edgartown and later noted in his diary: "We were ready to be offended that an Englishman . . . in the company spake not a word to us. But," he continued by way of explanation, "it seems he is deaf and dumb."

This Englishman was indeed deaf, as were two of his seven children. His is the first recorded case of what we now know to be a form of inherited deafness that was to appear consistently within this island population for more than 250 years and affect dozens of individuals. Probably one or several of the small number of settlers who originally populated the area brought with them a trait for hereditary deafness. As long as the "gene pool" remained limited in the small island population, this trait appeared with high frequency in subsequent generations. Put another way, the founders of this isolated society had a greater likelihood of perpetuating the trait for congenital deafness than if they had been part of a larger, changing population.

Martha's Vineyard offers what I feel to be a good example of the way in which a community adapts to a hereditary disorder. Lying some five miles off the southeastern coast of Massachusetts, the island was first settled by Europeans in the early 1640s. The population, of predominantly English stock with some admixture of indigenous Wampanoag Indian, expanded rapidly, owing to a tremendously high birthrate. Families that had fifteen to twenty children were not uncommon and twenty-five to thirty not unheard of. Although several hundred households are listed in the census records of the mid-eighteenth century, only about thirty surnames are to be found, and during the next century and a half only a handful more were added to the original group of names.

After the first generation, marriage "off-island" was rare. While Vineyard men sailed around the world on whaleships, merchantmen, and fishing vessels, they almost invariably returned home to marry local girls and settle down. Women married off-island even less frequently than did the men. Contact with the mainland was said to be more sporadic than with foreign countries. In the nineteenth century, islanders claimed that more of their men had been to China than to Boston, only eighty miles away. Even today, many islanders have never been to the island of Nantucket, barely eight miles to the east.

Throughout the seventeenth, eighteenth, and nineteenth centuries, marriage patterns on the island followed the customs of any small New England community. Most of the islanders, however, could trace their descent to the same small nucleus of original settlers, indicating that although they were unaware of it, considerable "inbreeding" took place. The result was that during these two and a half centuries, within a population averaging little more than 3,100 individuals, hereditary deafness occurred at a rate many times that of the national population. For example, in the latter part of the nineteenth century, an estimated one out of every 2,730 Americans was born deaf. On Martha's Vineyard the rate was closer to one out of every 155. But even this figure does not accurately represent the distribution of deafness on the Vineyard.

Marriages were usually contracted between members of the same village, creating smaller groups *within* the island's population characterized by a higher frequency of deafness. The greatest concentration occurred in one village on the western part of the island where, by my analysis, within a population of 500, one in every twenty-five individuals was deaf. And even there the distribution was not uniform, for in one area of the village during this time period, one out of every four persons was born deaf.

The high rate of deafness on the island brought only occasional comment from island visitors over the years. Because most of the island deaf lived in the more remote areas of the island, few off-islanders were aware of their presence. Vineyarders themselves, used to a sizable deaf population, saw nothing unusual in this, and many assumed that all communities had a similar number of deaf members. Almost nothing exists in the written records to indicate who was or was not deaf, and indeed, only a passing reference made by an older islander directed my attention to the fact that there had been any deaf there at all.

While most of my information on island deafness has been obtained from the living oral history of islanders now in their seventies, eighties, and nineties, part of my genealogical data was acquired from the only other study of this deaf population. I came to know of it when an 86-year-old woman I was interviewing recalled that her mother had mentioned a "teacher of the deaf from Boston" at one time taking an interest in the island deaf. This "teacher of the deaf" turned out to be Alexander Graham Bell, who, having recently invented the telephone, turned his attention back to his lifelong interest in deafness research. Concerned with the question of heredity as it related to deafness, Bell began a major research project in the early 1880s, which was never completed.

Nineteenth-century scholars, without the benefit of Mendel's concept of unit factor inheritance (which only received widespread circulation at the turn of the century, although it had been published in the 1860s), were at a loss to explain why some but not all children of a deaf parent were themselves deaf. Selecting New England because of the older and unusually complete records available, Bell believed that by tracing back the genealogy of every family with two or more deaf children, he could establish some pattern for the inheritance of deafness. He soon found that practically every family in New England with a history of deafness was in some way connected with the early settlers of Martha's Vineyard, but he was unable to account for the fact that a deaf parent did not always have deaf children and so he abandoned the study. Although Bell never published his material, he left dozens of genealogical charts that have proved invaluable for my research—particularly because they corroborate the information I have been able to collect from the oral history of the older islanders.

Since Bell's time, scientists have found, through the construction and analysis of family pedigrees and the use of mathematical models, that congenital deafness may result from several causes: spontaneous mutations involving one or more genes; an already established dominant or recessive inheritance, as Mendel demonstrated; or factors otherwise altering normal development of the ear and its pathways to the brain. Human populations, of course, cannot be studied with the same exactness as a laboratory experiment. However, the appearance of apparently congenitally deaf individuals is far too frequent on Martha's Vineyard to be mere coincidence, and the evidence collected thus far points to a recessive mode of inheritance.

While the genetic nature of a hereditary disorder in small populations is something that both anthropologists and geneticists have studied, there is another question, rarely addressed, that is of equal importance: How does the population of a community in which a hereditary disorder exists adjust to that disorder—particularly one as prominent as deafness? In modern society the emphasis has been on having "handicapped" individuals adapt to the greater society. But the perception of a handicap, with its associated physical and social limitations, is tempered by the community in which it is found. The manner in which the deaf of Martha's Vineyard were treated provides an interesting example of how one community responded to this type of situation. "How," I asked my informants, "were the island deaf able to communicate with you when they could not speak?" "Oh," I was told, "there was no problem at all. You see, everyone here spoke sign language."

From the late seventeenth century to the early years of the twentieth, islanders, particularly those from the western section where the largest number of deaf individuals lived, maintained a bilingual speech community based on spoken English and sign language. What is of particular interest is that the use of sign language played an important role in day-to-day life.

Islanders acquired a knowledge of sign language in childhood. They were usually taught by parents, with further reinforcement coming from the surrounding community, both hearing and deaf. For example, recalling how she learned a particular sign, one elderly woman explained:

> When I was a little girl, I knew many of the signs, and the manual alphabet of course, but I didn't know how to say "Merry Christmas," and I wanted to tell Mr. M. "Merry Christmas." So I asked Mrs. M., his wife. She could hear and she showed me how. And so I wished Mr. M. "Merry Christmas" —and he was just so delighted.

This women then described how she taught her son, now in his late seventies, how to speak the language.

When my son was perhaps three years old, I taught him to say in sign language "the little cat and dog and baby." This man, who was deaf, he used to go down to our little general store and see people come and go. One day when I went down there, I took my son there and I said to him, "Go over and say 'how-do-you-do' to Mr. T.," the deaf man. So he went right over, and then I told him to tell Mr. T. so-and-so—a cat, a dog, and whatever. And wasn't Mr. T. tickled! Oh, he was so pleased to know a little bit of a boy like that was telling him all those things, and so he just taught my son a few more words. That's how he learned. That's how we all learned.

Particularly in the western section of the island, if an immediate member of the family was not deaf, a neighbor, friend, or close relative of a friend was likely to be. Practically all my "up-island" informants above the age of seventy remembered signs, a good indication of the extent to which the language was known and used. In this section, and to a lesser extent in the other villages on the island, sign language formed an integral part of all communications. For example, all informants remembered the deaf participating freely in discussions. One remarked:

> If there were several people present and there was a deaf man or woman in the crowd, he'd take upon himself the discussion of anything, jokes or news or anything like that. They always had a part in it, they were never excluded.

As in all New England communities, gathering around the potbellied stove or on the front porch of what served as a combination general store and post office provided a focal point for stories, news, and gossip. Many of the people I have talked to distinctly remember the deaf members of the community in this situation. As one man recalled:

> We would sit around and wait for the mail to come in and just talk. And the deaf would be there, everyone would be there. And they were part of the crowd, and they were accepted. They were fishermen and farmers and everything else. And they wanted to find out the news just

as much as the rest of us. And oftentimes people would tell stories and make signs at the same time so everyone could follow him together. Of course, sometimes, if there were more deaf than hearing there, everyone would speak sign language—just to be polite, you know.

The use of sign was not confined to small-group discussions. It also found its way into assembled crowds. For example, one gentleman told me:

They would come to prayer meetings; most all of them were regular church people, you know. They would come when people offered testimonials, and they would get up in front of the audience and stand there and give a whole lecture in sign. No one translated it to the audience because everyone knew what they were saying. And if there was anyone who missed something somewhere, somebody sitting near them would be able to tell them about it.

The deaf were so integral a part of the community that at town meetings up-island, a hearing person would stand at the side of the hall and cue the deaf in sign to let them know what vote was coming up next, thus allowing them to keep right on top of things.

The participation of the deaf in all day-to-day work and play situations contrasted with the manner in which those handicapped by deafness were generally treated in the United States during the same time period.

Sign language on the island was not restricted to those occasions when deaf and hearing were together, but was used on a regular basis between the hearing as well. For example, sign language was used on boats to give commands and among fishermen out in open water to discuss their catch. I was told:

Fishermen, hauling pots outside in the Sound or off Gay Head, when they would be heaven knows how far apart, would discuss how the luck was running—all that sort of thing. These men could talk and hear all right, but it'd be too far to yell.

Indeed, signs were used any place the distance prohibited talking in a normal voice. For example, one man remembered:

Jim had a shop down on the shore of Tisbury Pond, and his house was a ways away, up on the high land. When Trudy, his wife, wanted to tell Jim something, she'd come to the door, blow a fish horn, and Jim would step outside. He'd say, "Excuse me, Trudy wants me for something"; then she'd make signs to tell him what she needed done.

On those occasions when speaking was out of place, such as in church, school, or at some public gatherings, the hearing communicated through signs. Such stories as the following are common: "Ben and his brother could both talk and hear, but I've seen them sitting across from each other in town meetings or in church and telling each other funny stories in sign language."

Island people frequently maintained social distance and a sense of distinct identity in the presence of tourists by exchanging comments about them in sign language. The occurrence of what linguists call code switching from speech to sign also seems to have been used in certain instances. For example, I was told:

People would start off a sentence in speaking and then finish it off in sign language, especially if they were saying something dirty. The punch line would often be in sign language. If there was a bunch of guys standing around the general store telling a [dirty] story and a woman walked in, they'd turn away from her and finish the story in sign language.

Perhaps the following anecdote best illustrates the unique way island sign language was integral to all aspects of life:

My mother was in the New Bedford hospital—had an operation—and father went over in his boat and lived aboard his boat and went to the hospital to see her every night. Now the surgeon, when he left him in her room, said they mustn't speak, father couldn't say a word to her. So he didn't. But they made signs for about half an hour and mother got so worked up, they had to send father out, wouldn't let him stay any longer.

Sign language or rather sign languages—for even within this country there exist a number of distinct languages and dialects—are languages in their own right, systems of communication different from the spoken languages used by hearing members of the same community. It has often been noted that American Sign Language, the sign system commonly used among the deaf in the United States today, is influenced by French Sign Language, introduced to America in 1817. The data from Martha's Vineyard, however, clearly support the hypothesis, made by the linguist James Woodward, that local sign language systems were in use in America long before this. By 1817 (the year the American School for the Deaf was founded in Hartford, Connecticut), deaf individuals on Martha's Vineyard had been actively participating in island society for well over a century. Because they were on an equal footing, both socially and economically, with the hearing members of the community, and because they held town offices, married, raised families, and left legal and personal documents, there must have existed some sort of sign language system that allowed full communication with family, friends, and neighbors.

It may prove difficult to reconstruct the original sign language system used on the island during the seventeenth and eighteenth centuries, but study of this question is currently under way. Whatever the exact nature of the original language, we know that it later grew to acquire many aspects of the more widely used American Sign Language, as increasing numbers of deaf island children were sent to the school in Hartford during the nineteenth century. This combination of the indigenous sign system with the more standardized American Sign Language seems to have produced a sign language that was, in many respects, unique to the island of Martha's Vineyard. The most common remark made by islanders who still remember the language is that they find it very difficult or are completely unable to understand the sign language spoken by off-islanders or the translations for the deaf that are beginning to be seen on television.

The use of sign language as an active system of communication lessened as the number of individuals in the community with hereditary deafness gradually disappeared, the last few dying in the 1940s and early 1950s. This decrease in the number of deaf can be attributed to a shift in marriage patterns that began in the latter part of the nineteenth century, when both hearing and deaf islanders began to marry off-islanders. The introduction of new genes into the once small gene pool has reduced the chance of a reappearance of "island deafness."

As the number of islanders born deaf dwindled, younger generations no longer took an interest in learning sign language, and the older generations rarely had the need to make use of it. Today, very few people are left who can speak the language fluently, although bits and pieces of it can be recalled by several dozen of the oldest islanders. A few signs are still kept alive among those who knew the language and on a few of their fishing boats. As one gentleman, well along in his seventies, told me recently:

> You know, strangely enough, there's still vestiges of that left in the older families around here. Instinctively you make some such movement, and it means something to you, but it doesn't mean anything to the one you're talking to.

The Revolution of the Deaf

Oliver Sacks

Wednesday morning, March 9: "Strike at Gallaudet," "Deaf Strike for the Deaf," "Students Demand Deaf President"—the newspapers are full of these happenings today; they started three days ago, have been steadily building, and now are on the front page of The New York Times. It looks like an amazing story. I have been to Gallaudet College in Washington a couple of times in the past year, and have been steadily getting to know the place. Gallaudet is the only liberal arts college for the deaf in the world, and, moreover, it is the core of the world's deaf community—but, in all its 124 years, it has never had a deaf president.

I flatten out the paper and read the whole story: the students have been actively campaigning for a deaf president ever since the resignation last year of Jerry Lee, a hearing person who was president since 1984. Unrest, uncertainty, and hope have been brewing. By mid-February, the presidential search committee narrowed the search to six candidates—three hearing, three deaf. On March 1, three thousand people attended a rally at Gallaudet, to make it clear to the board of trustees that the Gallaudet community was strongly insisting on the selection of a deaf president. On March 5, the night before the election, a candlelight vigil was held outside the board's quarters. On Sunday, March 6, choosing between three finalists, one hearing, two *deaf*, the board chose a former dean of students at the University of South Carolina, Elisabeth Ann Zinser, the hearing candidate.

The tone, as well as the content, of its announcement caused outrage: it was here that the chairman of the board, Jane Bassett Spilman, made her comment that "the deaf are not yet ready to function in the hearing world." The next day, a thousand students marched to the hotel where the board was cloistered, then the six blocks to the White House, and on to the Capitol. The following day, March 8, the students closed the university and barricaded the campus.

Wednesday afternoon: The faculty and staff have come out in support of the students and their four demands: 1) that a new, *deaf*, president be named immediately; 2) that the chairman of the board, Jane Bassett Spilman, resign immediately; 3) that the board have a 51 percent majority of deaf members (at present it has seventeen hearing members and only four deaf); and 4) that there be no reprisals. At this point, I phone my friend Bob Johnson. Bob is head of the linguistics department at Gallaudet, where he has taught and done research for seven years. He has a deep knowledge of the deaf and their culture, is an excellent signer, and is married to a deaf woman. He is as close to the deaf community as a hearing person can be.[1] I want to know how he feels about the events at Gallaudet. "It's the most remarkable

---

1   One can be very close to if not actually a member of the deaf community without being deaf. Perhaps the most important prerequisite besides the knowledge of and sympathy for deaf people is being a fluent user of American Sign Language: the only hearing people who are ever considered full members of the deaf community are the hearing children of deaf parents for whom Sign is a native language. This is the case with Dr. Henry Klopping, the much-loved superintendent of the California School for the Deaf. One of his former students, talking to me at Gallaudet, signed, "He is deaf, even though he is hearing."

thing I've ever seen," he says. "If you'd asked me a month ago, I'd have bet a million dollars this couldn't happen in my lifetime. You've got to come down and see this for yourself."

When I visited Gallaudet in 1986 and 1987, I found it an astonishing, and moving, experience. I had never before seen an entire community of the deaf, nor had I quite realized (even though I knew this theoretically) that sign language might indeed be a complete language—a language equally suitable for making love or speeches, for flirtation or mathematics. I had to see philosophy and chemistry classes in Sign; to see the absolutely silent mathematics department at work; I had to see deaf bards, Sign poetry, on the campus, and the range and depth of the Gallaudet theater; I had to see the wonderful social scene in the student bar, with hands flying in all directions as a hundred separate conversations proceeded—I had to see all this, see it for myself, before I could be moved from my previous "medical" view of deafness (as a "condition," a deficit, which had to be treated) to a "cultural" view of the deaf as forming a community with a complete language and culture of its own. I had felt there was something very joyful, even Arcadian, about Galluadet—and I was not surprised to hear that some of the students were sometimes reluctant to leave its warmth and seclusion and protectiveness, the coziness of a small but complete and self-sufficient world, for the unkind and uncomprehending big world outside.

But there were also tensions and resentments under the surface, which seemed to be simmering, with no possibility of resolution. There was an unspoken tension between faculty and administration—a faculty in which all the teachers sign, and many are deaf. The faculty could communicate with the students, enter their worlds, their minds; but the administration (so I was told) formed a remote governing body, running the school like a corporation, with a certain "benevolent" caretaker attitude to the "handicapped" deaf, but little real feeling for them as a community or as a culture. It was feared by the students and teachers I talked to that the administration, if it could, would reduce still further the percentage of deaf teachers at Gallaudet, and further restrict the teachers' use of Sign there.

The students I met seemed animated, a joyous group when together, but often fearful and diffident toward the outside world. I had the feeling of some cruel undermining of self-image, even in those who professed "Deaf Pride." I had the feeling that some of them thought of themselves as children—an echo of the parental attitude of the board (and perhaps of some of the faculty). I had the feeling of a certain passivity among them, a sense that though life might be improved in small ways here and there, it was their lot to be overlooked, to be second-class citizens.

Thursday morning, March 10: A taxi deposits me on Fifth Street opposite the college. The gates have been blocked off for forty-eight hours; my first sight is of a huge, excited, but cheerful and friendly crowd of hundreds barring the entrance to the campus, carrying banners and placards, and signing to one another with great animation. One or two police cars sit parked outside, watching, their engines purring, but they seem a benign presence. There is a good deal of honking from the traffic passing by—I am puzzled by this, but then spot a sign reading HONK FOR A DEAF PRESIDENT. The crowd itself is at once strangely silent and noisy: the signing, the Sign speeches, are utterly silent; but they are punctuated by curious (to my ears and eyes) applause—an excited shaking of the hands above the head, accompanied by high-pitched vocalizations and screams. As I watch, one of the students leaps up on a pillar, and starts signing with much expressiveness and beauty. I can understand nothing of what he says, but I feel the signing is pure and impassioned—his whole body, all his feelings, seem to flow into the signing. I hear a murmured name—Tim Rarus—and realize that this is one of the student leaders, one of the Four. His audience visibly hangs on every sign, rapt, bursting at intervals into tumultuous applause.

As I want Rarus and his audience, and then let my gaze wander past the barricades to the great campus filled with passionate Sign, with passionate soundless conversation, I get an overwhelming feeling not only of another mode of communication, but of another mode of sensibility, another mode of being—unique, precious, complete in itself. One has only to see these people—even casually, from the outside (and I felt quite as much an outsider as those who walked or drove casually by)—to feel that in their language, their mode of being, they *deserve* one of their own, that no one not deaf, not signing, could possibly understand them. One feels, intuitively, that interpretation can never be sufficient—that the students would be cut off from any president who was not one of them.

Innumerable banners and signs catch the brilliant March sun: DEAF PREZ NOW is clearly the basic one. There is a certain amount of anger—it could hardly be otherwise—but the anger, on the whole, is clothed in wit: thus a common sign is DR. ZINSER IS NOT READY TO FUNCTION IN THE DEAF WORLD, a retort to Spilman's malapropos statement about the deaf. Dr. Zinser's own comment on *Nightline* the night before ("A deaf individual, one day, will . . . be president of Gallaudet") provoked many signs saying WHY NOT MARCH 10, 1988, DR. ZINSER? The papers spoke of "battle" or "confrontation" which gives a sense of a negotiation, an inching to-and-fro. But the students said: 'Negotiation'? We have forgotten the word "'Negotiation' no longer appears in our dictionaries." Dr. Zinser kept asking for a "meaningful dialogue,"

but this in itself seemed a meaningless request for there was no longer, there had never been, any intermediate ground on which "dialogue" could take place. The students were concerned with their identity, their survival, an all-or-none: they had four demands and there was no place for "sometime" or "maybe".

Indeed Dr. Zinser is anything but popular. It is felt by many not only that she is peculiarly insensitive to the mood of the students—the glaring fact that they do not want her, the university has been literally barricaded against her—but that she actively stands for and prosecutes an official "hard line." At fist there was a certain sympathy for her: she had been duly chosen and she had no idea what she had been thrown into. But with the passing of each day this view grew less and less tenable, and the whole business began to resemble a contest of wills. Dr. Zinser's tough, "no-nonsense" stance reached a peak yesterday, when she loudly asserted that she was going to "take charge" of the unruly campus. "If it gets any further out of control," she said, "I'm going to have to take action to bring it under control." This incensed the students, who promptly burned her in effigy.

Some of the placards are nakedly furious: one says ZINSER—PUPPET OF SPILMAN, another WE DON'T NEED A WET NURSE, MOMMY SPILMAN. I begin to realize that this is the deaf's coming of age, saying at last, in a very loud voice: "We're no longer your children. We no longer want your 'care.'"[2]

I edge past the barricades, the speeches, the signs, and stroll onto the large and beautifully

2   This resentment of "paternalism" (or "mommyism") is very evident in the special edition of the students' newspaper (The Buff and Blue) published on March 9, in which there is a poem entitled "Dear Mom." This starts:
Poor mommy Bassett-Spilman,
How her children do rebel.
If only they would listen
To the story she would tell
and continues in this vein for thirteen verses. (Spilman had appeared on television, pleading for Zinser, saying "Trust us—she will not disappoint you.") Copies of this poem had been Xeroxed by the thousand—one could seem them fluttering all over the campus.

green campus, with its elegant Victorian buildings setting off a most un-Victorian scene. The campus is buzzing, silently, with conversation—everywhere there are pairs or small groups speaking. There is conversing everywhere, and I can understand none of it; I feel like the deaf, the voiceless one today—the handicapped one, the minority, in this great signing community. I see lots of faculty as well as students on the campus; one professor is making and selling lapel buttons (FRAU ZINSER, GO IIOME!), which are bought and pinned on as quickly as he makes them. "Isn't this great?" he says, catching sight of me. "I haven't had such a good time since Selma. It feels a little like Selma—and the Sixties."

A great many dogs are on the campus—there must be fifty or sixty on the great greensward out front. Regulations on owning and keeping dogs here are loose; some are "hearing" dogs, but some are just—dogs. I am struck by the unusual intimacy of the deaf in their relationship with their dogs: perhaps because dongs aren't verbal, and don't discriminate. I see one girl signing to her dog: the dog, obediently, turns over, begs, gives a paw. This dog itself bears a white cloth sign on each side: I UNDERSTAND SIGN BETTER THAN SPILMAN. (The chairman of Gallaudet's board of trustees has occupied her position for seven years while learning hardly any Sign.)

Where there was a hint of something angry, tense, at the barricades, there is an atmosphere of calm and peacefulness inside the campus; more, a sense of joy, and something like festivity. There are dogs everywhere, and babies and children too, friends and little families everywhere, conversing silently in Sign. There are little colored tents on the grass, and hotdog stands selling frankfurters and soda—dogs and hotdogs: it is rather like Woodstock, much more like Woodstock than a grim revolution.

Earlier in the week, the initial reactions to Elisabeth Ann Zinser's appointment were furious—and uncoordinated; there were a thousand people on the campus, milling around, tearing up toilet paper, destructive in mood. But all at once,

as Bob Johnson said, "the whole consciousness changed." Within hours there seemed to emerge a new, calm, clear consciousness and resolution; a political body, two thousand strong, with a single, focused will of its own. It is the astonishing swiftness with which this organization emerged, the sudden precipitation, from chaos, of a unanimous, communal mind, that astonished everyone who saw it. And yet, of course, this was partly an illusion, for there were all sorts of preparations—and people—behind it.

Central to this sudden "transformation"—and central, thereafter, in organizing and articulating the entire "uprising" (which was far too dignified, too beautifully modulated, to be called an "uproar")—were the four remarkable young student leaders: Greg Hlibok, the leader of the student body, and his cohorts Tim Rarus, Bridgetta Bourne and Jerry Covell. Greg Hlibok is a young engineering student, described (by Bob Johnson) as "very engaging, laconic, direct, but in his words a great deal of thought and judgement." Hlibok's father, also deaf, runs an engineering firm, and he has two deaf brothers, one an actor, one a financial consultant. Tim Rarus, also born deaf, and from a deaf family, is a perfect foil for Greg: he has an eager spontaneity, a passion, an intensity, that nicely complement Greg's quietness. I saw, we all saw, more of these two than of the others, but all four worked closely, in absolute harmony, as beautifully coordinated as a string quartet.

The four had already been elected before the uprising—indeed while Jerry Lee was still president—but took on a very special, unprecedented role during the months that followed President Lee's resignation.

Hlibok and his fellow leaders never incited or inflamed students—on the contrary, they were always calming, restraining, and moderating in their influence, but were highly sensitive to the "feel" of the campus and, beyond this, of the deaf community at large, and felt with them that a crucial time had arrived. They started to organize the students to press for a deaf president, and to seek support from deaf leaders and communities all around the country. Thus, much calculation, much preparation, preceded the "transformation," the emergence of a communal mind. It was not an order appearing from total chaos (even though it might have seemed so). Rather, it was the sudden manifestation of a latent order, like the sudden crystallization of a supersaturated solution—a crystallization precipitated by the naming of Zinser as president on Sunday night. This was a qualitative transformation, from passivity to activity, and in the moral no less than in the political sense, it was a revolution. Suddenly the deaf were no longer passive, scattered, and powerless; suddenly they have discovered the calm strength of union.

I talk in the afternoon with a couple of deaf students. A young woman of about twenty tells me:

> I'm from a hearing family . . . My whole life I've felt pressures, hearing pressures on me— "You can't do it in the hearing world, you can't make it in the hearing world"—and right now all that pressure is lifted from me. I feel free, all of a sudden, full of energy now. You keep hearing "you can't, you can't," but I can now. The words "deaf and dumb" will be destroyed forever; instead they'll be "deaf and able."

These were very much the terms Bob Johnson had used when we first talked, when he spoke of the deaf as laboring under "an illusion of powerlessness," and of how, all of a sudden, this illusion had been shattered.

Many revolutions, transformations, awakenings, happen as a response to immediate (and intolerable) circumstances. What is so remarkable about the Gallaudet strike of 1988 is its historical consciousness, the sense of deep historical perspective that informed it. This was evident on campus; as soon as I arrived I spotted a picket saying LAURENT CLERC WANTS DEAF PREZ. HE IS NOT HERE BUT HIS

SPIRIT IS HERE. SUPPORT US. I overheard a journalist say, "Who the hell's Laurent Clerc?" But his name and his persona unknown to the hearing world, are known to virtually everyone in the deaf world. Clerc is a founding father, a heroic figure, in deaf history and culture. The *first* emancipation of the deaf—their achievement of education and literacy, of self-respect and the respect of their fellows—was largely inspired by the achievement and person of Laurent Clerc, a French writer and teacher who was himself born deaf.[3]

Clerc not only founded the American Asylum in Hartford in 1817, with Thomas Gallaudet, who wife was deaf, but he introduced a sign language ("French" sign language). Clerc was, in effect, the spiritual leader of the world community of the deaf until his death fifty-two years later. It was immensely moving, then, to see the placard bearing his name, and one could not help feeling that Clerc *was* here, on the campus, and that he was, albeit posthumously, the authentic spirit and voice of the revolt. (Clerc did indeed visit Gallaudet College in 1867, and in a stirring speech to the students encouraged them to aspire boldly, and to feel that no academic or professional position was "above" them).

The French sign system imported by Clerc rapidly amalgamated with the indigenous sign languages here—the deaf generate sign languages wherever they are; it is for them the easiest and most natural mode of communication—to form a uniquely expressive and powerful hybrid, American Sign Language (ASL).

Given this strong sign language, the previously despised and illiterate deaf of America now found that a full school education was open to them, as well as a new and more generous understanding by the general public; and with this, the deaf became literate, self-respecting, ar-

---

3   Indeed, Harlan Lane uses the life and voice of Laurent Clerc as the vehicle for his history of the deaf, *When the Mind Hears* (Random House, 1984). A visiting professor at Gallaudet this year, Lane took an active part in helping the student movement in March.

ticulate. By 1830 a generation of deaf had arisen that could hold its own in society, in a way that could not have been imagined a dozen years earlier. (This was a recapitulation of events in France, in the previous century, when the introduction and use of Sign in education, by the Abbé de l'Epée in the 1750s, had within a generation transformed the lives, the status, of the deaf in France).

Other residential schools for the deaf soon opened throughout the United States, all using the Sign that had evolved at Hartford. Virtually all the teachers in these schools were educated at Hartford and most had met the charismatic Clerc. They contributed their own indigenous signs and later spread an increasingly polished and generalized ASL in many parts of the country, and the standards and aspirations of the deaf continually rose. By the 1850s it had become clear that higher education was needed—the deaf, previously illiterate, now needed a college. In 1857, Thomas Gallaudet's son, Edward, only twenty-four but uniquely equipped through his background (his mother was deaf, and he learned Sign as a primary language), his sensibilities, and his gifts, was appointed principal of the Columbia Institution for the Instruction of the Deaf and the Dumb and the Blind,[4] conceiving and hoping from the start that it could be transformed into a college, with federal support. In 1864 this was achieved, and what was later to become Gallaudet College received its charter from Congress.

Edward Gallaudet's own full and extraordinary life[5] lasted well into the present century, and spanned great (though not always admirable) changes in attitudes to the deaf and their education. In particular, gathering force from the 1860s, and promoted to a large extent in the US by Alexander Graham Bell, was an attitude that opposed the use of signing, and sought to forbid its use in schools and institutions. Gallaudet himself fought against this, but was overborne by the climate of the times, and by a certain ferocity and intransigence of mind that he was too reasonable to understand.[6]

By the time of Gallaudet's death, his college was world-famous and had shown once and for all that the deaf, given the opportunity and the means, could match the hearing in every sphere of academic activity—and for that matter, in athletic activity, too (the spectacular gym at Gallaudet, opened in 1880, was one of the finest in the country; and the football huddle was actually invented at Gallaudet, for players to pass secret tactics among themselves). But Gallaudet himself was one of the last defenders of Sign in an educational world that had turned its back on signing, and with his death the college lost—and because the college had become the symbol and aspiration of the deaf all over the world, the deaf world also lost—its greatest and last proponent of Sign in education.

With this, Sign, which had been the dominant language at the college before, went underground, and became confined to a colloquial use. The students continued to use it among themselves, but it was no longer considered a legitimate language for formal discourse or teaching.[7]

---

4 There was soon a division of the ways, with blind pupils being educated separately from the "deaf and dumb" (as the congenitally deaf, with little or no speech, used to be called). Among the two thousand deaf students at Gallaudet now, there are about twenty students who are both deaf and blind. These students, of course, must develop astonishing tactile sensibility and intelligence, as Helen Keller did.

5 See Edward Miner Gallaudet, *History of the College for the Deaf*, 1857-1907 (Gallaudet University Press, 1983).

6 The contestants in this struggle, Bell and Gallaudet—both the sons of deaf mothers (but mothers with completely different attitudes to their own deafness), each passionately devoted to the deaf in his own way—were about as different as two human beings can be. See Richard Winefield, *Never the Twain Shall Meet: Bell, Gallaudet, and the Communications Debate* (Gallaudet University Press, 1987).

7 There exists a condition *diglossia* at Gallaudet, and in other deaf communities, where the deaf use ASL among themselves, but instantly switch to a signed form of English if they have to speak in the presence of the nondeaf.

Thus the century between Thomas Galluadet's founding of the American Asylum and Edward Gallaudet's death in 1917 saw the rise and fall, the legitimation and delegitimation, of Sign in America. The suppression of Sign in the 1880s had a deleterious effect on the deaf for seventy-five years, not only on their education and academic achievements but on their image of themselves and on their entire community and culture. Such community and culture as did exist remained in isolated pockets—there was no longer the sense there had once been, at least the sense that was intimated in the "golden age" of the 1840s, of a nationwide (even worldwide) community and culture.

But the last thirty years have again seen a reversal, and indeed a relegitimation and resurrection of Sign as never before; and with this, and much else, a discovery or rediscovery of the cultural aspects of deafness—a strong sense of community and communication and culture, of self-definition as a unique mode of being.

The scientific relegitimation of Sign began in the 1950s, when a young professor of English and Chaucer scholar, William Stokoe, came to Gallaudet. Stokoe thought he had come to teach Chaucer to the deaf; but he very soon perceived that he had been thrown, by good fortune or chance, into one of the world's most extraordinary linguistic environments. Sign language, at this time, was not seen as a "proper" language, sometimes not even by the demoralized deaf themselves, but as a sort of pantomime or gestural code, or perhaps a sort of broken English on the hands. It was Stokoe's genius to see, and prove, that it was nothing of the sort; that it satisfied every linguistic criterion of a genuine language, in its syntax and plentitude of operators,

its (Chomskian) capacity to generate an infinite number of propositions. In 1960 Stokoe published *Sign Language Structure: An Outline of the Visual Communication System of the American Deaf,* and in 1965 (with Casterline and Croneborg) *A Dictionary of American Sign.*

Stokoe's work led to the most refined linguistic analyses of Sign, including some of the special forms, such as Art Sign, that are an essential part of deaf culture. And this in turn has led to the immensely important studies of Ursula Bellugi and her colleagues at the Salk Institute (as well as of others at Gallaudet and elsewhere), which look at the neural basis of Sign, the powers of specially enhanced visual perception and organization that have long been recognized, if only anecdotally, in the deaf. It has been established that the "language areas" of the left cerebral hemisphere, where are associated with speech, are also crucial for Sign, and that destruction to these areas of the brain can cause an inability to understand Sign—a Sign aphasia. It has also been found in those who are born deaf, and most especially those who are exposed to Sign from the start, that what would normally be auditory areas of the brain associated with hearing can be "reallocated" for purposes of visual analysis; that with constant exposure to and use of a visual language, the entire brain of the deaf person can adapt itself for a special, supervisual sensibility and organization,[8]a special enhancement of visual powers that may not occur in any other situation.[9]

What neuroscientists have insufficiently regarded or respected, and have scarcely yet begun to explore, is the unusual quality of imagination and imagery in the deaf, particularities that the brain and mind have been taught through being exposed from the start to an exclusively visual

8   This fundamental work—part physiological, part behavioral—on "visual enhancement" in the congenitally deaf is now readily accessible in two fascinating recent students: Howard Poizner, Edward S. Klima and Ursula Bellugi, *What the Hands Reveal about the Bran* (MIT Press, 1987), and Helen Neville, "Cerebral Organization for Spatial Attention," in J. Stiles-Davis, M. Krichevsky, and U. Bellugi, eds., *Spatial Cognition: Brain Bases and Development* (Lawrence Erlbaum, 1988)

9   This applies also, though to a smaller extent, to the "hearing deaf," i.e., the hearing children of deaf parents who have learned Sign as a primary language.

sensibility.[10] The language and culture and rich differentness of the deaf (unlike those, say, of the Welsh) have a neurological basis. It is not just culture (the culturally transmitted) that is different in the deaf, but nature, the nature of their experiences, dispositions, and thoughts. Deaf culture is reared upon deaf nature, though at this point one almost has an impulse to drop the word "deaf," and replace it with "visual," and to speak rather of an intensely visual culture merging from a physiological enhancement of visuality.

Cognitive and behavioral studies at Galluadet and elsewhere have indicated that this unique form of visuality may in turn predispose the deaf to specifically "visual" (or logical/spatial) forms of memory and thinking; that, given complex problems with many stages, the deaf tend to arrange these, and their hypotheses, in logical space, whereas the hearing arrange them in a temporal (or "auditory") order.[11] Thus it is not only the form of language, but the form of perception and of thinking itself, that may be different in the deaf, especially those given full freedom to exploit their own way of being. This is fully recognized by the students and the staff at Gallaudet, and methods of teaching emphasizing visual and spatial forms are clearly respected.

This seems to be the case, for example, in the very strong mathematics department at Gallaudet, where a majority of the faculty is deaf.

The validation of Sign as a complete gestural language, with specific physiological correlates in the brain, over the past thirty years, cannot be wholly separated from its cultural aspects, for the phenomenon of Sign is at once biological and cultural. The last few decades have seen the development and rise of many art forms and cultural forms unique to the deaf—most notably those of deaf theater and Sign poetry—Sign arts that have no correlate in other languages, and cannot be translated satisfactorily into speech. Indeed, this is true of the entire deaf experience; it cannot be conveyed or comprehended properly without Sign. There has been a proliferation of research, some by the deaf themselves, on the cultural aspects of Sign, on all that goes into the making of a deaf culture and community.[12]

This leads to the political aspects of deafness; the need for full recognition of the unique deaf community and culture; for full autonomy, for the power to decide and to legislate for themselves; the need for the deaf to be considered the equals of the hearing in every way, and given identical rights.[13] As the linguistic and cultural run to-

---

10   This early adaptation of the brain to the visual in general and visual signs in particular may be the reason why the congenitally or "prelingually" deaf who learn Sign in infancy, as their first language, achieve an inimitably fluent and graceful signing, which the "postlingually" deafened (who grew up in an aural-oral mode, dominated by auditory sensibilities and speech) find it difficult or impossible to achieve. It is as if the brain has to be molded from the start to the "super" visuality needed for perfect signing. Highly gifted polyglots, who may speak a dozen languages, may not find it nearly as easy to learn Sign, because their nervous systems are already "set" in such an auditory mode. Deaf signers, in contrast, can usually acquire other sign languages with relative ease; this may in part be due to the sharing or similarity of various linguistic conventions, but it suggests, also the peculiar visual giftedness that all native signers have.

11   There is a considerable and somewhat controversial literature on the character of cognitive functions among the deaf. See, for example, John Belmot, Michael A. Karchmer, and James W. Bourg, "Structural Influences on Deaf and Hearing Children's Recall of Temporal/Spatial Incongruent Letter Strings," *Educational Psychology*, Vol. 3, Nos. 3 and 4 (1983), pp. 259-274.

12   Much of this work has been published by the Linstok Press, set up by William Stokoe, as well as by Gallaudet University Press and the National Association of the Deaf. See especially *Sign Language and the Deaf Community: Essays in Honor of William Stokoe* (NAD Press, 1981).

13   For example, few of the deaf sought or obtained higher degrees twenty years ago—there were fewer than half-a-dozen deaf Ph.D.'s in the world. But the number of deaf scholars and administrators has steadily risen; now there are hundreds with much experience and Ph.D.'s—such as Harvey Croson, superintendent of the Louisiana School for the Deaf, and I. King Jordan, dean of the Gallaudet School of Arts and Sciences, the two deaf finalists considered—but rejected—for the position of president of Gallaudet by the board.

gether, so both of these run into the political. Along with the rising status of sign language and deaf culture has come an increasing awareness of the deaf in our midst, and an increasing awareness on their part of their autonomy and power. But all of this has been gathering under the surface; it did not become clear (at least to the outside world, and even to many within the deaf community) until it exploded, in March of this year.

To understand the spirit of that explosion one has, I believe, to go back to Clerc. His teachings, until his death, had the effect of widening the nineteenth-century view of "human nature," of introducing a relativistic and egalitarian sense of great natural range, not just a dichotomy of "normal" and "abnormal."[14] We speak of our nineteenth-century forebears as rigid, moralistic, repressive, censorious, but the tone of Clerc's voice, and of those who listened to him, conveyed quite the opposite impression; that this was an age very hospitable to "the natural"—to the whole variety and range of natural proclivities—and not disposed (or at least less disposed than our own) to make moralizing or clinical judgements on what is "normal" and what is "abnormal."[15] A sense of this openness is suggested in the title of Harlan Lane's book on the deaf, *When the Mind Hears*; and its relative absence today, at least

among the administrators of Gallaudet, was given the same form in reverse when (on *Nightline*) the deaf actress Marlee Matlin said (of the hearing administration), "You people are deaf in the mind." Lane's title, consciously, and Matlin's outburst, consciously or not, both echo the words of Victor Hugo to a deaf friend, Ferdinand Berthier: "What matters deafness of the ear, when the mind hears? The one true deafness, the incurable deafness, is that of the mind."

The accusation that the Gallaudet authorities were "deaf in the mind" implies no malevolence, but rather a misdirected paternalism, which, the deaf feel, is anything but benign—based as it is on pity and condescension, and on an implicit view of them as "incompetent," if not diseased. Special objection has been made to some of the doctors involved in Gallaudet's affairs, who, it is felt, tend to see the deaf merely as having diseased ears, and not as whole people adapted to another sensory mode.[16] In general, it is felt that this offensive paternalism hinges on a value judgement by the hearing: their saying, "We know what is best for you. Let us handle things"—whether this is in response to the choice of language (allowing, or not allowing, Sign) or in judging capacities for education or jobs. It is still sometimes felt, or again felt—after the more

---

14   This sense of the range of nature, and our respect (even if uncomprehending) for this range, is apparent again and again in Clerc's brief *Autobiography*. "Every creature, every work of God, is admirably made. What we find faulty in its kind turns to our advantage without our knowing it." Or, again, "We can only thank God for the rich diversity of his creation, and hope that in the future world the reason for it will be explained."
   Clerc's concept of "God," "creation", "nature"—humble, appreciative, mild, unresentful—is perhaps rooted in his sense of himself, and other deaf, as different but nonetheless complete beings. It is in great contrast to the half-terrible, half-Promethean fury of Alexander Graham Bell, who constantly sees deafness as a swindle and a privation and a tragedy, and is constantly concerned with "normalizing" the deaf, "correcting" God's blunders, and, in general, "improving on" nature. Clerc argues for cultural richness, tolerance, diversity. Bell argues for technology, for genetic engineering, hearing aids, telephones. The two types are wholly opposite but both, clearly, have their parts to play in the world.

15   This hospitality to a wide range of proclivities and dispositions, this lack of labeling and stigmatizing, persists as continuing tolerance and civility among the deaf. I had occasion to see one expression of this on my visit—for I went to Gallaudet with a friend of mine who has Tourette's Syndrome of some severity, a condition which, with its convulsive movements and tics, nearly always attracts negative attention in New York. At Gallaudet there was no staring, no "diagnosing", no "reaction" at all—simply an immediate accepting of him as another human being.

16   See *How you Gonna Get to Heaven If You Can't Talk with Jesus: On Depathologizing Deafness* by James Woodward (T.J. Publishers, 1982).

spacious opportunities offered in the mid-nineteenth century—that the deaf should be printers, or work in the post office, do "humble" jobs, and not aspire to higher education. The deaf, in other words, felt they were being dictated to, that they were being treated as children. Bob Johnson told me a typical story:

> It's been my impression, after having been here for several years, that the Gallaudet faculty and staff treat students as pets. One student, for example, went to the Outreach office; they had announced there would be an opportunity to practice interviewing for jobs. The idea was to sign up for a genuine interview and learn how to do it. So he went and put his name on a list. The next day a woman from the Outreach office called and told him she had set up the interview, had found an interpreter, had set up the time, had arranged for a car to take him, and she couldn't understand why he got mad at her. He told her, "The reason I was doing this was so that I could learn how to call the person, and learn how to get the car, and learn how to get the interpreter, and you're doing it for me. That's not what I want here." That's the meat of the issue.

Far from being childlike or incompetent, as they were "supposed" to be (and as so often they supposed themselves to be), the students at Gallaudet showed high competence in managing the March revolt. This impressed me especially when I wandered into the communications room, the nerve center of Gallaudet during the strike, with its central office filled with TTY-equipped telephones. Here the deaf students contacted the press and television—invited them in, gave interviews, compiled news, issued press releases, around the clock—masterfully; here they raised funds for a "Deaf Prez Now" campaign; here they solicited, successfully, support from Congress, presidential candidates, union leaders. They gained the world's ear, at this extraordinary time, when they needed it.

Even the administration listened—so that after four days of seeing the students as foolish and rebellious children who needed to be brought into line, after years of seeing things in hard, inflex-

ible, authoritarian terms, Dr. Zinser was forced to pause, to listen, to reexamine her own long-held assumptions, to see things in a new light—and, finally, to resign. She did so in terms that were moving and seemed genuine, saying that neither she nor the board had anticipated the fervor and commitment of the protesters, or had seen that their protest was the leading edge of a burgeoning national movement for deaf rights. "I have responded to this extraordinary social movement of deaf people," she said as she tendered her resignation on the night of March 10, and spoke of coming to see this as "a very special moment in time," one that was "unique, a civil rights moment in history for deaf people."

Friday, March 11: The mood on campus is completely transformed. A battle has been won. There is elation. More battles have to be fought. Placards with the students' four demands have been replaced with placards saying "3½," because the resignation of Dr. Zinser only goes halfway toward meeting the first demand, that there be a deaf president immediately. But there is also a gentleness that is new, the tension and anger of Thursday have gone, along with the possibility of a drawn-out, humiliating defeat. A largeness of spirit is everywhere apparent—released now, I partly feel, by the grace and the words with which Zinser resigned, words in which she aligned herself with, and wished the best for, what she called an "extraordinary social movement."

Support is coming in from every quarter: three hundred deaf students from the National Technical Institute for the Deaf arrive, elated and exhausted, after a fifteen-hour bus ride from Rochester, New York. Deaf schools throughout the country are closed in total support. The deaf flood in from every state—I see signs from Iowa and Alabama, from Canada, from South America, as well as from Europe, even from New Zealand. Events at Gallaudet have dominated the national press for forty-eight hours. Virtually every car going past Gallaudet honks now, and the streets are filled with supporters as the time for the march on the Capitol comes near. And yet, for all the honking, the speeches, the banners, the pickets, and extraordinary atmosphere of quietness and dignity prevails.

Noon: There are now about 2,500 people, a thousand students from Gallaudet and the rest supporters, as we start on a slow, joyful walk to the Capitol. As we walk a strange and wonderful sense of quietness grows, which puzzles me. It is not wholly physical (indeed, there is rather a lot of noise in a way—the earsplitting, but to them inaudible, yells of the deaf, as a start), and I decide it is, rather the quietness of a moral drama. The sense of history in the air gives it this strange quietness.

Slowly, for there are children, babies, and some physically disabled among us (some deaf-blind, some ataxic, and some on crutches), slowly, and with a mixed sense of resolve and festivity, we walk to the Capitol, and there, in the clear March sun that has shone the entire week, we unfurl banners and raise pickets. One great banner says WE STILL HAVE A DREAM, and another, with the individual letters carried by fourteen people, simply says HELP US CONGRESS.

We are packed together, but there is no sense of a crowd, rather of an extraordinary camaraderie. Just before the speeches start, I find myself hugged—I think it must be someone I know, but it is a student bearing a sign ALABAMA, who hugs me, punches my shoulder, smiles, as a comrade. We are strangers, but yet, at this special moment, we are comrades.

There are many speeches—from Greg Hlibok, the student body president, from some of the faculty, from congressmen and senators. I listen for a while:

> It is an irony (says one, a professor at Gallaudet) that Gallaudet has never had a deaf chief executive officer. Virtually every black college has a black president, testimony that black people are leading themselves. Virtually every women's college has a woman as president, as testimony that women are capable of leading themselves. It's long past time that Gallaudet had a deaf

president as testimony that deaf people are leading themselves.

I let my attention wander, taking in the scene as a whole: thousands of people, each intensely individual but bound and united with a single sentiment. After the speeches, there is a break of an hour, during which a number of people go in to see congressmen. But most of the group, who have brought packed lunches in on their backs, now sit and eat and talk, or rather sign, in the great plaza before the Capitol—and this, for me, as for all those who have come or chanced to see it, is one of the most wonderful scenes of all. For here are a thousand or more people signing freely, in a public place—not privately, at home, or in the enclosure of Gallaudet, but openly and unselfconsciously, and beautifully, before the Capitol.

The press has reported all the speeches, but missed what is surely equally significant. They failed to give the watching world an actual vision of the fullness and vividness, the unmedical life, of the deaf. And once more, as I wander among the huge throng of signers, as they chat over sandwiches and sodas before the Capitol, I feel the utter naturalness and sufficiency of their lives, and the sense of them as necessarily, but passionately and beautifully, other, unique, separate from yet integral to us. I find myself remembering the words of a deaf student at the California School for the Deaf, who had signed on television:

> We are a unique people, with our own culture, our own language (American Sign Language, which has just recently been recognized as a language in itself), and that sets us apart from hearing people.

I walk back from the capitol with Bob Johnson. I myself tend to be apolitical, and have difficulty even comprehending the vocabulary of politics. Bob, a pioneer Sign linguist, who has taught and researched at Gallaudet for years, says as we walk back:

> It's really remarkable, because in all my experience I've seen deaf people be passive and

accept the kind of treatment that hearing people give them. I've seen them willing, or seem to be willing, to be "clients," when in fact they should be controlling things . . . Now all at once there's been a transformation in the consciousness of what it means to be a deaf person in the world, to take responsibility for things. The illusion that deaf people are powerless—all at once, now, that illusion has gone, and that means the whole nature of things can change for them now. I'm extremely enthusiastic about what I'm going to see over the next few years.

"I don't quite understand what you mean by 'clients,'" I say.

"You know Tim Rarus (Bob explains)—the one you saw at the barricades this morning, whose signing you so admired as pure and passionate—well, he summed up in two words what this transformation is all about. He said, "It's very simple. No deaf president, no university," and then he shrugged his shoulders, looked at the TV camera, and that was his whole statement. That was the first time deaf people ever realized that a colonial client-industry like this can't exist without the client. It's a billion-dollar industry for hearing people. If deaf people don't participate, the industry is gone.

Saturday has a delightful, holiday air about it. It is a day off (some of the students have been working virtually nonstop from the first demonstration on Sunday evening), and a day for cookouts on the campus. But even here the issues are not forgotten. The very names of the food have a satirical edge; the choice lies between "Spilman dogs" and "Boardburgers." The campus is festive, now that students and schoolchildren from a score of other states have come in (a little deaf black girl from Arkansas, seeing all the signers around her, says in Sign, "It's like a family to me today"). There has also been a influx of deaf artists from all over, some coming to document this unique event in the history of the deaf, and some to celebrate it (in lyrical paintings and poems).

Greg Hlibok is relaxed, but still very vigilant: "We feel that we are in control. We are taking things easy. We don't want to go too far." Two

days earlier, Dr. Zinser was threatening to "take control." That would have been an imposed, foreign control. What one sees today is self-control, that quiet consciousness and confidence that come from inner strength and certainty.

Sunday evening, March 13: The board met today, for nine hours. There were nine hours of tension, waiting, . . . no one knowing what was to come. Then the door opened, and Philip Bravin, one of the four deaf board members and known to all the deaf students, came out. His appearance—and not Spilman's—already told the story, before he made his revelations in Sign. He was speaking now, he signed, as chairman of the board, for Spilman had resigned. And his first task now, with the board behind him, was the happy one of announcing that King Jordan had been elected the new president.

King Jordan, deafened at the age of twenty-one, had been at Gallaudet for fifteen years; he was dean of the School of Arts and Sciences, a popular, modest and unusually sane man, who had at first supported Zinser when she was selected. Greatly moved, Jordan, in simultaneous sign and speech, said:

I am thrilled to accept the invitation of the board of trustees to become the president of Gallaudet University. This is a historic moment for deaf people around the world. This week we can truly say that we together, united, have overcome our reluctance to stand for our rights. The world has watched the deaf community come of age. We will no longer accept limits on what we can achieve. The highest praise goes to the students of Gallaudet for showing us exactly even now how one can seize an idea with such force that it becomes a reality.

With this, the dam burst, and jubilation burst out everywhere. When everyone then returned to Gallaudet for a final, triumphal meeting, Jordan said, "They know now that the cap on what they can achieve has been lifted. We know that deaf people can do anything hearing people can except hear." And Greg Hlibok, hugging Jordan, added,

"We have climbed to the top of the mountain, and we have climbed together."

Monday, March 14: Gallaudet looks normal on the surface. The barricades have been taken down, the campus is open. The "uprising" has lasted exactly one week—from last Sunday evening, March 6, when Dr. Zinser was forced on an unwilling university, to the happy resolution last night, that utterly different Sunday evening, when all was changed.

But has all been changed? Will there be a lasting "transformation of consciousness"? Will the deaf at Gallaudet, and the deaf community at large, emboldened by the events of this week, indeed find the opportunities they seek? Will we, the hearing, allow them these opportunities? Allow them to be themselves, a unique culture in our midst, yet admit them as coequals to every sphere of activity? One hopes the events at Gallaudet will be a beginning.

Postscript

"It took seven days to create the world, it took us seven days to change it"—this was the joke of the students, flashed in Sign from one end of the campus to another. And with this feeling they took their spring break, going back to their families throughout the country, carrying the euphoric news and mood with them.

But objective change, historical change, does not happen in a week, even though its first prerequisite, "the transformation of consciousness"

may happen, as it did, in a day. "Many of the students," Bob Johnson told me, "don't realize the extent and the time that are going to be involved in changing, though they do have a sense now of their strength and power . . . The structure of oppression is so deeply ingrained."

And yet there are beginnings. There is a new "image" and a new movement, not merely at Gallaudet but throughout the deaf world. News reports, especially on television, have made the silent deaf articulate and visible across the entire nation. But the profoundest effect, of course, has been on the deaf themselves. It has welded them into a community, a worldwide community, as never before. There has already been a deep impact upon deaf children. One of King Jordan's first acts, when the college reconvened after the spring break, was to visit the grade school at Gallaudet, and talk to the children there, something no president had ever done before. Such concern has to affect their perception of what they can become. (Deaf children sometimes think they will "turn into" hearing adults, or else be feeble, put-upon creatures if they do not.)

All sorts of changes, administrative, educational, social, psychological, are already beginning at Gallaudet. But what is clearest at this point is the much-altered bearing of its students, a bearing that conveys a new, wholly unself-conscious sense of pleasure and vindication, of confidence and dignity. This new sense of themselves represents a decisive break from the past, which could not have been imagined just a few months ago.[17]

---

17   I am deeply grateful to Robert Johnson and Harlan Lane for their great help to me during my visit to Gallaudet and thereafter. I could not have written this piece without them.

CHAPTER 3

The Structure of American Sign Language

Students are often unaware that linguists have questioned whether American Sign Language is truly a language. Until recently, some language scholars raised this question seriously. The sign language used by deaf persons has been the target of prejudice as has people's race, creed and cultural differences. William C. Stokoe, a former professor of English at Gallaudet University, was among the first in the academic world to suggest that American Sign Language is not pantomime or "English-on-the-hands," but a separate and distinct language with its own structure and vocabulary.

Human languages have three similar features: symbols, grammar and syntax. In all languages, concepts are represented by symbols. These symbols may be written, spoken, pictorial or manual. Language scholars call the symbols of a language a lexicon. Grammar is the agreement among the symbols in a language. In English, the sentence "the boat are floating" sounds peculiar because there is not agreement between the subject of the sentence (boat) and the verb (are floating). Syntax involves the order in which the symbols of a language occur in the course of communication. The words of this passage, while intelligible in themselves, would make no sense to the reader if they were printed in random order.

American Sign Language is unique among human languages. While most languages are oral (spoken) and aural (heard), American Sign Language is visual, spatial and gestural. These features make ASL ideal to study by videotaping. One of the pioneers in sign language research is Dr. Ursula Bellugi, a linguist at the Salk Institute for Biological Studies. She studied native signers by means of videotaped interviews. A native ASL user is an individual who is born deaf of deaf parents and whose first language is American Sign Language. Through videotapes, Dr. Bellugi was able to document the non-manual features of American Sign Language which are essential to the grammatical and syntactical structures in the language. Her research has been augmented by other language scholars in the United States and around the world. These studies continue to prove that ASL is a language with unique and fascinating features not found in spoken languages. The work of some of these researchers is featured in the articles in this chapter.

They Finally Listened

Bart Barnes

Two decades ago when William C. Stokoe first proposed a linguistic analysis of sign language, his colleagues thought he was crazy. Although sign language had been the primary means of communication among the deaf for more than 150 years, it was strictly barred in some schools for the deaf and discouraged or neglected in most others. While its use by students out of class was tolerated, sign language was almost universally ignored by educators of the deaf and there were few who took it seriously as a legitimate language.

The reaction at Gallaudet College for the Deaf in Washington, D.C., where Stokoe had just been hired as chairman of the English department, was much the same.

"They told me my job was to teach them English," recalled Stokoe. "Even some of the deaf people on the faculty thought I was out of my skull. All the experts were saying, 'Sign language can be ignored. It is not a language.' "

Now, almost 20 years later, there has been a 180-degree turnaround.

Despite his colleagues' skepticism, Stokoe pressed ahead with his idea and in 1960 produced the first linguistic analysis of sign language.

For most of the past 19 years, supported by grants from the National Science Foundation and the Center for Applied Linguistics, he has continued his research, on his own at first and later as director of Gallaudet's linguistics research lab.

"What Bill and his colleagues have been saying and proving is that sign language is a language," says Raymond Trybus, dean of the research institute at Gallaudet. "It has everything a language has. It has vocabulary, grammar and syntax. It is a language which defines a community and it is worthy of respect just like any other language.

"Not long ago, sign language was looked down on as something deaf people did because they couldn't do any better. Now it is a legitimate topic of academic investigation. All of that can be attributed to the work started by Bill Stokoe."

When Stokoe, 59, came to Gallaudet in 1955, his only previous contact with the deaf had been a deaf blacksmith in the town where he grew up.

"I didn't know any sign language, but when I brought in a piece of farm machinery, he was able to communicate to me whether or not he could fix it," said Stokoe.

One of the first things Stokoe did after arriving at Gallaudet was to take a crash course in sign language. He had not been on the campus long before he became fascinated with sign language as a potential topic of serious academic scrutiny, but his was a lonely effort at first.

"I used to feel like somebody standing alone on the beach shouting, 'Hey, I've got something interesting here!' but nobody was listening. It felt like the things I was studying and researching were of no interest to anyone."

Gradually, during the 1970s, it all began to change. Deaf pride and deaf awareness groups organized. Other scholars, at Gallaudet and elsewhere, began studying the linguistics of sign language.

Stokoe began publishing a quarterly journal called "Sign Language Studies." Increasingly, hearing people began to develop an interest in learning sign language.

"It is a very sophisticated languageage," said Stokoe. "Sign language is not English any more than French is English. People used to think there were certain features it didn't have. Now researchers are discovering those features all the time."

Unlike other handicapped people, Stokoe observed, the deaf constitute a special community not unlike a separate ethnic group, in large measure because they have their own language.

"Having a common language joins people with the strongest of bonds," he wrote in a recent article. "One of the most important uses of language is the formation and preservation of social groups. . . . The deaf constitute a social group both by the difference of not hearing, but even more by the social working of language."

To study the intricacies of sign language, Stokoe has spent thousands of hours examining sign language conversations in minute detail.

"The signs in a sign sentence may occur in the same order as the words in an English sentence or they may occur in different order," he writes.

"A sign sentence may seem to omit signs for words that are essential in the English sentence. Again, the sign sentence may have signs for which the English sentence has no equivalent word.

"Sign language grammar has its own rules as well as its own lexicon, or vocabulary of signs; and rules and lexicon of sign differ from the rules and lexicon of English. . . . There is a unique set of rules for making sign language constructions just as there is for making standard English constructions . . . or the constructions of any language."

While current research tends to build a case for recognition of sign language as a separate language, it also has uncovered common similarities between sign language and all spoken language.

Stokoe, for example, has found that persons of the same age groups or the same sex tend to sign alike. Other researchers studying the sign language patterns of black and white deaf people in the South have found signing differences comparable to different dialects of a spoken language. They have also found that sign language is different in different countries, just as spoken language is different.

Moreover, says Stokoe, "it is more than a hand language —it is body, face and eyes."

The simple sentence, "I saw what he was doing," Stokoe noted, could mean, with the eyes focused differently, "*he* saw what *I* was doing."

And, like any other language, sign language is always changing. "There is evidence of rapid and widespread change in the 200 years since the sign language behavior of the deaf was recognized and partially recorded," Stokoe said last year in a revised version of his first linguistic analysis of American Sign Language.

Most of Stokoe's work has focused on American Sign Language or Ameslan. But there are two other forms of manual communication commonly used by deaf people in the United States. One is finger spelling; the other is interpretation of spoken English into manual signs. But unlike Ameslan, neither form has an independent linguistic base.

At Gallaudet, Stokoe no longer teaches English but has developed a course in "socio-linguistics," which he describes as the ethnography of speaking. "We try to look at what kinds of social factors, nonlinguistic factors influence the way we use language," he said.

"The study of sign language is basic to the study of all language. Babies communicate with their faces, and their eyes and their bodies long before they use words."

The Roots of Language in the Sign Talk of the Deaf

Ursula Bellugi and Edward S. Klima

Almost anyone who watches a deaf person use sign language can tell only that the person is moving his hands rapidly; he cannot be sure when one sign ends and another begins; for that matter, he cannot distinguish between the making of a sign and some irrelevant hand movement. One cannot even infer the subject of the conversation. Just as one cannot infer the meaning of the Spanish word *hermano* from its sound alone, so one could not guess the meaning of the hand sign for *brother* in the sign language of the deaf.

We are interested in the biological basis of language, its structure, and the structure of human thought as expressed in language. Our research group includes Susan Fischer, a linguist, and Bonnie Gough, a deaf woman who is very articulate in sign language. One way to learn about these universals is to study the communication that persons develop when they are born unable to hear and therefore do not speak. To do so, we first learned sign language, and now we are exploring how deaf children of deaf parents learn sign as a native language; how the form and structure of spoken and sign languages differ, and how they may be alike.

To begin our investigation of the language we use studies of spontaneous signing, of paraphrase, of folk art, and experiments in memory for signs.

See. Sign and speech differ fundamentally in the organs that perceive them: the eye and the ear. The deaf cannot communicate unless they can see each other; they analyze language by sight whereas we analyze language by sound. As a result, sign language is not simply parallel to or derivative of spoken English. In its deepest and most interesting respects, sign seems to be a language in its own right, with properties that are different from spoken languages in general and from English in particular.

There are several kinds of hand language. Most of us are familiar with fingerspelling: a symbol for each letter of the alphabet, with words being spelled in the air. This is like writing in the air and is based on English. Another variety of hand language, also based on English, combines fingerspelling and signs. One version, called *Seeing Essential English,* used in some teaching and in formal situations, is close to written English in word order and morphology.

But the language that most of the deaf in this country use with each other is called American Sign Language (ASL) and is the object of our study. *(A Dictionary of American Sign Language on Linguistic Principles* by William C. Stokoe *et al.* presents more than 2,000 signs.) American Sign Language is the language that deaf children usually learn from their deaf parents, and it is not based on English. It has its own processes of word formation, its own methods of incorporating semantic variation into the basic units—the sign, and sign phrase. It is a self-contained, largely arbitrary system, not a universally understood language or pantomime. For example, deaf persons in Britain use a sign language that is radically different from the sign language used by the American deaf.

Differ. In our studies we have begun to ask about the structure of signs. How are the basic units or elements of a language that is produced by hands different from a language that is produced by the vocal apparatus? In Stokoe's system, each sign is made up of three parameters that occur simultaneously: a) a particular hand configuration; b) the place of articulation in relation to the body; c) the movement of the hands. For example, the sign for *home* calls for the hand to shape a tapered *O* on the cheek, with movements that include touching the cheek near the side of the mouth, moving away slightly, and touching again on the upper cheek. A change in any of the parameters may transform the sign *home* into a different sign. If one closes the hand with the thumb and little finger extended and touches the cheek with the same motion, it is *yesterday*. If we change the location and make the sign on both sides of the nose, it is *flower*. If we make a small circular motion on the cheek with the hand in the same tapered *O*, it is *peach*.

Share. In our early studies of the language, we began to notice that these parameters are recombinable in various ways and that some semantic families of signs share a common parameter. (However, as in sound segments of spoken languages, the parts may recombine in ways that are semantically related or in ways that are purely arbitrary.) Since we are interested in language regularities, we have begun to study semantically and formationally related signs in more detail.

Some signs are alike in one parameter and different in others. Thus some signs that have to do with emotion (*e.g., heart, terrible, hate, feel, sick, excited, pity, discouraged*) share a common handshape. The placement of the hand and its accompanying motion distinguish each sign.

Other signs are identical except for place of articulation. Many male-female sign pairs—e.g., *father/mother, man/woman, brother/sister, husband/wife* and even *male cousin/female cousin*—are identical except that the one sign is made near the forehead and the other sign on the lower cheek.

Use. The third parameter is movement. Signs take shape in the physical space in front of the signer's body between signer and addressee. The use of space, direction, movement, are all crucial in sign language and give it a different character from spoken language. Signs may be made with one or both hands, and on occasion two different signs may be made at once. Signers often use the space in front of their bodies to locate objects, persons, the subjects of their discourses, and (perhaps because our memory for spatial arrangements is so well developed) they can then continue to refer to these topics in the allocated direction or space.

Space and movement in space have other functions in sign:

1. Space can provide intonational cues. A signer's hands may be seen, in slow motion, to come to rest in front of the body at the end of a sentence or clause. When they pause in midair, or move slightly toward the addressee, they may indicate a question; these are subtle differences that the uninitiated may not notice.

2. A change in direction of movement may turn one sign into its opposite. A simple reversal of hand motion turns *join* into *disconnect; thrilled* into *discouraged; appear* into *disappear; with* into *without.*

3. Change in movement may add negation to a sign. The sign for *know* is a bent hand, fingers together, with fingertips touching the head. The sign for *dont-know* is the same handshape, also touching the forehead, but followed by a movement of the fingertips downward and away from the signer. This same downward movement marks the negation of *like, want* and *good.*

4. Movement may signal the tense. Signs for the future move forward from the signer, usually at the level of the face; signs for the past generally move toward the signer and in the direction of over the shoulder. The sign for *look,* when it is made in a forward arc, means *prophecy;* the same sign, made in an arc that moves back across the ear, means *reminiscing.* Other such pairs are *will/past; tomorrow/yesterday; next year/last year.*

5. Motion may distinguish singular from plural or collective nouns. The sign for *forest* is

identical to that for *tree,* but the wrist motion is repeated several times—literally many trees.

6. Finally, movement may indicate the subject and/or object of a sentence. Since signs are made in the space between signer and addressee, direction of hand or movement often indicates the subject or object of a verb. The signs for *I-inform-you* and *you-inform-me, I-inform-him, he-informs-me* are the same except for direction of movement; the same process works for other verbs such as *teach, copy, invite, look-at, arrest* and *help.* (There are, as in all languages, many exceptions to this rule. Among signs that do not change are *chase, follow, lead* and *fire*).

Err. American Sign Language uses these parameters productively to express semantic variations and grammatical relations. We have been looking for clues to regularities in sign. We find them not only in what deaf people sign but in the mistakes that they sometimes make in conversation.

In certain kinds of anticipatory errors (called "spoonerisms" in speech) we find clues to formational rules of sign language. Spoken spoonerisms have a tightly structured economy that frequently produces two nonsense words, as in "this nipper is zarrow." The process is apparently the same in sign: some parameter of two signs are exchanged, the result being nonexistent signs that are nevertheless physically possible.

One young woman was signing to a friend about putting pennies in a parking meter and found that she did not have the correct change. She intended to make a sign that means *I'm-sick-of-it* and then *I'm-reluctant* (to go looking for change). Instead of making the signs correctly, she used the hand configuration of *I'm-reluctant* in the place of articulation for *I'm-sick-of-it* and vice versa. This seemed funny to her companion just as many spoonerisms sound funny to us. The important point to a linguist is that the inadvertent switch resulted in two possible signs (because they use parameters of the language), that are nevertheless nonexistent signs in American sign language.

Recall. In a series of experiments in short-term memory for signs, we have been finding unexpected evidence for a kind of psychological reality to these parameters of sign. In one memory study, we showed lists of videotaped signs to congenitally deaf persons and asked them to sign them back to us as soon as a list was completed. (In another condition we asked deaf subjects to write down what they remembered in the English-word equivalents for the signs they had seen.) When we looked at the errors that occurred more than once in their ordered recall of signs, we found that the errors nearly always shared some properties in common with the original sign. These errors occurred when the response was written as well as when it was signed. The errors, then, resembled the correct stimulus, sharing most of its properties but differing on one or more parameters. For example, one subject saw the sign for *time* but remembered it as *potato.* These signs differ only in that the handshape for *time* uses one finger while the one for *potato* uses two. Another subject saw *tea* but remembered *vote;* the difference is that the motion for *tea* is a small circle, while the one for *vote* is a direct motion. Still another subject saw the sign for *onion* and remembered it as *key;* the two are the same in hand and motion but one is made at the forehead and the other on the palm of the hand. (In each case the subjects had named the original signs correctly.) The parameters we have been using to analyze signs appear as features of these errors.

Look. We find differences between sign language (ASL) and English at the level of vocabulary and not just differences in the way signs, words or sentences are formed. In some parts of its lexicon, American sign is perhaps limited in comparison with English; the deaf have to finger-spell many technical English words or invent signs for them. But sign language has domains that are more highly differentiated than English is. Absence of hearing and reliance on vision characterize the world of the deaf. We find that the vocabulary of sign language makes many more discriminations about ways of looking and seeing than spoken English does.

Many single signs require several English words for translation. Some indicate tense or aspect: *have-already-seen, to-look-forward-to, to-look-continually.* Other signs define the number of persons and the direction of looking. *I-look-at-you, two-look-at-each-other, everyone's-looking-at-me.* Still others describe ways of looking, or objects of looking: *to-look-away-in-disdain, to-do-a-double-take, sight-seeing, to-window-shop, to-gaze-at-one-another-like-lovers, to-make-eyes-at-someone.*

There are also many single colloquial signs that do not readily translate into single English words, such as *I-didn't-mean-that, to-flop-in-under-the-covers, rolling-in-the-aisles-with-laughter, dutch-treat, to-capture-for-love,* and *to-fall-asleep-with-boredom.*

We have been examining the differences between a spoken language and a gesture language. Our basic study also includes research on how one acquires this different language.

Change. What can we find out about the general process of language learning by studying its acquisition in another modality? We began our studies with a deaf child of deaf parents. Pola's sign vocabulary seems to cover the full range of concepts expressed by hearing children of comparable age. Among the signs she used spontaneously before the age of three were: *name, stay, tomorrow, will, where, who, what, how, dead, know, understand, none, nothing, don't-know,* and letters of the hand alphabet. We find in Pola's early combinations of signs the full range of semantic relations expressed by hearing children. We also find a steady increase in the length of her signed sequences that matches the increase found in hearing children. It does seem that, in spite of the change in modality, the milestones of language development may be the same.

In a previous article on language learning, Bellugi reported that "children are systematic, regular and productive in their language . . . Children seem to develop rules of maximal generality, often applying them too broadly at first and only later learning the proper restrictions on them" ["Learning the Language," PT, December 1970]. We now have at least some evidence that this is true for deaf children learning sign language as well as for hearing children who are learning spoken language. We have suggested that the principles underlying regularities in sign language may be quite different from those in spoken language. It seems evident that sign language has its own rich morphology, but is based in part on movement and position of the hands in space, place of articulation, hand configuration, etc.

We already have some evidence of overgeneralization on the part of deaf children based on the parameters and regularities of the sign language itself. Pola seemed to extract the common component of certain negative signs, and use that as a negative indicator in the period when negative forms were first emerging in her language (*not, don't-want, bad, don't-know, none, nothing, can't*). She also sometimes changed the direction of movement of a sign to mean "you do something to me," when the sign was one of the set that does not change in the sign language of adults. This is analogous to the hearing child's use of *holded, digged* and *bringed.* The child may have discovered the general possibility in sign for changing direction of a sign to indicate subject and object relations, and extended this to cases where an adult signer would not.

Pun. We have been describing regularities within a language system. Knowledge of the rules of formation and combination governs one kind of creativity in language—the ability to construct and understand an infinite number of sentences from a finite vocabulary. There are other kinds of creativity in sign language—the kind involved in puns or in wit, and the kind involved in simple songs and poems. Bonnie Gough has been the source of many of the witticisms we have found in the language. Most of them are hard to translate into words. Consider the sign for *clever*, an open, cupped hand with the thumb touching the forehead. One time Gough signed that one person was clever, another was . . . (and she added another cupped hand to the one already at her forehead to double the effect and make it "super clever"). She herself was . . . (she made the sign for *clever* on the back of her head instead of on her forehead). This gesture violated the clearly defined space in front of the body that is used for signing, and created a nonexistent sign that means the reverse or negation of the real one. It was a pun on the sign for *clever*.

Another time we went to a captioned film for the deaf. We were sitting behind a large man and our son had to move his head from side to side to read the captions. Someone suggested that he move, but he preferred to stay near us. "Well," the person signed, "the only thing you can do is . . ." and he made the sign for *look-at* the movie, with one change. Starting the sign with both hands in front of the eyes, he traced a path for the eyes that would diverge, move around the obstacle in front of them, and come together again on the side.

The deaf occasionally use fingerspelling for special effect. One deaf woman told us about a girl who was very interested in boys. To describe the girl's preoccupation, she put her hands on her forehead, palms facing away, and spelled with two hands *b-o-y-s*—to indicate, literally, "boys on the mind."

Play. What is a song? We think of poetry as based on rhyme and meter, on structural patterning of words; we think of a song as a poem set to music. In a hand language, there is nothing immediately analogous to rhyming, nothing like a melody.

To find the sign language equivalents of spoken poetry and sung melodies, we have begun to explore children's songs, lullabies, and early rhythmic play among the deaf. A deaf woman signed us a lullaby that her mother used to sign

to her every night; she said she thought it was the best song in the world when she was a child. We may translate it as follows, including periods to indicate pauses:

Sleep . . . sleep . . . sleep.
Wake-up.
Eat . . . cake.
Ride . . . beautiful . . . white . . . horse.
Sleep . . . sleep . . . sleep.

In this little song, the signs are somnolent, slow, deliberate and rhythmical, with long pauses between. The song has a hypnotic quality for deaf and hearing alike.

Another young deaf adult, from a large deaf family, signed a song that her brother had made up in sign language at the age of seven. It is a little love song about the boy's first girl friend. We tried to render it in English as follows:

Everybody needs to know
Who my sweetheart is,
Everybody—you, you, you—should know
Who my sweetheart is.
Everybody needs to know
Who my sweetheart is.

Know what?
She has blonde hair,
Like the sun shining down on me.
And has blue eyes,
Like the skies above.

Don't don't be jealous,
Don't don't be jealous,
Don't be envious.
No, no, no, no,
I'm very understanding.

As we watched the young woman sign, we felt very clearly that it was a "song." She began with a dance rhythm: her body moved and swayed with a clear beat, evident in her knees, hips and shoulders. Four beats preceded her signing, and four beats separated each stanza of the song. We recorded her performance on videotape, slowed it down, and found that we could easily count the number of beats per line. It was perfectly rhythmic and regular: eight beats a line in the first stanza, with one or two beats to a sign; *sweetheart* has four beats. She would elongate the sign for *sweetheart* and move it through space to the rhythm of her dancing motion. The middle stanza has a slightly different beat, with alternate lines in parallel rhythm. There were other parallels as well in the formation of signs themselves. The signs for colors are usually initial-letter handshapes: *yellow* is made with a "Y" handshape, *blue* with a "B." Here she modified the signs by moving them from their normal position closer to the nouns they modify: she signed *yellow* next to the line of her hair, and *blue* near her eyes, instead of in front of her. And, instead of signing *sun* or *sunshine* where they normally would have been (close to the body), she made an enlarged, slow poetic sign-hands open and above her, face looking upward—which we interpret as *sun-shining-down-on-me*.

A 12-year-old deaf boy made up a brief poignant poem in sign language, which his teacher translated into English as: "Deafness means my mother cries and I can't hear her. Why?"

Beyond such folk art, there are more highly developed art forms. The National Theater of the Deaf, a superb group of actors, has done opera, classical plays, haiku, children's theater and original works-entirely in sign.

Attest. Many researchers, ourselves included, used to think that sign language lacked inflections and grammar. We have come to believe now that sign language indeed has a rich surface structure, quite different from English, and based on totally different principles from that of any spoken language. For instance, spatial relations in sign have no counterpart in English, but they certainly have grammatical properties; we have seen how a change of direction or movement reverses subject and object in a sentence. We do not yet know the limits of this use of directionality. We can suggest that while the surface structure of sign and speech vary widely, the language-learning process may be the same.

Sign language, it is clear, is far more than mystical hand-waving. Its range and diversity permit humor and pun, song and poetry, whimsy and whispering. What it lacks in comparison with spoken English it amply compensates for in other ways. The study of sign gives us insight into the structure of language and the universality of communication, but even more it attests to the richness of human intelligence and imagination.

The Facial Behavior of Deaf Signers: Evidence of a Complex Language

Charlotte Baker-Shenk

Contrary to popular assumptions, American Sign Language is not simply a manual language, and the signer's face does much more than show emotions. A review of the major findings of linguistic research on the nonmanual components of ASL shows that the signer's face, head, torso, and eyegaze have important linguistic roles. The author's study illustrates how different combinations of facial and head movements signal different kinds of questions: yes-no, wh-, and rhetorical. Awareness of these nonmanual signals may help teachers communicate their questions more effectively to students and understand their students' questions better. Learning how to distinguish linguistic facial behaviors from affective facial behaviors may also help teachers avoid misunderstandings.

Many, perhaps even most, descriptions of American Sign Language (ASL) say that it is a manual language—one produced with the signer's hands. Some descriptions remark that the face is important too, because it shows the signer's emotions (e.g., Walker & Pearson, 1979). However, linguistic research on ASL, in particular the studies of the last decade, has found that some important parts of the language are produced with other parts of the signer's body. These other parts include the signer's eyes, face, head, and torso (Baker, 1976, 1979, 1980a & b; Baker-Shenk, 1983; Baker & Cokely, 1980; Baker & Padden, 1978; Bellugi & Fischer, 1972; Fischer, 1973; Liddell, 1978, 1980; Stokoe, 1960; Stokoe, Casterline, & Croneberg, 1965; Woodward & Erting, 1975).

Similar research on signed languages in other countries indicates that these languages also use the signer's face and head, etc., as well as hands and arms (Bergman, 1983; Lawson, 1983; Sorenson, 1979; Vogt-Svendsen, 1981; Volterra, 1984; Washabaugh, Woodward & DeSantis, 1978; Woll, 1981). Thus, though it may be true that the "manual" codes for spoken/written languages, such as Signed English and Signed Swedish, are indeed manual, the signed languages of deaf communities use the signer's body much more fully. These languages are more appropriately described as visual-gestural languages—where *gesture* is a generic term referring to body movement.

In these languages, movements of the signer's eyes, face, and head help form signs, act as adverbs and adjectives, and serve as grammatical signals. For example, some signs are made solely with the face: the sign *don't-know* in Swedish Sign Language is made by puffing out one cheek and letting the air pop out; the sign *to-like-something* in Providence Island Sign Language is made by raising the eyebrows, pursing the lips, and sucking in air; the sign *yeah-I-know-that* in ASL is made by a repeated twitching of one side of the nose.

Other movements of the eyes, face, and head form adverbs and adjectives, which modify the co-occurring manual signs (Baker, 1979; Baker & Cokely, 1980; Baker-Shenk, 1983; Liddell, 1980). There appear to be at least 20 such modifiers in ASL. For example, making the sign *write* with the nonmanual adverb that means *inattentively* or *without control* can produce the combined meaning *write down any old thing,* or *write something carelessly.* Similarly, if the nonmanual adverb that means *normally* or *regularly* is made with the verb *write* the result is a combined meaning like *write at a regular/expected pace.*

When the nonmanual adverb changes, the form of the verb also changes. This is one of several verb agreement rules in ASL where the form of the facial behavior and the form of the manual behavior agree.

Other movements of the signer's eyes, face, head, and torso play an important role in the syntax of signed languages (Baker, 1980a & b; Baker-Shenk, 1983; Baker & Cokely, 1980; Baker & Padden, 1978; Liddell, 1978, 1980). Combinations of these movements form grammatical signals indicating whether a sentence is a question, an assertion, a command, or if it is conditional and whether the sentence is negated, has a topicalized segment, or includes a relative clause.

These grammatical signals appear immediately before the sentence begins and generally continue until the sentence or segment ends. For example, the signal telling the receiver that the sentence is conditional is composed of a brow raise and head and/or body tilt to one side. These nonmanual movements usually begin immediately before the first sign in the conditional segment and continue until the end of the condition. A different grammatical signal then appears to indicate what type of clause the result segment is. For example, in the ASL sentence *If it rains, are you going?* the conditional signal occurs during *If it rains* (the condition), and the yes-no question signal occurs during *are you going?*

Although there are signs that can also indicate that a sentence is conditional (e.g., *suppose, if*), they do not have to be used in the sentence. The nonmanual conditional signal is sufficient. However, even when these signs are used (e.g., *suppose rain),* the signer still uses the nonmanual signal during the condition. Similarly, the signer can negate a sentence with a negative sign like *not,* but can also negate the sentence with the

nonmanual, negation signal (which includes headshaking) In addition, more than one nonmanual grammatical signal can occur at the same time. For example, signing *remember you* with the yes-no question and negation signals yields the meaning *Don't you remember?*

As would be expected, expressions of the signer's emotion may also occur with each of the grammatical signals as well as with the nonmanual adverbs and adjectives. For example, the signer might combine the yes-no question and negation signals with the jaw drop for surprise (Ekman & Friesen, 1978b) while signing *you* to communicate *Not you?!* as in "You weren't one of the people offered the teaching position?!".

Research on the exact form of these nonmanual linguistic signals and how they combine with facial expressions of emotion is still very new. One problem in this research has been the difficulty of finding precise and reliable means of coding what ASL signers are doing with their faces as well as their head, eyes, and body.

Lacking such a means of precise description, researchers have more than once come to different conclusions. For example, Coulter (1979) claims that the nonmanual signals for yes-no questions and topics are the same—i.e., they both have a brow raise. But Liddell (1980) shows that these signals are different: Yes-no questions involve head movement forward, and topics involve head movement backward.

McIntire (1980) also observed only the brow raise in rhetorical and yes-no questions and concludes that these two signals are the same. However, Baker-Shenk (1983) found that the corresponding head movements are different in these two signals, and that an upper eyelid raise also occurs in the yes-no questions but not in the rhetoricals or the topics.

For hearing researchers and teachers who are not native signers, these differences in eyelid movement or head position are often initially hard to see. And it may be hard to believe that such differences are really linguistically significant.

However, to native ASL signers, for whom vision is a finely tuned and continuously used sense, differences in facial and head position are "loud." In fact, since the addressee looks at the signer's face (not hands) during ASL conversations, the face is the area of highest visual acuity (Siple, 1978). This fact enables the face, a highly versatile articulator, to carry much lexical, grammatical, and affective information in Sign Language conversations.

In response to the need for a reliable means of describing signers' facial behavior, Baker-Shenk (1983) recommends the Facial Action Coding System and illustrates its use in an ethnographic study of ASL questions.

Method

Coding Procedure

The Facial Action Coding System (FACS), developed by psychologists Ekman and Friesen (1978a) provides a tool for the precise description of facial behavior. FACS uses 44 numbers (called Action Units, or AUs) to identify all possible facial movements. With a few exceptions, the AUs have a one-to-one correspondence with single muscles. Ekman and Friesen (1978b) have used FACS to identify the facial movements that occur universally when people experience one of six basic emotions: surprise, fear, happiness, sadness, disgust, and anger.

FACS also enables the coder to identify when a facial action begins (A), when it reaches its highest intensity (B), when it starts to decrease from that apex (C), and when it is no longer visible (D). It also enables the coder to determine

the relative intensity level of the facial action during its apex (see Figure 1).

Categories for coding eyegaze, head movement and position, and torso movement and position were developed by Baker-Shenk (1983), including 9 locations of eyegaze, 11 head movements, and 4 torso movements. Manual signs and other hand/arm movements were coded using English glosses and/or phrases, noting when the movements began and ended.

All movements and positions of the signer's (1) eyegaze, (2) face, (3) head, (4) torso, and (5) hands and arms were coded separately and then put together on a timeline. The coding indicates both what happened and when it happened. This full coding took approximately 6.25 hours per 1 second of discourse data, with slightly under half of that time spent on the transcription of facial behavior.

Subjects and Data

The primary data base consisted of eight one-hour videotapes of four deaf native signers (two male, two female) engaging in dyadic free conversation. The signers ranged in age from 19 to 28 and were from California (one southern, one northern), Michigan, and North Carolina. As each conversation took place, four different videotapes synchronized with a digital clock were made. They included full-face closeups and a long shot of the full bodies of both signers. Later, a numerical marking was added to each tape on each videofield—i.e., every 1/60 second.

From these tapes, 40 segments ranging in length from 1.3 to 13 seconds were selected to include approximately 65 questions and 40 statements. Three types of questions were used: yes-

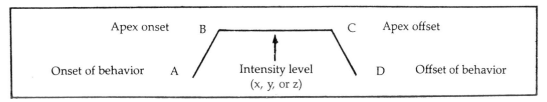

Figure 1. Temporal locations within a given behavior.

Table 1. Predominant Behaviors with each Question Type.

Question Type	yes-no	wh-	rhetorical (wh)
AU 1+2			+
AU 1+2+5	+		
AU 4		+	
Head forward/ (downward)	+		
Head back/(to side)			+
(No prediction for head)		(+)	
' + ' Eye gaze	+	+	+

no questions (e.g. "Did you do that?"), wh-questions (e.g. "Why did you do that?"), and rhetorical questions ("Why did I do it? I don't know"). A written description of the context in which each segment occurred and a translation of each segment were provided by two bilingual individuals, one deaf and one hearing.

Analysis

Patterns of manual and nonmanual activity during and surrounding each question were noted, observing both what occurred and when it occurred with respect to the manual signs and other co-occurring nonmanual behaviors. As patterns emerged for each type of question, the contexts in which questions appeared with atypical nonmanual combinations were examined.

Results

Distinct Signals

Specific combinations of nonmanual behaviors were found to occur regularly with each question type. These combinations differ from each other, as seen in Table 1.

Affect-Related Variations

The affect of the signer can alter the form of the grammatical signal so that the signal is still recognizable but is different from its characteristic form. For example, characteristically, the brow raise in yes-no questions is at a medium level of intensity and the upper eyelid is slightly raised. However, when the signer is surprised and asks a question, the brow raise and the eyelid raise increase in intensity and the jaw drops open.

Distress in a signer was found to alter the characteristic shape of the brow raise in several of the rhetorical questions. The resultant shape matched that which Ekman & Friesen (1978b) describe as an expression of sadness—the brows are drawn together as the inner portions of the brows are raised.

Manual Signs

No specific manual signs or types of signs necessarily occurred to signal a particular question type. That is, wh- questions appeared that did not include a wh- sign (e.g., *what, who, how*). For example, one signer simply made the sign *quote* with the non-manual wh- question signal to ask "What was the title?" Similarly, the rhetorical question "Who'd he get [to be on the team]? His two sons." was asked with a two-handed alternation of the sign *get* accompanied by the nonmanual rhetorical question signal. The pronoun *you* occurred at the end of several yes-no questions; and in 50% of these questions, some form of sign repetition occurred (e.g., *have same-as your same-as*). However, again there were no particular manual signs indicating that the sentence was a yes-no question. The only consistent marker of question type in each sentence was the co-occurring nonmanual signal.

Conclusion and Implication

In ASL, grammatical signals composed of head and/or facial movements can indicate (a) that a sentence is a question and (b) what kind of question it is—yes-no, wh-, or rhetorical.

Kluwin (1983) has observed that hearing teachers in classrooms with deaf students often experience difficulty in getting the students to recognize that a question has been asked and to respond appropriately to it. Since most hearing teachers do not know ASL, it is reasonable to assume that they may not be using the grammatical signals described above. Though we do not yet know the source(s) of this problem with questions in the classroom, it is certainly possible that teachers' inclusion of the appropriate nonmanual signals may aid students' understanding and hence their ability to respond appropriately.

Anecdotes by deaf adults suggest that, as students, they felt they were often misunderstood by their hearing teachers. Some of these anecdotes focused on the deaf person's face—the teacher said the student was misbehaving, expressing an inappropriate emotion, and the student said she or he was not. It is certainly possible that the root of this misunderstanding lies in the different ways deaf signers and hearing speakers use their faces. For example, the brows of a deaf signer who is asking a wh- question and the brows of a hearing speaker who is angry look the same. In both cases, the brows are drawn together into a squint.

Linguistic studies of deaf signers' faces are just beginning to discover the complex ways in which movements of facial muscles serve linguistic functions in signed languages. They serve as signs, as components of signs, as modifiers, and as grammatical signals. These studies are also finding that other nonmanual behaviors, such as movements of the signer's head, play an important role in the syntax of signed languages and that these behaviors interact in complex ways with each other. For these reasons, the signed languages of deaf communities are appropriately described as visual-gestural, rather than manual languages.

Such studies also demonstrate the inaccuracy of calling ASL or other signed languages condensed or abbreviated. Instead, what these studies (and other research on manual movements) show is that the information was there all along; we just did not know the right place to look for it.

References

Baker, C. (1976). What's not on the other hand in American Sign Language. *Papers from the Twelfth Reigional Meeting of the Chicago Linguistic Society.* Chicago: University of Chicago Press.

Baker, C. *(1979). Nonmanual components of the sign language signal.* Paper presented at the NATO Advanced Study Institute, Copenhagen.

Baker, C. (1980a). On the terms "verbal" and "nonverbal." In I. Ahlgren & B. Bergman (Eds.), *Papers From the First International Symposium on Sign Language Research* (pp. 41-52). Swedish National Association of the Deaf, Leksand, Sweden.

Baker, C. (1980b). Sentences in American Sign Language. In C. Baker & R. Battison (Eds.), *Sign language and the deaf community: Essays in honor of William C. Stokoe* (pp. 75-86). Silver Spring, MD: National Association of the Deaf.

Baker-Shenk, C. (1983). *A microanalysis of the nonmanual components of questions in American Sign Language.* Unpublished doctoral dissertation, University of California, Berkeley.

Baker, C., & Cokely, D. (1980). *American Sign Language: A teacher's resource text on grammar and culture.* Silver Spring, MD: T.J. Publishers.

Baker, C., & Padden, C. (1978). Focusing on the nonmanual components of American Sign Language. In P. Siple (Ed.), *Understanding language through sign language research* (pp. 27-57). New York: Academic Press.

Bellugi, U., & Fischer, S. (1972). A comparison of sign language and spoken language: Rate and grammatical mechanisms. *Cognition,* 1, 173-200.

Bergman, B. (1983). Verbs and adjectives: Morphological processes in Swedish Sign Language. In Kyle & Woll (Eds.). *Language in sign* (pp. 3-9). London: Croom Helm.

Coulter, G. (1979). *American Sign Language typology.* Unpublished doctoral dissertation, University of California, San Diego.

Ekman, P., & Friesen, W. (1978a). *Facial action coding system.* Palo Alto, CA: Consulting Psychologists Press.

Ekman, P., & Friesen, W. (1978b). *Facial action coding system: Investigators guide, part two.* Palo Alto, CA: Consulting Psychologists Press.

Fischer, S. (1974). Sign language and linguistic universals. In Rohrer & Ruwet (Eds.), *Conference Proceedings, Collogue franco-allemand sur la grammaire transformationelle du francais.* (pp. 187-204). Tübingen: Max Niemeyer.

Kluwin, T. (1983). Discourse in deaf classrooms: The structure of teaching episodes. *Discourse Processes,* 6, 275-293.

Lawson, L. (1983). Multi-channel signs. In J. Kyle & B. Woll (Eds.), *Language in sign, An international perspective on sign language,* (pp. 97-105). London: Croom Helm.

Liddell, S. (1978). Nonmanual signals and relative clauses in American Sign Language. In P. Siple *(Ed.), Understanding language through sign language research* (pp. 59-90). New York: Academic Press.

Lidell, S. (1980). *American Sign Language syntax.* The Hague: Mouton.

McIntire, M. (1980). *Locatives in American Sign Language.* Unpublished doctoral dissertation, University of California, Los Angeles.

Siple, P. (1978). Visual constraints for sign language communication. *Sign Language Studies, 19,* 95-110.

Sorensen, R. (1979). Rhythms, "intonation," and sentence markers in Danish Sign Language. In Ahlgren & Bergman (Eds.). *Papers From the First International Symposium on Sign Language Research* (pp. 263-281). Swedish National Association of the Deaf, Leksand, Sweden.

Stokoe, W. (1960). *Sign language structure: An outline of the visual communication systems of the American deaf.* University of Buffalo, Occasional Papers, 8 (revised 1978), Silver Spring, MD: Linstok Press.

Stokoe, W., Casterline, D., & Croneberg, C. (1965). *A dictionary of American Sign language on linguistic principles.* Washington, DC: Gallaudet College Press. Second Edition, Silver Spring, MD: Linstok Press, 1976.

Vogt-Svendsen, M. (1981). Mouth position and mouth movement in Norwegian Sign Language. *Sign Language Studies, 33,* 363-376.

Volterra, V. (Ed.). (1984). *La Lingua Italiana dei Segni: LIS.* Roma: Istituto di Psicologia del Consiglio Nazionale delle Richerche.

Walker, B., & Pearson, H. (1979). *Signfest: Teacher resource manual.* Washington, DC: Model Secondary School for the Deaf.

Washabaugh, W., Woodward, J., & DeSantis, S. (1978). Providence Island Sign Language: A context-dependent language. *Anthropological Linguistics, 20,* 95-109.

Woll, B. (1981). Question structure in British Sign Language. In B. Woll, J. Kyle, & M. Deuchar (Eds.). *Perspectives on British Sign Language and deafness,* (pp. 136-149). London: Croom Helm.

Woodward, J., & Erting, C. (1975). Synchronic variation and historical change in American Sign Language. *Language Sciences, 37,* 9-12.

ASL: Adjective Before Noun or After Noun?

M. J. Bienvenu

With all the research on American Sign Language (ASL) during the past 25 years, we have discovered many important things that have helped us to recognize it as a language and to recognize the existence of Deaf Culture. Although much work has been done, research on ASL is still in its beginning stages and promises many more years of exciting studies and discoveries.

One of the areas that is least studied is adjectives in ASL. People generally know some of the rules in the English language related to adjectives—for example, that you can add small word parts that can change nouns to adjectives, like the suffixes "-ive" and "-ful." You can add "-ful" to the noun "beauty" and get the adjective "beautiful." You also have probably learned in your English classes that you must put adjectives before nouns and that if you put it after nouns, you have to add a copula (is, are, am, etc.) between the noun and the adjective.

One study related to adjectives was done by Ursula Bellugi, of the Salk Institute in San Diego, California. It studied how changes in movement of the addition of another hand can make a difference in the meaning of the adjective. Bellugi found those changes cannot be made on all adjectives, and not all adjectives can be made with two hands. For example, you can sign SILLY to mean one thing, but when you add another hand with circular, alternating movement, you will get a different meaning. (*The Signs of Language*, Bellugi & Klima, Chap 11, pp 243-271).

What other rules are there related to adjectives in ASL? Is there any specific movement to show an adjective? Is there any specific movement that can make a noun in ASL an adjective? How many types of adjectives are there in ASL? Where do we put adjectives in ASL sentences? Should we sign an adjective before or after a noun? Is there any specific facial expression that will show the sign is an adjective; what I mean is if there is a specific facial expression that fits only with adjectives, but cannot occur with nouns, verbs, etc.? Some people have said that the older ASL signers will sign adjectives after nouns and younger ASL signers will sign them before nouns. For example, "GIRL PRETTY[1] . . . " as compared to "PRETTY GIRL . . . " However, to my knowledge, there has not been any substantive research on this.

Overwhelmed by all those questions, I began to do a basic, beginning kind of research on adjectives in ASL. I decided to try to find if there is more than one function of adjectives in ASL. I believed this could help further analysis, such as sign order in ASL, when using adjectives.

That was where my basic analysis began. After hiring a native[2] informant, I asked her to watch 20 sentences that I signed her and to tell me whether or not they were grammatical[3]. Those 20

---

1   I used capital letters to show a "rough" English equivalent word(s) for the sign, one way to transcribe ASL signs/sentences that helps us record them, including non-manual behaviors, e.g. facial expression.

2   A native signer, him/herself fluent in ASL, is a person who acquired ASL from his/her Deaf parents/family before attending any school.

3   Grammaticality: a sentence used or accepted by native users of the language. For example, it is grammatical to use a topic marker at the beginning of an ASL sentence but ungrammatical if at the end of a sentence.

sentences included 20 different adjectives, for example, GREEN, WHITE, FAT, and HAPPY. I topicalized the nouns, and then signed adjectives after them. For example,

$$\overline{\quad}^{t} \qquad \overline{\qquad}^{t}$$
CAR, GREEN and GREEN, CAR.

When a noun is topicalized, it is signed at the beginning of a sentence with a specific facial expression and head movement, a "rule" in ASL to show what topic is being talked about.[4]

The informant was to answer which sentences were acceptable and which seemed to be complete sentences. For this person, all sentences with topicalized nouns at the beginning of the sentence were acceptable. However, none of the sentences with topicalized adjectives at the beginning of the sentences were acceptable.

This study shows that those ASL adjectives function as, what linguists call, "predicate adjectives," meaning they function similarly to a verb, making sentences complete.

I then tested to see if there are adjectives that could function as, what linguists call, "descriptive adjectives," meaning they function to describe the nouns. Sentences that include nouns with descriptive adjectives still require the addition of a verb. For example, in English, "The pretty girl is eating."[5] In this study, I added a verb and asked my informant which were acceptable. For example,

$$\overline{\qquad\qquad}^{t}$$
CAR GREEN, ME KISS-FIST or

$$\overline{\qquad\qquad}^{t}$$
GREEN CAR, ME KISS-FIST

Both were acceptable, but when I changed sign order for example,

ME KISS-FIST CAR GREEN or
ME KISS-FIST GREEN CAR[6]

only the second order was acceptable. This showed me that if the noun phrase with the adjective at the beginning of the sentence is topicalized either order is acceptable, but if it is signed at the end of the sentence only the 'adjective + noun' order is acceptable.[7]

From those two analyses, it was found that adjectives in ASL can function in two ways and that partially answered the question why some adjectives come after nouns and some before. Let me add that for many years people have overlooked the importance of facial expression in ASL, for example, the facial expression that marks topics. It makes a difference in those sentences and it requires nouns before predicate adjectives. It is probably parallel to rules in English requiring a copula in between when putting an adjective after the noun. ASL has its own, separate rule that requires topicalization when using predicate adjectives.

With better understanding of two types of adjectives in ASL, I moved on to do a basic analysis on older signers. I collected videotapes from a Senior Citizens Banquet in Detroit, in 1980, and studied them. I looked for sentences that seemed to have adjectives in them. I transcribed 25 sentences, from 4 native signers and two near-native (meaning they have hearing parents, but acquired fluency in ASL from residential schools for the Deaf). After transcribing

---

4   A note here on the transcription symbols: A line over the word or words with a letter "t" signals that the eyebrow is raised to topicalize that part of the sentence. In another instance, lines over a word or phrase would signal something non-manual is occurring that would add specific meaning to the sentence. The word "nod" over the line which is over a phrase or a word means the head is nodding either for emphasis or affirmation.

5   The underlined word is a descriptive adjective (in English).

6   Please note that those two sentences (with adjective at end of sentence) do not have a topic marker. This will probably make a difference in my analysis and I intend to go back and test those sentences again.

7   A personal note: Although the informant said they were acceptable, we had a brief discussion afterwards where we both agreed that we had some intuitive feeling that probably the sentences were more 'Englishy' and probably the reason why the adjective has to be before the noun.

sentences, I looked for a pattern to see if there was similarity in sign order when using adjectives. My method of getting sentences from them was asking them questions mostly related to their families, educational background and their life experiences, with hope that they would use adjectives in their sentences. They then could answer me freely, using their own words, either a few sentences or a short story.

From my analysis, I discovered their sign order was similar to the younger informant—if a noun phrase with a descriptive adjective occurs at the end of a sentence, it will have an 'adjective + noun' sign order. However, when the noun phrase is signed at the beginning of a sentence, it's usually a 'noun + adjective' sign order. An example sentence with 'adjective + noun' sign order below:

MUST FINGERSPELL, KEEP <u>GOOD</u> LANGUAGE[8]

and with 'noun + adjective' order below:

<u>   t</u>
MY FATHER MOTHER DEAF, ENTER THAT SCHOOL

The older signers also used predicate adjectives. I found it interesting that they do not always use topicalization. If they did not use topicalization, they instead used a head nod/nodding or body shift on adjectives. Examples below:

       ⊥
(with topic) ME, CAREFUL

       <u> nod </u>
(w/o 't') OLDER GIRL, DEAF

SEEM MOTHER KNOW INSTITUTE IN F-L-I-N-T SCHOOL THROUGH

           <u>body shifts to rt</u>
MY COUSIN,   DEAF

So with better understanding of ASL's adjectives functioning in two ways and comparative study between younger and older signers, we can see there are sign order rules in ASL related to adjectives. Another difference I noted is that it is

always adjective after nouns for older signers when signed first in sentences and with younger signer, it is either order. Another example is:

MY SISTER OLDEST HEARING, SELF EXPERT SIGNING

Both groups need to sign adjectives before nouns when the noun phrase is at the end of the ASL sentence. However, I have one unanswered question—why the difference? I recall that not one older signer I used in my research ever attended Gallaudet and the younger informant is presently a student. Does collegiate education encourage 'code-switching'? Is sign order in ASL going through some historical change, especially when using adjectives in noun phrases? (But, see footnote 7).

Here I would like to add that I faced some problems in my analyses. There was a variety of sentences, of adjectives and of number of sentences. The older signers, were free to sign anything while the younger informant answered to a set of sentences. Although there is a difference in methodology from both age groups, the results seem to be the same. Also, what I wanted to find out from both groups was different: from the informant, functions of adjectives; and with older signers, I looked closer to sign order when using adjectives.

One important thing I believe, is that we can now say adjectives in ASL function in two ways—predicate and descriptive. And, we have some better understanding of the sign order in ASL when using adjectives. We should look closely in future studies as to why there is a difference when using adjectives inside noun phrases between older and younger signers, when in the first part of the sentence. I hope this basic research will help some of you understand your first language better, and those of you who are studying ASL, understand your second (or third) language better.

---

8   The underlined gloss is an adjective (in ASL).

The Transparency of Meaning of Sign Language Gestures

Harry W. Hoemann

Breger (1970) has presented evidence that the meaning of 30 signs from the American Sign Language lexicon is transparent to persons with no prior experience with the language. In a 30-item multiple choice test administered live by a deaf person, 31 of Breger's 35 Ss made correct responses in more than half the trials, and all but four of the items were correctly identified at better than chance levels.

These results might have both theoretical and practical implications, if confirmed. On a theoretical level, Breger's findings suggest that the trend from iconic to "formal" signs described by Tervoort (1961) has not proceeded very far from the signs' original motivations. They suggest, further, that historical trends in the formation of signs described by Bellugi and Klima (in press) have left the imitative, ideographic component of the signs fairly well intact.

Breger's results have practical significance, since the opinion has sometimes been expressed that the ideographic lexicon of American Sign Language makes it an inferior language (Myklebust, 1964). This opinion may have to be revised, since there is evidence from translations into and out of Sign Language that Sign is able to preserve all of the meanings and nuances of an original text in English (Hoemann & Tweney 1973; Tweney & Hoemann 1973). On the other hand, if the meaning of signs is relatively transparent even to persons unfamiliar with the language, Myklebust's reservations may need to be taken seriously.

Breger's results, however, must be viewed with considerable caution, since the difficulty level of a multiple choice test is affected by the test composer's selection of incorrect alternatives for each item. From the one example presented in Breger's paper and from the "most frequent errors" reported, it appears that almost all of the incorrect alternatives for each item appeared elsewhere in the test as response choices for other stimulus signs to be identified. No explanation is given for constructing the test in this manner. Moreover, there is reason to question whether the thirty items used in Breger's test are representative of the Sign Language lexicon. Three of the items are socially restricted (breast, penis, feces). While socially restricted signs are present in American Sign Language, they do not comprise ten percent of the lexicon. Again, no explanation is given for the manner in which stimulus items were chosen for the test.

In view of the questionable methods used by Breger to assess the transparency of meaning of signs and in view of the theoretical and practical implications that such findings might have for evaluating the American Sign Language as a communicative channel, a replication was conducted which sought to overcome the major limitations of the Breger study and to quantify more precisely the extent to which the meaning of the American Sign Language lexicon is transparent to persons who have had no experience with the language.

Method. Fifty-two undergraduate students at Bowling Green State University were recruited from courses which required participation as Ss in psychological experiments. The sex division was approximately equal. None had any prior knowledge of Sign Language.

One hundred Sign Language gestures were drawn randomly from a deck of 500 sign language flash cards (Hoemann & Hoemann 1973). Although there is no way to verify whether the 500 items in the deck are the most frequently used signs in American Sign Language, the contents of the deck are very similar to the contents of other published dictionaries of Sign Language (for example, O'Rourke 1973).

The Ss were tested anonymously in small groups of six to twelve Ss in sessions lasting about 25 minutes. They were informed that they would see examples of signs from the American Sign Language of the Deaf. They were told that the meaning of some signs may be guessed from the manner in which the sign is executed and that the purpose of the study was to determine how many signs could be guessed by persons who had no previous experience with Sign Language. They were advised to provide a response to each item, even though it might be a guess. The signs were executed one at a time by the author. Appropriate body and facial cues were supplied, as, for example, in *sleep, smile, awkward, awful,* etc., but without exaggeration. Items were repeated on request.

Results. Since scoring the guesses of Ss involved some subjective judgments, two scoring procedures were adopted, one of which was likely to yield a conservative estimate of Ss' ability to guess the meaning of the signs and the other of which was likely to yield a liberal estimate. The conservative scoring criterion was provided by a deaf informant, who was asked to generate a scoring key by writing down all of the meanings which each stimulus sign might have in various contexts. Responses were scored as correct if they were identical to or synonymous with the items in the key. The liberal scoring criterion was prepared by adding to the conservative criterion all words which were listed by a conventional thesaurus as synonyms of the words in the conservative key. Responses were scored

as correct if their meaning was the same or synonymous with the items in the expanded key. The scoring was done by four judges working independently, two using the conservative criterion and two using the liberal criterion. Interjudge agreement was 98% between judges using the conservative criterion and 92% between judges using the liberal criterion.

The data were first inspected to determine how many of the 100 signs might be considered to have a transparent meaning and to identify, which signs they were. It was decided that if any of the four judges considered the meaning of a sign to have been guessed correctly by 25% of the Ss, it would be considered transparent. The signs identified by this criterion are listed in Table 1. Some of the signs were guessed correctly far more frequently than others; therefore, in order to provide an estimate of relative transparency of meaning, the scores of the four judges were averaged, and the signs were ranked in Table 1 from high to low.

Twenty-nine signs (29% of the total) satisfied this relatively liberal criterion for transparency. If the mean of the four judges were taken as the basis for identifying signs guessed correctly by 25% of the Ss, 18 of the signs would be considered transparent. If Breger's criterion were used, requiring correct responses in more than half the trials, the number of transparent signs would be seven according to the most conservative judge and 13 according to the most liberal judge. A conservative estimate of the number of transparent signs in the present list would be 10 to 15 percent. A liberal estimate would be from 20 to 30 percent.

Three of the signs in Table 1 have conventional meanings in American Sign Language which were not guessed correctly (your, school, red). They are included because the Sign Language informant who prepared the conservative scoring key listed the natural meaning of the signs as permissible (stop, clap, lips).

The data were also examined to discover whether any items resulted in considerable agree-

Stimulus	Flash Card No.	Mean No. Correct
hear	224	52
Your (stop)	410	49
pray	436	45
house	154	42
walk	293	40
school (clap)	277	28
smile	51	28
sleep	32	24
stand	188	24
around	433	20
to	240	20
spread	245	19
about	39	18
pepper (season)	267	17
letter	139	15
my	307	15
lipread	465	15
red (lips)	425	13
know	14	12
near	163	12
airplane	1	11
learn	217	10
abandon	276	10
steal	130	8
praise	57	6
from	16	4
light	462	4
conscience	486	4
quit	211	4

Table 1.
Signs Identified as Transparent Ranked on the Basis
of Mean Number Correct

ment among the Ss but in guesses that were wrong. It was reasoned that if up to one-third of the Sign Language lexicon has a meaning that is somewhat transparent to persons who have had no experience with the language, this result might be partly or wholly offset by items whose appearance misleads observers so that they are likely to be mistaken in their guesses. Signs for which the same incorrect meaning was guessed by at least 25% of the Ss are listed in rank order in Table 2. The frequency count includes responses whose meaning was the same as the erroneous word cited in the Table; for example, think, thinking, idea, thought. There are 36 items in Table 2, seven more than in Table 1. While none of the erroneous meanings was guessed as unanimously as some of the correct meanings (52, 49, 45, 42), it appears that for many signs the same incorrect meaning was inferred more frequently than the correct one.

Figure 1 was prepared to permit comparison of meanings correctly guessed and erroneous meanings inferred with some consistency. In addition, the extent to which the most conservative and the most liberal judge differed in their scoring was taken into account. Correct responses scored by the most conservative and the most liberal judges are presented in the histograms with the higher frequencies at the left. Incorrect responses frequently given are presented with the higher frequencies at the right. (Each histogram was based on a different ranking; hence, the base line implies merely that there were 100 signs in the list without identifying them as to location on the base line.)

Two outcomes are apparent. First, while the most conservative and the most liberal judge generated slightly different histograms, they do not lead to opposite conclusions. A few signs are apparently relatively transparent to persons with no experience with Sign Language, but both histograms are characterized by a sharp decline from a high consensus, and they reach the zero point well below the end of the base line. Secondly, the somewhat larger area under the histogram on the right suggests that the outward appearance of a large number of signs was likely to be misleading.

Table 1 and 2, which include signs which were more or less transparent and signs which were

Stimulus	Flash Card No.	Most Frequent Error	Frequency of Most Frequent Error
count	461	climb	40
Call	29	slap	37
true	291	quiet	35
government	256	think	34
except	330	pick up	34
miss	175	catch	31
important	343	join	31
kill	450	down	27
what?	298	cut	26
bird	111	talk	26
warm	356	speak	25
autumn	299	brush away	25
thank	246	speak	25
funny	376	nose	24
awkward	455	walk	24
number	305	turn over	22
begin	124	screw	22
both	395	catch	21
grandmother	341	throw away	20
train	25	rub	20
some	60	cut	20
because	318	think	19
sit	206	grasp	18
machine	105	together	18
signature	427	punish	18
abandon	276	throw	18
star	108	rub	17
smile	51	mustache	15
emphasize	431	turn	15
measure	316	touch	15
person	18	straight	15
conscience	486	heart	14
electricity	89	hit	14
make	210	pound	13
show	247	push	13
which	333	run	13

Table 2.
Signs for Which The Same Incorrect Response Was Given by at Least 25% of the Subjects

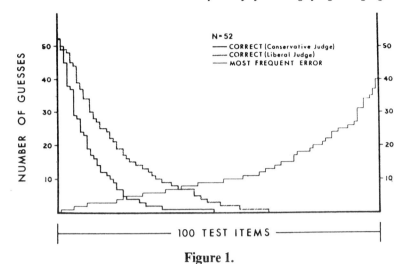

Figure 1.

Correct guesses and most frequent errors for 100 signs with correct responses ranked from left to right and most frequent errors ranked from right to left in order of their frequency of occurrence.

more or less misleading in appearance, account for 65 of the signs. The remainder, approximately one-third of the items in the list, led to a wide range of guesses on the part of the Ss. Apparently the outward appearance of these signs suggested nothing that the Ss could use as a basis for guessing the meaning of the signs. Thus, approximately one-third of the signs were more or less transparent based on a liberal criterion, one-third were misleading in their appearance, and one-third were opaque.

Finally, the results were analyzed for information on individual differences between Ss' ability to recognize the signs. It was of interest whether some Ss were able to guess a rather large number of signs correctly or whether the performances were relatively homogeneous. Means and standard deviations for the judges using the conservative key were Mean = 9.86, Standard Deviation = 2.50 for Judge 1 and Mean = 10.02, Standard Deviation = 2.76 for Judge 2. The same statistics for judges using the liberal key were Mean = 12.83, Standard Deviation = 2.58 for Judge 3 and Mean = 18.46, Standard Deviation = 3.38 for Judge 4. The small standard deviations indicate

that the Ss performed very similarly to one another. The 95% Confidence Intervals around the means for Judge 1 through 4, respectively are $9.10 < \mu < 10.62$, $9.33 < \mu < 10.71$, $12.10 < \mu < 13.52$, and $17.53 < \mu < 19.39$.

Discussion. The opinion that the meaning of signs is relatively transparent may have arisen from an awareness that a sizeable percentage of the lexicon of the American Sign Language consists of motivated signs, that is, the form of the gesture symbol is influenced by the form of the referent (Tervoort 1961). For example, the sign for *man* is said to be derived from the custom of men to tip their hats, while the sign for *woman* is said to be derived from bonnet strings tied beneath the chin. The probable origin of signs is sometimes specified in Sign Language dictionaries (Stokoe, Casterline, & Croneberg 1965), and the motivation behind signs is often exploited for pedagogical purposes, since knowing the motivation for a sign may assist students in remembering its meaning (Watson 1964).

The motivation behind some signs is relatively obvious. *House* traces the outline of the roof and walls, *car* turns an imaginary steering wheel, and *throw* is a natural gesture whose execution is influenced by the size and weight of the object and the direction or force of the action. On the other hand, the particular aspect of a referent that a sign imitates is not always predictable. For example, *house, tree,* and *airplane* represent the physical appearance of the entire object, but *cat, policeman,* and *letter* imitate a specific part of the referent, the cat's whiskers, the policeman's badge, and the letter's stamp. Some signs range far afield for their motivation. *Coffee* imitates the turning of the handle of a coffee grinder, *black* touches the eyebrow as an example of something that is sometimes black, and *word* represents a small segment of hand-set type. The fact that a sign's motivation may be derived from a single, narrow aspect of its referent makes it an uncertain clue as to the meaning of the sign.

Moreover, the meaning of a sign may generalize during the course of time so as to be applied to a broader field of meaning than its original motivation. Tervoort (1961) cites an example of a name sign for a school principal in The Netherlands which was motivated by her dimples. By the time she retired, the sign "Ms. Dimples" had become attached to her office as principal as well as her person, and her successor was referenced by the same sign even though she had no dimples. In a similar fashion the name sign for the school nurse at the Western Pennsylvania School for the Deaf, a "B" on the forehead, has come to mean any hospital or infirmary in the city of Pittsburgh. Schowe (1955) reports that at the Ohio School for the Deaf the sign for Negro generalized to all fire trucks in Columbus, Ohio, from an all-Negro fire company that once manned the station house across the street from the school. The motivation behind these signs would have surely been lost to posterity except for the interest of the scholars whose curiosity was aroused by the signs they observed and who recorded their origins.

The original motivation for a sign may also become obscure if the formation of the sign changes over time. Signs requiring elaborate or cumbersome movements may be shortened. Fre-

quently used signs may be influenced by a tendency, which seems to exist in all languages, for frequently used words to be short. Zipf's law (Zipf 1949) notes that there is an inverse relation between the length of a word and the frequency of its occurrence in a language. It is reasonable to consider that signs, too, may have a tendency to become truncated with frequent use over time. The current sign for *woman* may be executed by briefly brushing the right jaw with the thumb of the clenched right hand. A person with no knowledge of Sign Language would never guess that the hand is clenched because it once held an imaginary bonnet string about to be tied to its counterpart under the chin. Bellugi and Klima (1975) have studied some of the historical changes that have occurred in the formation of signs, reviewing films and publications dating back fifty years or more and interviewing elderly informants whose memory of sign language use goes back many years. They have concluded that there is a tendency for iconic signs to come to resemble more and more the rest of the Sign Language lexicon. Signs tend to lose idiosyncratic features characteristic of pantomime and gradually take on the formational parameters found in conventional signs.

Another factor which may account for the obscurity of meaning of many signs is the relationship that exists between American Sign Language and English. Deaf persons growing up in the United States are taught English in school at more or less the same time that many of them are learning Sign Language from deaf associates. The ease with which they learn to draw on fingerspelled English to supplement their Sign Language vocabulary is well known to anyone who is acquainted with deaf people. In fact, there are no signs for months of the year, makes of cars, brand names of merchandise, and many other referents for which English provides a technical vocabulary. This absence of symbols for large numbers of referents is sometimes cited as a deficiency in American Sign Language (cf. Fusfeld 1958), but it is more parsimonious to assume that a technical vocabulary has failed to emerge in Sign Language because the availability of English words has made parallel vocabularies unnecessary. The intimacy of the relation between American Sign Language and English can be seen in the many signs which incorporate a letter of the alphabet as the hand configuration of the sign, a letter which is often the first letter of a cognate English word. Some of the items in the present test were initialized in this manner *(law, wine, brown, nation)*. None of the 52 Ss guessed the meaning of any of these signs. It is highly unlikely that the meaning of any initialized signs would be guessed correctly by persons who had no knowledge of the manual alphabet.

Five factors, then, account for the difficulty experienced by the Ss in the present study in guessing the meaning of a hundred signs drawn at random from a standard source. First, the motivation of a sign is not a certain clue as to its meaning; since the sign may imitate a narrow aspect of the referent rather than the entire field of meaning. Second, the field of meaning of a sign may generalize over time and go beyond the constraints of the original motivation. Third, signs may become shortened over time or a difficult movement modified so that it is easier to execute, with the result that the original motivation becomes increasingly difficult to recognize in the gesture. Influences from English have supplemented and modified the American Sign Language lexicon so that many signs are virtually impossible to identify from their outward appearance. Finally, it is likely that the outward appearance of many signs will bear a superficial resemblance to a number of possible referents, most of which will not correspond to the meaning or meanings of the sign.

The present data indicate that only a small percentage of the signs in the American Sign Language lexicon have transparent meanings for persons who have had no prior experience with the language, 10 to 15 percent based on a conservative estimate and 20 to 30 percent based on a liberal estimate. The outward appearance of many signs is rather misleading, and more of them are likely to lead to a consensus that is wrong than to one that is correct. Under these circumstances it is permissible to say that certain signs are transparent as to their meaning, but it is inappropriate to ascribe transparency of meaning to the Sign Language lexicon as a whole.

References

Bellugi, U. and Klima, E. S. (1975) Aspects of Sign Language and its Structure, in *The Role of Speech in Language*, J. Cavanagh and J. Cutting, eds. (Cambridge, Mass., M.I.T. Press).

Breger, I. (1970) Perceptions of Sign Language of the Deaf, *Perceptual and Motor Skills*, 31, 426.

Fusfeld, I. S. (1958) How the Deaf Communicate: Manual Language, *American Annals of the Deaf*, 103, 255-263.

Hoemann, H. W. and Hoemann, S. A. (1973) *Sign Language Flash Cards* (Silver Spring, Md. National Association of the Deaf).

Hoemann, H. W. and R. D. Tweney (1973) Is the Sign Language of the deaf an adequate communicative channel? *Proceedings: 81st Convention, American Psychological Association*, Vol. II., 801-802.

Myklebust, H. (1964) *The Psychology of Deafness*, Second edition (New York, Grune & Stratton).

O'Rourke, T. J. (1973) *A Basic Course in Manual Communication*. Revised edition (Silver Spring, Md., National Association of the Deaf).

Schowe, B. M., Jr. (1955) Sign Language Development (Ohio State University master's thesis).

Stokoe, W. C., Jr., D. Casterline, and C. Croneberg (1965) *A Dictionary of American Sign Language on Linguistic Principles* (Washington, D.C., Gallaudet College Press).

Tervoort, B. (1961) Esoteric Symbolism in the Communication Behavior of Young Deaf Children, *American Annals of the Deaf*, 106, 436-480.

Tweney, R. D. and H. W. Hoemann (1973) Back Translation: A method for the analysis of manual languages, *Sign Language Studies*, 2, 51-72, 77-80.

Zipf, G. K. (1949) *Human Behavior and the Principle of Least Effort: An introduction to human ecology* (Cambridge, Mass., Addison-Wesley).

CHAPTER 4

Sign Language Systems

Is American Sign Language a universal language? Students ask this question frequently. They are astonished to discover that American Sign Language is not a universal language and that several *different sign languages* are in use in America today.

American Sign Language is the visual-manual language used by the majority of deaf persons in North America during the past two centuries. It has its own grammar and syntax. It is a language distinct from English. Fingerspelling, a system for representing English letters manually, is incorporated into sign language to spell proper nouns, names and technical vocabulary for which no signs exist. A popular myth is that deaf people spell messages on their hands as the principal means of communicating with each other. The manual alphabet and fingerspelling are adjuncts to ASL.

Confusing to students is the fact that several systems of representing English on the hands exist in America today. These forms of Manually Coded English (MCEs) arose in the late 1960s to address the perennial challenge facing educators—teaching English to deaf children. Three of the more prominent MCEs are Seeing Essential English (SEE 1) devised by David Anthony, Signing Exact English (SEE 2) created by Gerilee Gustason and Linguistics of Visual English (LOVE) constructed by Dennis Wampler. Three things are common to these Manually Coded English (MCE) systems. First, all represent English "word for word" on the hands by use of manual signals. Second, each was developed to facilitate the use and understanding of English by

deaf children. Third, all employ "lexical borrowing," that is, they make copious use of the signs contained in the lexicon of ASL. Introductory sign language students become frustrated and confused if they encounter a deaf person who uses MCE interchangeably with ASL. The article by Dr. McCay Vernon ("Controversy Within Sign Language") provides an excellent comparative analysis of these sign language systems.

Another form of manual communication currently in use is Pidgin Sign English (PSE). A pidgin is a method of communicating between two cultures with different languages. Pidgins share the features of the respective languages from which they come. PSE is a blend of American Sign Language and Signed English. Deaf children, who use English in the classroom and ASL in dormitories of residential schools or at home, often blend American Sign Language and English into Pidgin Sign English.

Efforts to develop international languages have been unsuccessful. The World Federation of the Deaf developed Gestuno, an international sign language, for use by deaf delegates from different nations at meetings of the World Congress of the Deaf. Apart from its limited use at the World Congress of the Deaf, Gestuno is rarely used. Foreign sign languages are found in hundreds of countries around the world. Some of the facts and myths about the fascinating field of foreign sign languages are explored in the article ("Cross-cultural communication with foreign signers: Fact and fancy") by Robbin Battison and I. King Jordan.

Controversy Within Sign Language

McCay Vernon

One of the most crucial issues in deafness today is that of which sign system to use with speech and speechreading in a Total Communication program (Rodda, in press 1986). At this time, research has not been done that demonstrates which system is superior. We are left with a complex array of facts from which to reach a conclusion .

This paper will address issues involved in the use of various manual communication systems, discussing the advantages and disadvantages of each. Concepts from bilingual education, existing research, language development and psychology will be brought into the evaluation of the major systems.

It took the field of deafness almost 100 years to accept the obvious fact that the lip movements of speech do not provide enough information for deaf people to understand what is being said (Barnum, 1984; Conrad, 1979; Pahz and Pahz, 1978). Under ideal one-to-one, face-to-face conditions, 40 to 60 percent of the sounds of English look the same on the lips or else they are invisible (Vernon, 1972 and 1975). In practice the best lipreader (or speechreader) understands 25 percent of what is said (Vernon, 1972). Incidentally, these superior lipreaders are usually hearing people who have the English skills most deaf children lack (Lowell, 1957-1958; Vernon, 1972). The average deaf person gets 5 percent of what is said through lipreading (Vernon, 1972). Obviously, if a deaf person only perceives 5 to 25 percent of what is said, he will be unable to understand or communicate effectively.

Thus, it is anxiomatic that some additional manual system is needed to supplement speech and lipreading for deaf people in educational settings. The issue is which system to use.

Corollary to the above axiom, research shows that presenting information bimodally (i.e., in speech and sign) improves understanding (Brooks, Hudson & Reisberg, 1981). Regardless of what manual system is used to supplement speech, the deaf child or adult understands more than when just speech is used.

Although it is hard to understand why, there are still people who advocate concealing lip movements and using no signs with deaf children in order that they may "hear" better (Gaeth, 1966; Gates, 1970).

Broadly categorized, there are four basic options to choose from in selecting a sign system. Two of these appear to have obvious flaws and will be discussed briefly. More attention will be devoted to the issues in selecting between a composite of American Sign Language (ASL), Pidgin Sign and Signed English versus forms of Manual English, including artificial signed systems (Seeing Exact English and Seeing Essential English).

Cued speech is a set of 12 hand positions designed to make clear the differences between sounds that look alike when formed on the lips (Cornett, 1967). For example, *b* and *p* as in *bad* and *pad* look alike on the lips. Therefore, when one of these sounds is spoken, a hand position or sign is made by the speaker to clarify whether the lip movement means *p* or *b*.

This system is deficient for several reasons. First, it is totally dependent on lipreading (Cornett, 1967). If you can't lipread, the cues have no meaning. One cannot communicate unless one is close to and facing the speaker. Group discussions are difficult if not impossible.

Even more importantly, it is hard to synchronize the hand movement with the lip movement for each homophenous sound. For example, a small word such as *before* has two sounds, *b* and *f*, which require separate cues. For the speaker, synchronizing all of this is difficult. However, the major problem is that the deaf person has to process all of this information, to make complex associations and then interpret them in order to understand what is said. This is impossible for many deaf youth.

Deaf adults have so much difficulty with Cued Speech that they often refer to it somewhat obscenely as "screwed speech." It is extremely difficult to understand Cued Speech even after one has mastered English. It is an almost impossible technique to use in teaching English, especially to a baby who simply cannot possibly make the perceptions and cognitive processes required in reading Cued Speech. Many parents and deaf children who start out with Cues later change to American Sign Language.

Fingerspelling every word that is spoken is possible. When this is done, the process is called the Rochester Method. It has many problems which combine to make it unsatisfactory. First, it is slow and tedious for both the "speaker" and the "listener." This is a major defect. People's speech when using the Rochester Method sounds as if it were tape recorded and played at half speed. In addition, fingerspelling is hard to read because it is small, executed quickly and some hand positions are difficult to distinguish from each other.

Educationally, the major disadvantage of fingerspelling is that it is actually reading. Cognitively, reading words fingerspelled on the hand is an even more complex task than reading print (Vernon & Coley, 1978). This being the case, fingerspelling is obviously an unsatisfactory way to teach English to a preschool child or infant. How many deaf preschool children can read, especially if they do not know English?

Another disadvantage of fingerspelling is that it makes the expression of human feelings extremely difficult. In parent-child relationships, this is a major deficit. The advantage of the Rochester Method is that it is English. Thus, as contrasted to many other systems, it provides relatively clear, exact English vocabulary and syntax. Fingerspelling, incidentally, is a basic part of the next two signed systems to be discussed.

When considering a choice among sign language systems, several key premises are basic. The first is that sign languages of deaf people developed as they did for some sound logical reasons (Armstrong, 1984; Armstrong and Katz, 1981; Kimura, 1981; and Woodward, 1985). These have to do with practical, functional factors. For example, deaf people have developed signs that are easy to perceive visually. A sign language that was full of hard-to-see or invisible hand positions would make no sense. Similarly, the signs developed by deaf people are easy to form manually. For example, there are no signs that require touching the thumb of the right hand to the right forearm because this would be painful and slow.

The same two facts hold for spoken languages. Their sounds must be clearly distinguishable and reasonably easy to make. For this reason, we have no sounds in any language that are formed by touching the tongue to the nose.

These facts may seem so obvious that you may wonder why they are even mentioned. However, remember that it has taken hundreds of years for spoken languages to develop to where they are today (i.e., to the point at which they are relatively easy to pronounce, hear and understand). The same is true of the sign languages. It has taken centuries for them to evolve to their present advanced state in which they are simple to form on the hands and easy to read visually.

With this in mind, imagine the awesome problems posed by having to devise an entirely new language with new sounds and a new grammar. The result would be sounds and combinations of sounds people could not make or learn to understand. If this new language were taught to a group of infants who had never spoken, they might learn it. However, as time passed, they would change it in ways that made it easier to use. After several generations the language which had been created would be dramatically improved from the cumbersome nonfunctional original system into one that fit both the anatomy and motor mechanism of vocalization as well as the perceptual needs of the human auditory system. These improvements would occur because the development of a language or communication method is a slow, evolving process.

A similar evolution would take place in any artificially designed sign language. If we tried to invent a sign language, it would have hand positions difficult to make which would not flow from one sign to another gracefully. If it were used by deaf people for generations, it would be gradually changed and improved to the point of being almost totally different from its original form.

There is another background fact of great relevance. Visual languages offer options that are not present in oral languages. Space can be used (e.g., to indicate who is speaking). One deaf child describing a television western to another in sign language might stand in one place to indicate the villain and in another to indicate the hero. This use of space denotes nouns and pronouns that is not possible in oral or written language.

Another example relates to word order. When describing a scene in American Sip Language, the tendency is to recreate the scene as it was perceived visually. The most vivid visual aspects would be signed first with mime, facial expression and body language having major linguistic functions that visually recreate the scene. This cannot be done in a spoken or written language.

Thus, visual langues develop a certain structure that is unique and markedly different from the structure of spoken and written languages.

A final background point to be made is that anytime a language is spoken and signed simultaneously, two things happen (Brooks, Hudson and Reisberg, 1981; Kluwin, 1983). One is that speech tends to slow down. The second is that parts of what is spoken are left out of what is said manually. For example, in speech you might say, "British Columbia is a beautiful area" and sign "British Columbia, beautiful." In this particular example, the main concept would be communicated (i.e., the beauty of British Columbia), but the full vocabulary and syntax of the spoken English would not. Often when speaking and signing at the same time even the concept is not always communicated or else is inadequately conveyed (Kluwin, 1983). Thus, although deaf persons get more information than would be obtained by speech and lipreading alone, they are not provided the complete English vocabulary and syntax. Nor do they always get the complete meaning of what is said. This is obviously a serious problem. At the same time, far more information is conveyed than is the case with oral only communication (Brooks, Hudson and Risberg, 1981).

Given this background data, let's now consider the two major categories of sign systems used in Total Communication.

Total Communication was adopted by most educational programs in the United States and by many in Canada, Britain, Isreal and all over the world once research demonstrated the inadequacy of speechreading as a means of receptive communication for deaf children and adults (Jordan, 1982; Jordan, Gustason and Rosen, 1979). However, instead of using the existing sign language systems of the deaf people of these respective countries, a number of educators invented sign systems that followed English grammar and vocabulary exactly (Barnum, 1984). In Canada and the United States, several different manual English systems were devised (e.g., Seeing Exact English [SEE] and Seeing Essential English [SEE]). In Britain there is the Piaget-Gorman System.

The theory behind these systems is simple (i.e., if a child sees English and nothing else he will learn English). Thus, by signing English, speaking English and writing English to a deaf child the child will master English in about the same way as a hearing child does.

There are serious problems with the implementation of the theory that may make it unworkable. First, in these manual English systems the hand positions and the movements needed to go from one sign to the other are essentially arbitrary. They did not evolve by being used for generations. Thus, they are difficult to execute and to read (Armstrong, 1984; Armstrong and Katz, 1981; Kimura, 1981; and Kluwin, 1983). For example, in ASL, anytime two hands are used to form a sign they are either in the same position as in the sign "play" or else one hand is stationary and the other hand moves (e.g., the sign "duty"). The manual English systems tend to ignore this rule. Thus, their signs are hard to execute motorically and are difficult to read.

Even more importantly, because manual English systems use a grammar and vocabulary designed for a spoken language, not for a visual language, their basic structure is ill-suited to their modality. It is a little like trying to write American Sign Language. It has been done, but it is so laborious and unsatisfactory nobody uses it.

By contrast, American Sign Language evolved over many years as a visual language. Its structure is ideally suited to sight and to the motor and visual functions of human beings. The antithesis is true of manual English systems. Thus, deaf children taught artificial manual English systems such as SEE tend to change them into versions more similar in structure and form to ASL. Teachers and parents find the artificial manual English systems awkward, slow and lacking in expressiveness.

Limited research shows that these systems tend to be used in abbreviated telegraphic form by teachers, parents and children (Kluwin, 1983; Bernstein and Saulnier, 1981). When this happens, the entire theory falls apart because what is presented to deaf children and received from them is not English.

One further clarification needs to be made about manual English as used in this paper. It includes manual systems such as SEE that invent totally new signs or use signs from ASL in strange or modified ways.

American Sign Language (ASL) is the form of sign language developed by deaf people in Canada and the United States over a period of several centuries. It is a totally visual language which has evolved into its present grammar and hand configurations because generations of deaf people through trial and error have found these to be the best (i.e., they are the easiest to form and to read). Fingerspelling is incorporated into ASL to express concepts for which there are no signs. Hence when people use ASL they sign primarily and fingerspell some.

There is no question that ASL is by far the best of the manual systems we are discussing for visual communication (Rodda, 1986, in press). The problems it poses educationally is that its syntax is different from English. If deaf children learn ASL, they may be taught mathematics, social studies, science, etc., in this language, but they will not learn English unless it is specifically taught to them.

When a hearing teacher or parents tries to use ASL and speech in a Total Communication program, two things generally happen (Bernstein, Maxwell, and Mathews, 1985; Ertig, 1985; and Kluwin, 1983). One is that they tend to change the ASL into a grammar more similar to that of Engush. This is called Pidgin Sign Language. For example, instead of saying "Me home," the ASL form of the concept, the teacher or parent might sign "I go home" and say " I am going home."

Another option which uses ASL as a frame of reference is Signed English. In Signed English "markers" are added to existing ASL signs. A marker, and there are 14 of them in Signed English, is a sign added to a sign in order to make it conform to English syntax (Bornstein, 1982). For example, to change "play" to "playing" the sign for "play" is made to which is added a second sign for "ing."

Another problem that exists almost anytime a person signs and talks at the same time, as is done in Total Communication, is that part of what they are saying orally is left out in what they sign (Ertig, 1985; and Kluwin, 1983). This occurs regardless of what sign system is used whether it be ASL, SEE, LOVE, fingspelling, Cued Speech, etc. This means that the deaf person is not only shortchanged in terms of information but also in linguistic quality and quantity.

Deaf people in oral English-speaking environment are going to be short-changed relative to communication. This is reality. It is inherent in deafness just as illness is inherent in being a mortal human. In both instances, the realistic goal is to minimize, not eliminate, the problem. For the deaf child we have two primary communicative goals. First is to maximize the information they are able to get through communication. Second is to increase their English competence.

It is obvious from what has been presented thus far and from extensive research that the least effective way to do this is by using speech and lipreadirig (oralism) only (Vernon, 1972).

The problems posed by fingerspelling and Cued Speech as a form of Total Communication show that while they are superior to just speech and lipreading (oralism), they are far less effective than Signed English, Pidgin Sign Language or ASL. The manual system most effetive in a Total Communication program is a combination of ASL, Pidgin Sign, and a few markers from Signed English used with speech and lipreading.

The rationale for using a combination of ASL and Pidgin Sign and a few markers from Signed English in Total Communication is complex. To my knowledge, no one has tried to develop this logic in a comprehensive way before.

Research data indicate that deaf children who know ASL well and were exposed to it early do the best in learning English and in terms of the amount of information and formal education they master through communication (Vernon, 1975). The findings on deaf children of deaf parents who learn ASL as children best illustrate this fact (Vernon, 1975).

A second rationale is that we know that almost any deaf child can master ASL and use it in life to learn and to communicate. Other than case history testimonials, this has not been demonstrated with signed or manual English systems (or with Cued Speech and fingerspelling). Thus, by using ASL we are not only guaranteeing a deaf child an effective communication system, we are also maximizing that child's chances of learning English. In fact, deaf children given the chance will be fluent in ASL by school age.

This leads to another point which is that once ASL is established a deaf child can be taught English using many of the existing approaches employed in bilingual education (Genesee, 1985). For example, ASL could be taught the first few years of school. Then English would be presented. This is analogous to what is being done in some classes with Spanish-speaking Mexican-American children. This has a strong appeal to sophisticated linguists, both hearing and deaf. However, it has never been tried nor has a program for its implementation been published (Quigley and Paul, 1984).

Another advantage of ASL is its affective quality. It uses facial expression and body language in ways that greatly facilitate the expression of emotion. This is important psychologically, and it facilitates learning. Manual English systems lack this affective dimension.

Finally, in using a proven visual language such as ASL (modified by Pidgin Sign Language and markers from Signed English) we know the language will effectively serve the purposes for which any language exists. With manual English systems, Signed English alone or Cued Speech, we lack this assurance.

A tangential factor that bears on the issue of using signs is the egocentricity and insensitivity of human beings to each other, or more specifically, hearing people's treatment of those who are deaf.

Sign language is the case in point. For years it was a repressed language. Deaf children were forbidden the right to use it and were punished if they did. There are many places in Canada and in the United States where this still happens (Jordan, Gustason and Rosen, 1979).

This repression of sign language is ironic because these same individuals demand sign language when they themselves are in settings where they cannot hear. In fact, hearing people use signs in all aspects of their life where they are precluded from using their hearing. This point is often overlooked. Thus, several examples will be given to illustrate iy.

In large sports stadiums where noise and distance preclude spectators from hearing the umpire or referee, these officials are required to use signs. In baseball, the umpire has signs for "safe", "strike," "ball," etc. In football, the officials use so many different signs that they have to print them in the program. What hearing people demand in these signs is that they be easy to read and quick and simple to make. Hearing people are not dependent on lip movements as with Cued Speech.

Another example occurs in orchestral music. The key person, the conductor, uses sign language because the musicians could not hear him if he spoke. His signs bear no relationship to English and are independent of lip movements.

Religion also exemplifies the issue. In medieval times, churches and temples were so large that all worshippers could not hear the minister, priest or rabbi. This problem was solved by inventing signs for basic concepts such as prayer, the cross and God. With microphones and amplification this is no longer necessary, although vestiges of the practice are still a part of certain masses. In some monastic groups where speech is forbidden sign language systems were devised and are used today.

When Navy frogmen work underwater, sign language is used. On deck when ships have to communicate with other ships, the sign language of semaphore is employed. We used to use signs when we drove a car and wanted to signal a turn. Indian and Hawaiian have developed an intricate sign language that narrates their dance because the audience could not hear them do this by speech. Even exotic dancers use signs, to be specific, bumps and grinds, to communicate concepts that could not be heard above the music or which might be censored. Certain hunting societies (aborigines in Australia and North American Indians), in which the use of speech would scare away the prey, invented sign languages for hunting.

The point to be made from these examples is that sign language is universal. Hearing people use it anytime they cannot hear or when speech is forbidden. In these circumstances hearng people demand a highly visible sign system that is easy to use and understand. They do not lip read or ask for cues added to lip movements, a restriction to fingerspelling or signs that are in complete English.

It is sadly ironic that for years deaf people, who, by virtue of their deafness, are not able to hear or speak, have been forbidden by hearing people to use signs. Even now, many hearing people who finally acknowledge the need of deaf children for some kind of sign system to support speech and lipreading are putting almost no priority on the visual quality of the sign language that is used (Armstrong, 1984). Instead, the emphasis is on its similarity to the language that the hearing people use.

Human egocentricity knows no bounds and is a major reason for man's inhumanity to man. When we select the sign system component to a Total Communication program, the primary priority should be its quality as a visual language.

Signing Exact English

Gerilee Gustason

Six years ago, in January 1969, a group consisting of deaf individuals, parents of deaf children, teachers of the deaf, interpreters, and children of deaf parents met in southern California to form the nucleus of the first organized venture in Seeing Essential English. From this group developed three published manual English systems: Seeing Essential English, now headed by David Anthony at the University of Northern Colorado in Greeley; Linguistics of Visual English, spearheaded by Dennis Wampler in Santa Rosa, California; and Signing Exact English.

The main concern of the original group was the consistent, logical, rational, and practical development of signs to represent as specifically as possible the basic essentials of the English language. This concern sprang from the experience of all present with the poor English skills of many deaf students, and the desire for an easier, more successful way of developing mastery of English in a far greater number of such students. An average reading level of graduates from schools for the deaf hovering around the fourth grade and the functional illiteracy of roughly one-third of the adult deaf population, as well as personal experience teaching English at various levels from elementary school through college, indicated that whatever had been done in the past with English had not been sufficiently effective.

Language studies of hearing children had brought to light some sobering facts: these children had mastered a great deal of the structure of English, including basic sentence patterns and inflections, by the age of three; their language was fairly stable by age six, and language habits were extremely difficult to modify after the age

of puberty. Children learned the language of their environment, whether that language was Chinese or French or standard English or nonstandard English. Deaf children, on the other hand, wrote simpler, more rigid sentences, used far fewer auxiliaries, and tended to be much stronger in the dictionary meanings of words than in deriving meaning from context or sentence structure. The message was clear: deaf children had to be exposed as young as possible to English if we wanted them to learn it well, and since input must precede output we had to be sure that their perception of the language was as unclouded as possible.

Since 40 to 60 per cent of the sounds of English look like some other sound on the lips, speechreading alone was rejected as an incomplete presentation of English. Fingerspelling alone was also rejected, as harder to perceive than the gross movements of signs would be for a very young child. Since everyone in the group was a member in some way of the deaf community, and familiar with sign language, this mode of communication was easy to accept. But signs as they were then generally used were incomplete English. There were no verb tenses, no word endings such as *-ment* and *-ness,* and while some signs represented several English words (such as *begin* and *start*), some English words could take several different signs (such as *right*).

Accordingly, the group developed a set of principles which are basic to an understanding of all three systems. The most important principle was: **English should be signed as it is spoken for the deaf child to have linguistic input that would result in his mastery of English.** This meant, for instance, that idioms such as "dry up" and "cut it out" would be signed as those exact words, rather than as "quiet" or "stop" or "finish." A second principle was that **a sign would be translated to only one English equivalent.** The use of initialized signs came into play here, providing synonyms such as *hurt, pain, ache* and so on. But this also meant that a common sign had to be found for English words such as *run* or *bear*, which had various sign translations. These two principles, an attempt to provide a visual mode of representing English, led to a number of problems and jokes. How did one sign "I *saw* you yesterday?" Or "I *left* home yesterday?" Or *right, rite,* and *write*? In an attempt to come to grips with these problems in a sensible way, more principles developed.

Words came to be considered in three groups: BASIC, COMPLEX, AND COMPOUND. Basic words meant words that can have no more taken away and still form a complete word: *girl, talk, the.* For these basic words, the three-point criteria of spelling, sound, and meaning evolved. According to this principle, if any two of these three factors were the same, the same sign would be used. Hence the same sign would be used for *run* in "The boy will run, the motor will run, your nose will run," and so on, since spelling and sound were the same. But a different sign would be used for *wind* in "the wind is blowing, I must wind my watch," since only spelling was the same.

Complex words were defined as basic words with the addition of an affix or inflection: *girls, talked.* Once such an inflection had been added to a word, the combination could not be used as a basic word. Accordingly, when the past tense was added to *leave* to make *left,* this was not the same as the basic word for the direction *left.*

Compound words were two or more basic words put together, and were the source of many jokes and misunderstandings. The rule was that if the meaning of the words separately was consistent with the meaning of words together, then and only then would they be signed as the component words. Thus *underline* would be signed as *under-line,* but *understand* having no relation to the meanings of the words *under* and *stand,* would NOT be signed *under-stand.*

Within the framework of these basic rules, sign development proceeded. When an existing sign was clear and unambiguous, with only one English translation (*girl, home, know,* etc.), it was retained. Many common English words had either no signs or ambiguous signs *(salad, adult, car,* etc.). Many signs were developed for affixes.

In the course of this sign development, however, disagreements occurred within the group over the extent of departure from traditional signs. Accordingly, the one original group split into three distinct groups. Signing Exact English attempts to stay as close as possible to traditional signs while following the principles outlined above. We hold that manual English is easier for hearing parents and teachers to learn (as opposed to Ameslan, which is a foreign language to them), closer to the language which they speak in their daily lives, and so more likely to be naturally used and accepted by these persons. We also believe that if a deaf child is exposed to consistent, continuous English in his home and school environment in a visual form, he will develop English as comfortably and naturally as a hearing child does. An acceptance of manual English opens the way for parents to utilize total communication, including mime, gestures, Ameslan, speechreading, and aural amplification with their deaf child. We have found this type of sign system also helpful in teaching English to junior high, high school, and college deaf students, especially when coupled with English as a second language technique.

Our interest in and development of signs for the signing of English has led many concerned individuals to believe that we wish to eliminate Ameslan. This we in no way wish to do. We consider Ameslan a beautiful and expressive language, and are delighted with the increased study it is receiving both by linguists and in sign language classes. We encourage those who work with the adult deaf to learn Ameslan rather than

Signing Exact English or any other manual English system. Our goal is for deaf children to be truly bilingual, at ease in both Ameslan and English. Ideally, we would like to see teachers trained in both who could combine or otherwise utilize the two in and out of the classroom in a variety of ways to enrich the language experiences of the students. Manual English we see as a teaching tool, a means of manual expression for those who are speaking English, and an introduction to the richness and variety of signs for the parents of young deaf children.

To date we have published one book, *Signing Exact English,* and one supplement, with revision planned for the spring of 1975. These two books are sold by the National Association of the Deaf, and are used throughout the country and in a number of foreign countries. Workshops have been held in such places as California, Alaska, Montana, and Kansas. We do not have a count of the number of schools using this book, but approximately 1000 copies a month are being sold throughout the country.

Since the main thrust of this endeavor is in the teaching of English, it is hardly surprising that the chief users of this form of manual English are parents and teachers. We would like to see many more deaf adults familiarize themselves with the rationale and principles of Signing Exact English and with the vocabulary of new signs which has developed, so they can provide helpful input to parents and schools and make this form of manual English as compatible as possible with the richness and expressiveness of Ameslan. We want the best of both languages, Ameslan and English, in the hands of as many people as possible.

Seeing Essential English

David Anthony

For years, non-productive controversy has raged between advocates of the oral-only method and the nonexistent manualists. The latter term is gratuitously bestowed by the former as a scare tactic: if your child signs, he'll never talk! They may as well have suggested with straight faces that if he crawls he'll never walk. While there never have been purely manual schools, there are a few purely manual deaf individuals who are nevertheless not at all dumb—that is, they're neither mute nor stupid. The inescapable fact is that they're products of the oral method. This system perpetrates—and its few successful products perpetuate—the myth that **all** deaf children will presto! have the gift of speech. The many who do not are untenably classified "oral failures," untenably because it is the system rather than the deaf individual that has failed. It is the so-called oral deaf who, by their often strange vocal utterances, give rise and risibility to the term "deaf and dumb."

Opposed to the oralists are **not** the manualists but those realists who recognize the value of manual communication (i.e., signing and fingerspelling) as a supplement to and not a supplant of speech therapy and lipreading and auditory training. This side now banners Total Communication: use all and every possible means to educate a deaf child. Unfortunately, in not a few instances Total Communication has become but a license to sign. Many of the schools in this camp have, or used to have, purely oral methods of instruction in the elementary grades.

Usually, when a deaf child reaches or is socially promoted to the secondary level, parents and teachers give up the unequal oral battle and permit the child to do what he has been doing all along: sign! And they join him in speaking, or attempting to speak, "with hearts **and hands** and voices."

And who rejoices? Certainly the deaf child and the deaf community. But not so the profession at large. The *Babbidge Report*, though it predates the advent of Total Communication, indicts with a succinct sentence that holds true today: "The American people have no reason to be satisfied with their limited success in educating deaf children and preparing them for full participation in our society."

At heart is the general inability of the deaf to master the English language. With non-existent or defective hearing, the spoken word, the normal channel of English acquisition, is unheard or distorted: "Oh my goodness!" comes out "Oh buy good it!," and "Oh, be quiet!" becomes "Ho be try it!" With lipreading, the noble art of which is not all it's cracked up to be, only a small percentage of English speech is visible on the lips; only the key words are seen, and even then BED = MAD = BAD = PAD = MAT = BAT = PAT = MET = BET = PET, and TEACHER = SISTER, and MARRY = BURY, and VARIETY = FRIED EGG, and WHERE'S THE LAVENDER SOAP = WHERE THERE'S LIFE THERE'S HOPE, and BACK TO PHOENIX = BAKERSFIELD, and YOU SUFFER MUCH = YOU SON OF A BITCH, and MOTHER = BOTHER (Oh, Mother!). With fingerspelling alone (the Rochester Method), we are in the position of requiring a deaf infant to spell S C I S S 0 R S (how many college graduates can?) while the hearing baby can blithely lithp "thithurth." And of course we and the deaf child are easily fazed when asked D O E S T H E F I S H S O A R T O F I N D T H E O C E A N T H E E A G L E P L U N G E T O F I N D T H E A I R.

And signing? Ameslan (the *American Sign Language,* ASL; and for this paper pertinent only to the United States) has been a real force and a real success in educating the deaf—by the deaf themselves. It is this means, more out-of-school than in the classroom, that has enabled the American deaf to keep themselves up with American society as a whole, a phenomenon unsurpassed by any nation.

SEEING ESSENTIAL ENGLISH (SEE) was conceived in Denver in the spring of 1962 when I first came across mention of the system of Basic English in *Life* magazine. It gestated in the Deaf Research Project at Lapeer State Home and Training School, Michigan. It was delivered as *Signing Essential English,* the title of my master's paper, at Eastern Michigan University, Ypsilanti, in the summer of 1966. During its weaning period in California educators there, fearful of any mention of signing, suggested a name change. Thus SEEING ESSENTIAL ENGLISH: In keeping with my whimsy that the SEE acronym be retained.

SEE started creeping and crawling in Denver at two symposia, fall 1970 and spring 1971, attended by interested persons from the Community College of Denver, Colorado State University, Denver University, University of Colorado, University of Northern Colorado and the deaf community. It took its first faltering steps with the publication of the *SEEING ESSENTIAL ENGLISH Manual,* January 1972. It is fed a steady diet by the *SEEING ESSENTIAL ENGLISH Report,* an occasional paper that makes corrections and changes to signs published in the *Manual,* disseminates new signs developed since the publication of the *Manual,* and serves as a forum for news, views, criticisms, suggestions, brick-bats, and bouquets.

Today, SEE is a lusty two-year-old, going on three, that has been taken to many places across the nation and found to be well-liked. Its favorite place after Colorado is Iowa, though it is at home anywhere English is spoken.

SEE is the offspring of a marriage (shot-gun, perhaps) between the necessity of the English language and the utility of the sign language. Sometimes considered an Ugly Duckling by the less discerning, the more perspicacious see it taking on the beauty of both parents.

SEEING ESSENTIAL ENGLISH is the child of my belief that it is quite possible for deaf children to acquire English manually. That many people share this belief is evident in the number of new manual English systems that have sprung up **since** SEE became known, including a rival using the same acronym. With the emergence of SEE has also developed a burgeoning interest in Ameslan.

One sad fact about the appearance of SEE is that it has somewhat polarized both educators of the deaf and the deaf community into an outbreak of factions, jack-straw fashion. Consider:

- Gregg M. Brooks writes in *The Deaf Western* (November 1974): "This (the deaf acquiring English) cannot be done." Period! One has to admire Mr. Brooks' courage in coming right out with a statement that has to be subscribed to *sotto voce* by countless teachers and administrators. Ameslan is the way, the only way.

- *Signs for our times* (November 1974) reports a professional group's conclusion that "codes that purport to represent English (as SEE does) completely and accurately (SEE does not so claim) morpheme-by-morpheme need to be taken with a grain of salt." It offers no alternative other than, presumably, the, hmm, idea that the, you know, language of the deaf, er, deserves to be preserved as an, ah, interesting object of study, you know, er, esoterica.

- A linguist, circulating a paper with the request that it not be used or quoted without the author's permission, from a lofty perch pontificates on why the various manual English systems, including SEE particularly, are likely to disappoint adherents. Included were attributions to SEE that were non-SEE! No practical alternatives were offered.

- An administrator of a residential school for the deaf circulates a position paper saying that SEE cannot be accepted at the school in question because, *inter alia,* it is not the common language of the deaf. This decision was reached following one early SEE workshop.
- A superintendent of a school for the deaf indicates his willingness to testify in Court that SEE is detrimental to the education of deaf children. In his school, many of the SEE signs are in use.
- A PhD in a university counters my protest that SEEING ESSENTIAL ENGLISH and "Signing Exact English" should not be confused (I wanted credit for SEE since the latter is a copy of the former) with the specious argument that one is distinguished from the other by the use of periods: S.E.E.; SEE; see?

Amid all the havering and palavering is a multiplying interest in Ameslan and other forms of manual communication, including SEE, in our schools, colleges, universities, church groups, social and rehabilitation agencies, and parent organizations. This is all to the good. The more the public sees of signs, no matter the system, the less of a novelty will signs be. And the more the deaf will be recognized as a group.

People have asked if there will be a Tower of Babel situation in the deaf community when Ameslan users and users of other sign systems meet. Certainly! I And of course not! Such a situation has been prevalent even before SEE. In schools for the deaf on the Atlantic and Pacific seaboards, there are dialects of Ameslan. In every oral school, protestations to the contrary, a sign system exists and has existed. When Ameslan users, east and west, and products of the various

oral schools meet, as at national sporting events or the first week of fall at Gallaudet College, there's confusion. This confusion is always resolved by Ameslan and the more acceptable signs hold sway.

Today we see many new signs, mostly from SEE but often from elsewhere, taking root in Ameslan. We also see many deaf people, without benefit of classroom instruction, picking up SEE endings naturally, -ING, -S, -ED, -MENT, and so on. Through it all, we see one sign system accepting and adopting signs developed by another. And SEE itself has discarded some of its contrived signs in favor of some others.

The first thing that everyone has to get clear in his mind is that SEE is not, never was, a panacea but a possibility. As a possibility, it is the best so far and by far (if I do say so myself).

It has spurred interest in the acquisition of English by the deaf and in the idea of manual communication as a teaching tool. Other groups with the same goals in mind have started on different and more difficult tracks. Many have confused the use of SEE with the teaching of English to the deaf. SEE does not **teach** English; English (or any language) is not easily taught. SEE is an attempt to sign English, to **give** English, to make signs compatible with the English language as far as possible and as far as is practicable and practical.

Many manual English systems, conceding the cliche that English is the most difficult of all languages, underrate the intelligence of the deaf everywhere with the assertion that having one sign for one word (RIGHT as the opposite of *left*, RIGHT as the opposite of *wrong*, and RIGHT as in *all right*; BOX as in *fisticuffs* and BOX the gloves go in; this BEAR can't BEAR it!) is "too hard" for the deaf. Others suggest that, for example, signing BUTTER + FLY for "butterfly" will unhinge a deaf child but not a hearing one. Still another advises signing SICK + CAR for "ambulance."

SEE, on the other hand, insists that the deaf child is just as able as a hearing child to grasp the concept of a word from the context of English. And, what do you know? he is!

SEE is the only system that takes into consideration *both* English and Sign. An example (the only one, of many, to be discussed here) of the lack of consideration developers of new systems give to Amselan is the sign for the word THE—a most vital word in the English language. There is no sign for THE in Ameslan.

Deaf Americans have long used the palm-down Y handshape to show something definite, as a forceful downward stroke to say, "That's it!," or an up-and-down motion to suggest "Oh, I see." This last phrase can run the gamut from genuine-dawning-awareness to sarcasm through appropriate facial expression and speed of the arm movement.

In SEE, since we have embraced the one-word-one-sign-no-matter-the-meaning-of-the-word idea, we have signs for THAT and 'S and IT, and for OH and I and SEE. We took the palm-down Y handshape with a forceful downstroke to sign THE, the definite article. Emphatically placing this Y handshape on the palm of the other hand gives us THIS; extending the index finger of the Y handshape, thereby executing the ⅄ handshape (popularly known as the "I love you" handshape), and emphatically placing this ⅄ handshape on the palm of the other hand gives us THAT; sweeping the Y and the ⅄ handshapes from left to right across the palm of the other hand gives us THESE and THOSE respectively. Thus, the definite article and the demonstrative pronouns, vital words of English, have allied and yet discrete signs.

Now, in Ameslan, by raising a fist and twisting it out-and upward we say STRIKE or generally give the concept of REVOLT or DISOBEY. In certain new systems, THE is signed with the T handshape undergoing the STRIKE/REVOLT/DISOBEY movement—a wholly incongruous sign when Ameslan is to be considered. Furthermore, in many new systems the signs for THE, THIS, THAT, THESE, and THOSE are disparate from each other.

Why is this? Perhaps it is because practically all these other new sign systems are headed by hearing and/or deafened persons, whereas SEE is under the direction of a born deaf person.

Deafened persons are those who are postlingually deaf. They are hearing persons with deaf ears. Along with hearing people, their first language is English. They learned Ameslan from other deaf kids and adults. To their never-uttered but always apparent way of thinking, since the learning of Ameslan was so easy the learning of English must be equally easy. Hah!

They learned English, not in the classroom but in the home and in society, their everyday life. They learned Ameslan, not in the classroom but in the dorm-home and in the closed society of a residential school milieu, their everyday life. "Learned" is a misnomer here; they "picked up," or "acquired;" effortlessly.

What of the born deaf, the prelingually deaf? They come to a residential school, no matter at what age. If children of deaf Ameslan parents, a minuscule minority, they quickly fit in the Ameslan society and are bright and leaders. If children of hearing parents, the vast majority in this category, they soon pick up Ameslan from other children despite, in most cases, strictures and punishment on one side for signing—and on the other side the inability of their teachers and counselors and parents to communicate in Ameslan. Their English is confined to the classroom only. Thus, they pick up Ameslan effortlessly and look on English with real distaste.

By and large at school the prelingual deaf are up front where it counts with the best of the postlingual deaf in math and PE and voc. shop, but they fall farther and farther back academically (not really academically but "Englishically") and see their postlingual deaf peers spurting ahead painlessly.

Out of school and into adult life we see an unwitting (or is it?) collusion between the postlingual deaf and the hearing-who-work-with-or-for-the-deaf that extends into every facet of deaf life. In practically every deaf or deaf-related sphere of activity, the deaf person in a leadership or administrative capacity is a deafened one.

This is not a tirade against the deafened—the big fishes in small ponds, thank God for them!—but a pointer, a poser: What put them there? The one simple and clear answer: their English.

English in the classroom for the born deaf is a foreign language. Even in deaf education circles today some are embracing the idea of English as a second language. English will never be a second language unless it is in constant use.

Of the thousands of hearing students who have studied a foreign language in high school or college, how many are or become fluent in that language? Similarly, of the hundreds of prelingual deaf students who have studied English to death in pre, primary, elementary, middle, secondary, junior high, high, and prep schools and college, how many are fluent in English? Come on, how many?

Oh, yes, a few do manage: "David has good English, you know," followed by that damning palliative, "for a deaf person."

For the deafened and the hearing, Ameslan is a second language. Even while communicating in Ameslan (or very often in what they think is Ameslan) they are thinking in English. The more superior of them are able to watch an Ameslan presentation and mentally translate the whole thing into English. In reverse, they are able to present their own English-originated in Ameslan. Their bilingual ability comes from constant usage of both languages.

They are the people who do not need to acquire English (since, patently, they already have it) through SEE or some other new means. Many have an attitude that is condescending, patronizing, paternalistic towards the born deaf: "Worry not; English hard, you can't, me know; I for you help interpret will; OK." Some, conceding "true fact English important yes," suggest that to "improve English must read read read dictionary dictionary dictionary." (I tried to read read read

Spanish comics and Spanish children's books and Spanish dictionary dictionary dictionary—no, not a Spanish/English dictionary, a Spanish dictionary—to no avail. Me dumb?) Not a few of these people get their jollies from caricaturizing new sign systems but froth at the mouth when Ameslan is caricaturized!

Some have suggested that Ameslan is the **natural** language of the deaf. If this were so, then deaf people the world over would have a universal sign language. That they do not points to a linguistic truth: a language may be **native**, but it is never **natural**. A language does not come automatically with or at birth. All languages are contrived, and they are **acquired** and change through usage and usage alone. The **capacity** to acquire a language or languages, be it English or Ameslan or whatever or both or more, is inherent in each person, deaf or otherwise.

It is often claimed that SEE is harder and more confusing for the deaf child and his hearing parents, for the deaf adult and his hearing friends than the more common Ameslan. This is putting theory in place of fact. It has proven otherwise in practice. Whether deaf children acquire fluency in English via SEE remains to be seen, however.

Controversies such as the one between Ameslan and SEE, and internecinally among these two and other systems, do naturally make parents, teachers, and administrators apprehensive and pause. Resistance to change is natural. The proposals and techniques of SEE upset long-standing assumptions, deep-rooted habits, and possibly some vested interests.

SEE isn't perfect; it's a start. It is incumbent upon detractors and upon our hearing and deafened bilinguals in Ameslan-English to find out how and why SEE works; to find out if it can be bettered or if there is a better way; not to dissimulate reasons why it cannot, or is not supposed to, work!

In the current, if inelegant, catch-phrase, "Let's get with it!"

An Historical Sketch of the Manual Alphabets

Edward R. Abernathy

Manual communication takes two general forms which should be distinguished: one is by signs or manual motions to designate words or phrases; the other is the use of a manual alphabet for representation on the hand of letters of the alphabet and numerals. Signs do not depend on written language and indeed can be used between those who do not understand the written or spoken language of the other. The American Indians with many dialects used sign to communicate between tribes. Crude signs or gestures are of primitive origin and may well have preceded vocalization. As distinguished from these, the conventionalized signs of the deaf did not become established in use until the latter half of the 18th century and hence came after manual alphabets were in use as teaching-devices for the deaf. While some of the conventionalized signs of the deaf employ a manual letter in combination with a sign of exactness (such as "W" on the lips for water as distinguished from "V" on the lips for vinegar) generally signs are not dependent on written language. There are numerous experiences among the deaf of communicating through signs with foreign deaf persons where neither individual understood the written language of the other. By contrast, finger spelling is the spelling by individual letters, and, hence identified with a specific language.

Finger spelling or dactylology, is of uncertain but ancient origin. Best (1) states: "Such people as the Egyptians, Hebrews, Greeks, Romans, and others, seem to have made use of a finger notation or symbolization. Persons in enforced silence, notably monks of the Middle Ages, and to a less extent in later times, often resorted to some such

practice. Illustrations of the manual alphabet go back fairly far in the Christian era, most of the single-handed variety. Late in the seventh century the Venerable Bede . . . showed himself to be acquainted with the device, and refers (in *De Loquela per Gestum Digitorum*) to three different forms which were in existence before his time. In Latin Bibles of the tenth century pictures of dactylology are to be seen. Systems somewhat on the order of those now in use appear in the sixteenth century. In 1546 there appeared a brief work on the subject, with examples, called *Chiromantia*. It seems to have been Italy where these things largely emanated."

In a voluminous work on the dactylology of the ancients, Barrois (2) formulated a Prehellenic one-hand alphabet based on his highly fanciful interpretation of the position of the fingers in ancient statues, paintings and similar works. Much of his interpretation is based on imaginary Greek equivalents. He derives the letter U from the extended index and little fings, so in a bronze of Selenus from Herculaneum he imagines this to be Upsilon, standing for "hypnos" (sleep) and "hypar" (a vision); the statue of Apollo Belvedere shows the same formation which he interprets as "hybris" (wanton force); to be consistent he again interprets this formation as "hybris" in a fresco polychrome of St. Savin, of the 11th century. In the four armed god of ancient India, Vishnu, he sees two hands each with thumb to fourth finger as forming Mu or M (for the Greek "mater"); an open hand as Pi or P (for the Greek "pater"). Similarly, he interprets as a P the outstretched open hand of a figure of Pertinax, conveniently giving the initial of his name. By such Barrois derives an alphabet. He regards dactylology as the basis of Chinese writing, and in an ancient Phoenician papyrus he likens the characters to formations by the fingers. These absurdities are compounded with interpretations in Greek of Assyrian, Egyptian, ancient Mexican figures and continuing to an illustration in a French publication of 1686. While his imaginative alphabet is not to be credited, his work does raise a question as to the meanings intended by stylized but unusual finger formations found in ancient statues, vase paintings, bas-reliefs and the like. Barrois includes a plate of a 9th century bas-relief, "The Power of Charlemagne" wherein there are three arches, in each of which a hand is depicted giving some sort of finger spelling. Barrois observes (3) that some of the tombs or cenotaphs in the most ancient churches in Paris show effigies using the sign language.

A. Farrar (4) observes that "The earliest finger alphabets extant appear to have been founded on manual signs for numbers, as may be seen in the first chapter of Bede's *De Temporum Ratione* where a 'manual speech' is described. There is evidence that these manual alphabets were in common use in the Middle Ages for purposes of secret or silent intercourse."

It appears certain that some form of manual communication dating back over a thousand years came down through the Middle Ages, quite likely through religious orders under vows of silence and by those who desired secret or silent communication. It does not appear that any manual alphabet was used in instructing the deaf in that period. Farrar (5) notes that Jerome Cardan (1501-1576), an Italian mathematician and physician, urged the importance of teaching the deaf to read and write explaining ideas by the use of signs. Farrar (6) also states that there is no evidence of the use of a manual alphabet by the first regular instructor of the deaf, Pedro Ponce de Leon (1520?-1584), though apparently, he did use signs. Pedro Ponce de Leon, scion of the noble house of Arcos, is said to have been a native of Valladolid, Spain. Educated at the University of Salamanca, he joined the Benedictines and spent most of his life in their monastery at Oña. Hodgson (7) comments that "possibly the monk remote in his monastery at Oña never heard of this technique (of a manual alphabet) but was on the other hand used to to conventionalized signs for certain purposes within the community."

In 1579 Rossellio (8) in his *Thesaurus Artificiosae Memoriae* showed one-hand forms for the alphabet. For a majority of the letters he gave three forms presumably for three different alphabets, but for S, T, and V he gave two forms, and for X only one. No forms were given for J, K, R, U, W, Y, or Z. He also pictured a common device for manually indicating letters and figures by pointing to various parts of the body. We find both devices at later dates and, indeed, a combination of these (by pointing with the right hand to designated parts of the left hand). Pointing to parts of the body, for letters was grotesque and awkward, so gradually this gave way to more practical manual alphabet. Some of Rossellio's rather crudely drawn one-hand forms show similarity with present day forms for B, F, I, L, M, O, P, Q, and X.

The great contribution to the one-hand alphabet is that of Juan Pablo Bonet (d. 1629?). His *Reduccion de las Letras y arte para Enseñar a Ablar los Mudos* (simplification of the letters and the art of teaching deaf-mutes to speak) was published in Madrid in 1620. This is the earliest work extant on the education of the deaf. In Book II, Chapter III, he gives the "*Abecedario Demonstrativo*" (9), beautifully engraved reproductions of a one-hand alphabet. With some minor modifications this Spanish alphabet is the one widely used today in the United States and continental Europe. By comparison many of the letters are identical, a few similar and only D and R show marked differences. There is no J, as I was used instead, V and U are the same, and there is no K or W in Spanish. In the historical sketch given by Farrar (10) it is stated that of Bonet little is known. He was born in Jaca in Aragon in the latter part of the 16th century and filled various offices of state including that of secretary to the Constable of Castile. Farrar continues: "He was a man of the world rather than a cloistered teacher like Ponce de Leon, and, as a matter of fact, there is scarcely any evidence that teaching the deaf was at any time his vocation. Bonet, in the preface to his work, states that he was moved to write it from gratitude to the family of his master the Constable of Castile, who had a brother, Luis de Velasco, who lost his hearing at the age of two, and was made Marquis of Fresno by Philip IV in 1628. But he nowhere says anything of having educated this nobleman; on the contrary, we learn from other sources that this was done by Manuel Ramirez de Carrion, who was also tutor and secretary to another deaf-mute, the, Marquis of Priego. Ramirez de Carrion, in a work published in 1629 on another subject, himself states that he 'was occupied with the education of Luis de Velasco for four years, and though broken by such long intervals, that it hardly left three full years, I taught him to read, write, speak, and converse with such success, that he felt no other deficiency than that of hearing'. From his position in the Constable's household, Bonet must have been acquainted with Ramirez de Carrion; it is therefore the more remarkable that neither refers to the other in any way. All that can certainly be said on the point is that, whether or not Bonet had any share in Luis de Velasco's education, he has in his book described the method pursued."

Commenting on this, Harvey Peet (11), said "Bonet does not claim the merit of originating the widely used manual alphabet. . . . We are even left in doubt whether the alphabet given by himself which, as we have seen, differs essentially from those known to have been used by the ancients, was his own invention, or adopted by him, ready-made."

Incidentally, Bonet recommended that the alphabet be used to converse with a deaf person and not by other signs which would be less beneficial and the deaf person should reply by word of mouth. Bonet advocated the manual alphabet as a device in teaching speech.

Bonet (12), cited an older method of using parts of the body for letters, saying ". . . in antiquity it was considered the right thing to do to know how to use the demonstrations of the hands and other parts of the body in order to signify letters and figures. According to what Juan Bautista Porta (13), writes in his book *De Furtivis literarum*, bringing many examples they employed by hand and also demonstrations of many parts of the body that were touched to signify the letters, intending the

A. Auris—las orejas (ears)
B. Barba—la barba (chin)
C. Caput—la cabeça (head)
D. Dentes—los dientes (teeth)
E. Epar—el higado (liver)
F. Frontem—la frente (forehead)
G. Gutar—la garganta (throat)
H. Humeros—los ombros (shoulders)
I. Ilia—la hijada (cavity—small of the back)
L. Linguam—la lengua (tongue)
M. Manu—la mano (hand)
N. Nasum—la nariz (nose)
O. Oculos—los ojos (eyes)
P. Palatum—el paladar (palate)
Q. Quinquedigitos—los cinco dedos (the five fingers)
R. Renes—los riñones (kidneys)
S. Supercilia—sobre las cejas (eyebrows)
T. Tempora—el espacio de las sienes (temples)
V. Ventrem—la barriga (stomach)

Bonet notes that K, X, and Z were not used in the Latin language.

The Spanish alphabet was introduced into France by Jacob Rodriques Pereire (1715-1780), the first important teacher of the deaf in that country (14). Born at Berlanga in Spanish Estremadura, he belonged to a family of Spanish Jews who were driven through persecution to Portugal and then to Bordeaux, settling there in 1741. Pereire had a deaf sister whom he undertook to teach. Later—he instructed other deaf pupils. In 1749 he brought one of his pupils before the French Academy of Sciences in Paris. A commission appointed by the Academy to report on the value of Pereire's methods commented on the use of the manual alphabet. Subsequently, Pereire achieved even wider recognition. He kept his methods secret but through his most outstanding pupil, Saboureaux de Fontenay who also became a teacher of the deaf, we can gain some knowledge of Pereire's methods. The most distinctive feature was the use of Spanish manual alphabet which he enlarged and augmented to conform to French pronunciation and orthography. He used it as a means of teaching speech (as Bonet advocated).

Up until this time education of the deaf had been for the privileged few. Charles-Michel de l'Epée (1712-1789) was the founder of the first French school for the deaf irrespective of their social condition (15). He undertook the instruction of two deaf sisters in 1760. Later the school he founded and contributed to from his own private income, became in 1791 the National Institution at Paris. The Abbé de l'Epée was acquainted with the system employed by Pereire and used the manual alphabet in instruction (chiefly as a vehicle for the development of methodical signs rather than speech). Roch-Ambroise-Cucurron Sicard (1742-1822) became the head of the school in Paris after the death of the Abbé de l'Epée. The Abbé Sicard continued the use of the one-hand alphabet in conjunction with methodical signs. The manual alphabet employed by Sicard (16), was, with only slight differences, the same as that used in the United States today. It was brought to this country by Thomas Hopkins Gallaudet (1787-1851). In 1815, through a subscription of funds Gallaudet was sent to Europe for the purpose of qualifying himself to become an instructor of the deaf. He first went to London but due to a narrow monopolizing spirit he was rebuffed at the London Asylum. He next went to Edinburgh but the institution there was under obligation not to instruct teachers for a period of years. He had met Sicard in London and had been invited to Paris. So Gallaudet turned to Paris and the French system of instruction. He returned to the United States in August, 1816 bringing with him Laurent Clerc, a deaf teacher from Paris who had been, incidentally, an outstanding pupil under Abbé Sicard. Thus were signs and the Spanish manual alphabet brought to America. The American School for the Deaf, as it is now called, was opened at Hartford, Connecticut, on April 15, 1817—the first permanent school for the deaf in the United States. Dr. Gallaudet was the first head of this school and served in that capacity for fourteen years.

In Great Britain manual communication developed into a two-hand alphabet and remains as such today. After Bede, the earliest reference by any English writer to a manual alphabet was by John Bulwer, a physician. In 1644 he published in London, the *Chirologia or the Natural Language of the Hand Composed of the Speaking Motions, and Discoursing Gestures thereof whereunto is added Chironomia or the Art of Manuall Retoricke*. Therein he relates how a deaf man, one Master Babington of Burntwood could converse with his wife at night by means of an alphabet contrived on the joints of his fingers. In this work Bulwer shows six manual alphabets (J and U are omitted) which are mixtures of one and two-hand forms but showing little relationship to the two-hand alphabet that eventually became established in Great Britain.

Dr. George Dalgarno (1626?-1687) of Scotland was the first English writer to advocate a manual alphabet for the deaf. In 1680 be published *Didascalocophus, or the Deaf and Dumb Man's Tutor*. Although he mentioned and rejected a two-hand alphabet somewhat similiar to the one commonly used in Great Britain today, he advocated an alphabet he devised. This latter, had letter points assigned to one-hand which were designated by touching with the thumb or finger of the other. The vowels were on the ends of the fingers (A on the tip of the thumb, E on the tip of the index finger, etc.) which is characteristic of the present two-hand alphabet. But unlike the present day alphabet the remaining letters were located by pointing to the phalanges of the fingers and the palm of the hand.

Critchley (17) cites the alphabets advocated by La Fin and Wilkins. In 1692 La Fin (18), one-time secretary to Cardinal Richelieu, proposed an alphabet incorporating the old device of pointing to the various parts of the body (reminiscent of the system referred to by Bonet quoting Porta and also shown by Rossellio) combined with Dalgarno's device of the vowels on the tips of the five fingers. Similar to the mnemonic arrangement reported by Porta, La Fin used B-brow; C-cheek; D-deaf ear; F-forehead; G-gullet; H-hair, etc. As this alphabet was associated with the English language only, La Fin developed another for use in Latin.

The other citation by Critchley to Bishop Wilkins (19) of Chester who, in 1694 advocated a manual alphabet similar to that of Dalgarno, using the tips of the fingers for the five vowels; the middle parts for the first five consonants; the bottom parts for the next five; the spaces between the fingers the next four; T- one finger laid on the side of the hand; V- two fingers; W- three fingers; X- the little finger crossed; Y- the wrist; Z- the middle part of the hand.

The two-hand manual alphabet that eventually came to prevail in Great Britain is first found in a rare booklet, *Digiti Lingua* (20) published in London in 1698, which the author says is: "The most compendious, copious, facile and secret way of silent Converse ever yet discovered Shewing how any two persons may be capable in half an hour's time to discourse together by their Fingers only, as well in the dark as the light." There is no indication that the alphabet devised would be of use to the deaf although the anonymous author says of himself: "By a person who has conversed no other wise in above nine Years." He mentioned another alphabet, in use that employed, A-arm, E-elbow, M-mouth, N-nose, with most of the consonants about the head. He regarded his own system as more facile. The illustration given shows the vowels on the tips of the fingers as Dalgarno employed them and

which are still used today. The consonants shown in *Digiti Lingua* are, with some modifications, very similar to those in the present day two-hand British alphabet. Farrar (21) notes that the alphabet in *Digiti Lingua* is also figured in Defoe's *Life of Duncan Campbell* and that de l'Epée speaks of a two-hand alphabet as being well-known to French schoolboys in his time. In connection with this latter comment, it is interesting to note that hearing children in the United States frequently used a manual alphabet among themselves but it is usually the two-handed English alphabet (except they do not employ the tips of the fingers for the vowels). This is curious, in as much as our schools for the deaf and the adult deaf in United States have always used the one-hand alphabet. Apparently, whatever may have been the origin, the two-hand alphabet among school children is passed down through succeeding generations of children.

Farrar (21) states: "Many other finger alphabets, chiefly syllabic or phonetic—of the former, the French Recoing's in the early part of the last century, and of the latter, Grosselin's at a later time may be instanced—were formed for the deaf but . . . none ever acquired any permanent vogue . . ."

In resumé, it may be noted that finger spelling was employed during the Middle Ages without any indication of use by the deaf. The early instruction of the deaf was by speech, then came the manual alphabet as an adjunct by some (but not used at all by many). Bonet intended the manual alphabet to be shown as a device for teaching speech to the deaf. Not until de l'Epée did the manual alphabet in conjunction with signs become a single method in France, with speech only as an auxiliary if used at all. At the same time elsewhere in Europe speech alone was the principal method. In Great Britain, Dalgarno in advocating his alphabet discarded the teaching of speech to the deaf (which was then being done by Wallis and Holder). Eventually oral instruction came to prevail in Great Britain. In the United

States the first instruction by Gallaudet was manual; later oral schools developed.

Today, particularly among the adult deaf, we find, with some modifications in each, the 1620 Spanish one-hand alphabet figured by Bonet in use in the United States and continental Europe, while in the British Isles the two-hand alphabet shown in the 1698 *Digiti Lingua* is employed. Although the one-hand alphabet is faster, the two-hand is somewhat more pronounced; each is firmly established in the respective areas of use.

Acknowledgments

The writer is indebted to Gallaudet College for the use of several of the references, especially the Rossellio and the rare *Digiti Lingua* which are part of the fine Baker Collection in the Edward Minor Gallaudet Library. Also appreciation is expressed to the New York School for the Deaf, White Plains, New York, for the generous loan of a fine copy of Bonet. Likewise to the Volta Bureau, Washington, D.C., for the use of the work by Barrios.

References

1. Best, Harry, *Deafness and the Deaf in the United States*, Macmillan, New York, 1943, p. 518
2. Barrois, J., *Dactylologie et Langage Primitif*, Paris, 1850, Planche III
3. Barrois, J., (cited above), p. 23
4. Farrar, A., *Arnold on the Education of the Deaf*, College of Teachers of the Deaf, London, 1923 (2nd Edition), p. 39
5. Farrar, A., (cited above), p. 6
6. Farrar, A.. (cited above), p. 9
7. Hodgson, Kenneth W., *The Deaf and Their Problems*, New York, 1954, p. 83
8. Rossellio, R.P.F. Cosma, *Thesaurus Artificiosae Memoriae*, Venice, 1579
9. Bonet, Juan Pablo, *Reduccion de las Letras y arte para Ensenar a Ablar los Mudos*, Madrid, 1620, (Plates between 130 and 131)
10. Farrar, A., (cited above), p. 9
11. Peet, Harvey P., "Analysis of Bonet's Treatise on the Art of Teaching the Dumb to Speak", *American Annals of Deaf*, July, 1851, Vol. III. No. 4, p. 204.
12. Bonet, Juan Pablo, (cited above), pp. 128-129.
13. Porta, J. B., *De Furtivis Literarum Notis Vulgo de Ziferis*, Neapoli, 1563.
14. Historical account of Pereire based on Farrar, A., (cited above), pp. 32-37
15. Historical account of the Abbé de l'Epée based on Farrar, A., (cited above), pp. 42-47
16. Chart in the Appendix to: Sicard, Roch-Ambroise, *Cours D'Instruction d'un Sourd-Muet de Naissance*, 2nd Edition, Paris, 1803.
17. Critchley, Macdonald, *The Language of Gesture*, Edward Arnold & Co., London, 1939, pp. 32-35.
18. LaFin, *Sermo Mirabilis, or the Silent Language*, London, 1692
19. Wilkins, J., "Mercury or the Secret and Swift Messenger" from the collected *Mathematical and Philosophical Works*. Vol. II, London, 1802
20. (Anonymous) *Digiti Lingua*, London, 1698
21. Farrar, A., (cited above) p. 40

Cross-Cultural Communication with Foreign Signers: Fact and Fancy

Robbin Battison and I. King Jordan

According to popular belief, sign language is very different from spoken language in several ways. Many people believe that the signs of sign language are always iconic; i.e. that sign language is a "picture language". Others believe that sign languages have no grammar, no "proper" ways of expressing things, but merely "throw together" gestures and pantomimic actions; or they believe that sign languages abridge and corrupt correct spoken language grammar. These myths have been treated in recent years by other researchers, who find that the formal structures and communicative functions of sign languages used by deaf people are comparable to those of spoken languages used by hearing people (Stokoe 1960, 1970; Woodward 1973; Battison 1974; Bellugi & Klima 1975; Baker 1975; Frishberg 1975; Klima & Bellugi 1975; Liddell 1975; Padden & Markowicz 1975; Stokoe & Battison 1975).

What we choose to examine in this study is the global and international nature of sign language. We shall examine briefly some popular beliefs or myths about sign language in the world, formulate some questions for study and research, discuss some past work, and present some of our own research findings relevant to these questions. We will deal with some very basic questions about the nature of sign languages used here in the U.S. and in other countries. We will certainly not exhaust the topic, since our own investigations are limited in scope and duration, and are still continuing.

Popular beliefs. There are two related popular beliefs about sign languages on a global scale: **(1)**

Sign language is universally the same throughout the world; (2) Deaf signers everywhere have little or no difficulty understanding each other. Naturally if the first statement is true, the second must be true also, but not vice-versa. What we would like to do is break down both these beliefs into statements which can be shown to be true or false.

These beliefs are directly evident in the things that people write and say when they discuss sign language, and indirectly in the manner of their discussions. Consider such innocent things as the word *the*. It was especially popular in the 19th century to include "the sign language" in titles of books and articles written on deaf communication, and the practice has even continued into the 20th century. We can cite Long (1918), *The Sign Language,* and Michaels (1923), *A Handbook of the Sign Language of the Deaf.* The misleading implications of these titles and many others like them is that there is only one sign language. A very observant writer of the 19th century, Garrick Mallery, even stated that the sign language of Indians and of deaf people and everyone else "constitute together one language—the gesture speech of mankind—of which each system is a dialect" (1881:323).

Berthier, another 19th century writer, who was deaf himself, made a statement typical of his time: "For centuries scholars from every country have sought after a universal language, and failed. Well, it exists all around, it is sign language" (1854:5).

Michaels proposed a somewhat more moderate position: "The sign-language is universally used by the deaf people, and though all nations do not use the same mode of signs, one having a knowledge of the signs herein delineated will experience little, if any difficulty in understanding other modes, and of being understood by those who use a different mode" (1923:6f).

Even in very recent years, scholars have made proposals that sign language could become a universal language for all of mankind (Mead 1975), although no concrete analyses or proposals have recently been made.

There is abundant evidence that deaf signers themselves believe in the universality of sign language or at least in its potential easily to become universal. One can cite the efforts of the World Federation of the Deaf in creating a 323-item list of signs, primarily designed for use during international meetings (Magarotto & Vukotic 1959), and the more recent international sign language Gestuno (1975). A list of signs designed by a committee, however, should not be confused with a sign language.

There are also many stories circulating among deaf people regarding communication with foreign signers. The main elements of these stories seem to be that: (1) Deaf people communicate with deaf foreigners better than hearing people do with hearing foreigners; (2) Deaf people throughout the world are united by one basic sign language; (3) Sign Language will eventually become a world language for everyone, both deaf and hearing.

Issues. Of course, there is also information which contradicts these beliefs, and this is one of the things that initially guided us into the present study. After considering the many things people say and write about the issue, we formulated a basic set of questions:

1. Do deaf people around the world use the same signs?
2. Can signers understand each other's sign languages?
3. Can signers from different countries communicate with each other even if they don't know each other's sign languages?
4. Do signers have a clear idea of the separateness of different sign languages, or do they feel and act as if they are all basically the same thing?
5. What attitudes do people have about their own sign language and about foreign sign languages?

While some of these questions seem to overlap, the distinctions will become clear in the discussion which follows.

Procedure. From a number of sources, we began to collect information on interaction with foreign signers, including: (1) published material on the subject; (2) Interviews with both American and foreign signers about their own language background and experiences; (3) Our own observations of and participation in sign conversations involving American and foreign signers; (4) Videotaping unstructured conversations among foreign signers; and (5) A referential communication experiment by Jordan & Battison (1976: pages 69-80, below).

Most of these activities took place in July and August of 1975, when several thousand foreign deaf signers visited Washington, D.C. primarily in order to attend the 7th Congress of the World Federation of the Deaf. We also had ample contact with foreign students attending Gallaudet College, which primarily serves deaf students, and with Americans who had travelled abroad or who had interacted with foreign signers during the W.F.D. meetings. Whenever possible the longer of these interviews were videotaped.

A total of 53 interviews were conducted with people from the following 17 countries: Australia, Canada, Denmark, Finland, France, Germany, Great Britain, Hong Kong, India, Italy, Malaysia, Mexico, Poland, Portugal, Sweden, U.S.S.R., and U.S.A.

Findings. The first question, concerning the uniformity of signs throughout the world, is easy to answer, because there is much published information on the specific individual signs used in various countries. Some of the many available dictionaries include: American (Stokoe et al. 1965), French (Oléron 1974), Australian (Jeanes et al. n.d.), British (British Deaf & Dumb Association 1960), Swedish (Bjurgate & Nilsson 1968), American Indian (Mallery 1881 [1972]). See also Bernstein & Hamilton(1972). From examining these dictionaries it is evident that there is a great variety of signs used by people to denote the same thing. Signs are not uniformly the same throughout the world, nor are they necessarily standardized within many countries.

One example we can offer to show this variety is from a comparison of French and American signs done by Woodward (1975). He performed a detailed comparison of the 872 signs in a recent French dictionary (Oléron 1974)[1] with current American signs. One would expect a high correspondence between these French signs and American signs for two reasons: (a) French and American Sign Languages are historically related—they share a common ancestor, and (b) Oléron purposely chose for his dictionary those signs which are most easily explainable in "iconic" and "pictographic" terms (Woodward, personal communication), and thus one would expect more correspondence between American and French signs simply because with the more "iconic" signs there would supposedly be less chance of arbitrary symbolism entering into the formation of the signs and creating a difference. What Woodward found in his comparative study was that in spite of these two conditions (the historical relationship and iconic signs), there was only 26.5% shared vocabulary; i.e. only 26.5% of the signs were highly similar or identical in both the French and the American versions.

Of course the question of mutual intelligibility does not depend solely on the amount of shared vocabulary, since mutually intelligible dialects of the same language may have a great many lexical differences, and vice-versa.

As a concluding note on this question, it should be noted that earlier researchers on these problems sometimes emphasized (and perhaps exaggerated) the similarities between sign languages rather than noting their (random or systematic) differences. Sometimes the nature of the similarity and the total number of signs involved in the comparison were vague. For example in speaking of deaf signs and Plains Indian signs, Mallery says simply, "Many of them show marked similarity, not only in principle[2] but often in detail" (1881:323).

Let us take up the next two questions simultaneously, for the evidence bears on both of them: Can signers understand each other's sign language? and Can signers from different countries communicate with each other even if they do not know each other's sign languages? We would like to keep these two questions separate, because communication can take place without sharing a natural language—through mime or nonverbal communication, for example.

We quoted Mallery earlier as saying that the signs of Indians, deaf people, and everyone else really made up one language; however, he later notes that not all Indians can understand each other's signs (1881: 82, 86-90 passim.). What Mallery meant by *language* in these contexts is hard to determine, as he never attempts a concise definition. Certainly he missed one of the basic distinctions between Indian and deaf sign languages—that deaf sign languages are learned by some deaf children as native or first languages, and must necessarily serve all the social functions

---

1   The signs in Oléron (1974) are taken from the same corpus of data Oléron examined twenty-two years earlier (1952).
2   We interpret Mallery's "in principle" to mean that the general image evoked by the sign is the same, but not necessarily the actual formation of the sign. This is another example of the notion of iconicity clouding the investigation of formational structure.

of a complete language; whereas Indians primarily used signs with people who did not speak the same language, and in limited social situations like hunting, trading, etc. Interestingly, though Mallery discusses at length the signs of both Indians and deaf people, nowhere does he mention *deaf Indians* and how they might have used signs.

Let us go back ninety-five years to an early experiment in sign communication that took place in Washington, D.C., on March 16, 1880.[3] Colonel Garrick Mallery brought seven Ute Indians to Gallaudet College, where they met with seven deaf students, the college's president, E. M. Gallaudet, and a number of the staff . A "testing procedure" was used in which the two groups, Indians and deaf signers, alternated telling each other individual signs and connected narratives. Mallery describes six of the short narratives and describes seven of the "signs" in detail.[4]

Interestingly, four of the seven "signs" he, describes were not understood. The six short narratives were understood without much difficulty, although it is apparent that much of it was simply miming scenarios involving hunting, gathering food, and eating specific foods. Two examples will illustrate the *ad hoc* nature of the communication on that day:

> Among the signs was that for *squirrel,* given by a deaf-mute. The right hand was placed over and facing the left, and about four inches above the latter, to show the height of the animal; then the two hands were held edgewise and horizontally in front, about eight inches apart (showing length); then imitating the grasping of a small object and biting it rapidly with the incisors, the extended index was pointed upward and forward (in a *tree*).

> This was not understood, as the Utes have no sign for the tree squirrel, the arboreal animal not being found now in their region (1881:321).

We need only point out two things: (a) The supposed "sign" was really a sequence of at least four separate mime elements; (b) The Utes probably did understand what was being described (not named)—a small arboreal animal which gathers and chews small objects.

The second example indicated another weakness in these experiments. Despite Mallery's expertise in observing, collecting, and describing gestural communication, he neglected to fully take into account the effects of social context on intelligibility:

> When the Indians were asked whether, if they (the deaf-mutes) were to come to the Ute country they would be scalped, the answer was given, "Nothing would be done to you; but we would be friends," as follows:

> The palm of the right hand was brushed toward the right over that of the left (nothing), and the right hand made to grasp the palm of the left, thumbs [sic] extended over and lying upon the back of the opposing hand.

> This was readily understood by the deaf-mutes (1881:322).

We are not given the details of the students' interpretations of these two signs, but we can reasonably assume that the Utes were expected to say something of a friendly nature, thus it is not

---

3   Mallery gave the date as March 6 (1881:321). It is identical of course in the facsimile reprint of 1972. The date, however, for this event given in E. M. Gallaudet's diary is March 16, undoubtedly the more reliable date.

4   Seeking corroboration of Mallery's account of the meeting, we looked in the Gallaudet College archives at the personal records of E. M. Gallaudet. Apparently the event was not as impressive to him, for his diary entry for that day is:
    March, Tuesday 16. 1880 Cold raw day, a little rain. We had a visit at the Inst. [itute] from Col Mallery & a party of Ute indians [sic]. I took a Fr. [ench] lesson. Called on Mr. W. K. Rogers the Pmts. [Pres. Rutherford B. Hayes'] Pri. Secretary. Rev. John Chamberlain of N.Y. arrived & was quartered at the inst. [itute].
    In his report of the event Mallery records the names of none of the deaf students but names five of the Indians.

surprising at all that the students "readily understood" them.

But now let us move to more recent events with other transported signers. From our interviews with deaf signers from America and other nations, we obtained a range of self-reports on communication with members of other deaf cultures. First, examining the question whether sign languages are understood by foreigners, we have the following information:

1. A German actor, whose company performs in mime (not in any variety of German Sign Language), complained that one of the reasons they could not perform a stage show in their own sign language was that they would not be understood when they travelled to other German cities.

2. A young woman from Lyons reported that she refuses to visit Paris without her friend who has been to Paris more often and understands the Parisians' sign language better—Lyons and Paris are 250 miles apart.

3. A standard story, repeated by travellers and natives alike, holds that if you travel 50 miles in Britain you will encounter a different sign language that cannot be understood in the region you have just left.

4. An Italian and a Pole who have both travelled widely were in a casual conversation with five Americans. They made no attempt to imitate or use American signs; they stated flatly that they did not understand American signs; and they relied the entire time on an American who was skilled in using international signs and signs from various European countries.

5. From Swedish, Danish, and Finnish informants we learned that the four Scandinavian countries have separate sign languages, but that people from Sweden, Denmark, and Norway can understand one another with only moderate difficulty. On the other hand, interaction between Danes and Finns frequently requires the use of an interpreter.

6. An American who has a reputation for being a highly skilled communicator reported that when he was with the Israeli groups during the W.F.D. Congress: "They signed so fast, I felt like I was hearing!"[5]

7. Both an Australian learning American signs and a Dane learning Finnish signs reported that their comprehension of the new language exceeded their abilities to express themselves correctly in it. The Dane said, "After many visits, I can understand it with almost no problem, but I can't sign it myself." The Australian said, "I don't feel comfortable using ASL; I can understand it, but not express myself."

What we conclude from these reports and others like them is that: (a) Not only do people use different signs in different parts of the world but also these signs are largely unintelligible to foreign signers when used in connected discourse; (b) Geographical boundaries of sign language intelligibility do not always correspond to the boundaries of spoken languages—while many of the deaf in Scandinavia can understand one another with only moderate difficulty, we also have the opposite situation, that cities or regions within small countries (e. g. Britain, Germany, France) determine linguistic boundaries;[6]

---

5   In other words, he was made to feel like an average hearing signer, who always has great difficulty following a normal deaf sign conversation.

6   One might begin to look for an explanation for these geographic discrepancies in national attitudes toward sign languages. The two groups of countries named are at extreme ends of a continuum as regards public and educational acceptance of signing among deaf people. Signing in public and in schools is becoming widely accepted in Scandinavia, while it is forbidden in schools and heavily stigmatized and suppressed in Britain, France, and Germany. One could argue that the public and institutional acceptance of signs has a *standardizing influence,* since people communicate more freely

(c) As with spoken languages that are learned informally (in a normal communicative situation rather than in a classroom), comprehension of a second sign language surpasses correct expressive usage of that language.

Now we shall again take up the question *Whether deaf signers can communicate with each other, and if so, how?*

Most of our non-American informants, *particularly the Europeans,* say that communication with foreign deaf people is not a problem. Depending on past experience and amount of interaction with the foreigners, most people say that after two or three days they can understand each other pretty well.

This does not at all contradict the previous findings that sign languages are unintelligible to foreigners, because, when asked specifically about *how* they communicate with foreigners, many of them say specifically that *they stop using their own sign language and start using mime and gesture.* Other features of such communication are that it is slower than signing, very repetitious, and involves a lot of back-and-forth bargaining and checking about the meanings of various gestures. Gradually, a shared meaning for various signs emerges through the conversation. The compositie description of cross-cultural communication matches Mallery's (1881) very insightful discussion of interaction among different tribes of Indians.

The general consensus of our well-travelled informants was that this type of communication is a skill that can be improved with the experience of a great deal of foreign interaction. The communication may be augmented by other means: e.g. using agreed-upon international signs, fingerspelling familiar words from a spoken language, speaking occasional words which are thought to be well known. In this preliminary report we shall not attempt a detailed description of how these cross-cultural communications take place, but we would like to consider briefly the factors of topic, situation, and motivation.

Many contacts between deaf foreigners take place when people are travelling, and are therefore concerned with the basic necessities of food and shelter. Also, when meeting foreigners for the first time, much basic personal and social information is exchanged—Where are you from? What do you do? Are you married? Is your husband with you? Where are you going next? etc. In other words, there is a high expectancy that certain topics will come up again and again before interaction is allowed to move to more intricate and less superficial interactions.

Motivation is higher in these interactions, partly because when one is tired, cold, hungry, or bored, one tries very hard to alleviate these situations by establishing communication with those who live in the area. A consensus among our informants was that it is difficult to discuss very weighty or "deep" subjects with foreigners. Politics, religion, and philosophy are difficult, while travel, food, school, jobs, family, and entertainment are much easier. Also, it is much easier to discuss things in a dyad than in a larger group. One other motivational factor which may contribute to successful communication is the patience and perseverance of deaf people, most of whom have a great deal of practice dealing with weak communicative situations involving hearing people.

Moving to the fourth question: "Do signers have a clear idea of the separateness of different sign languages, or do they feel and act as if they are all basically the same? "—most of the evidence says they *do* keep languages separate in spite of the fact that a teriffic mixing of languages and styles takes place when in contact with foreigners.

The evidence regarding this separateness is of five kinds:

---

under these conditions and tend to interact over social and regional differences and in a greater variety of situations.

1. When native signers (those with deaf parents) are asked what their first language was, they almost always answer, "Sign Language" —not Swedish Sign Language or French Sign-Language, or any other national or regional type. It seems as if they are under-differentiating or confusing various sign languages that they know (or know about), but when pressed further, they make it clear that it is a sign language as opposed to a spoken language that they learned first.

2. Some signers in America tend to think of all European sign languages as being vaguely the same entity and are often surprised at the complexity and differences among European sign languages; while Europeans themselves are more experienced with languages. We have two illustrations of this contrast: (a) In the course of introducing a Dane to some Americans, the Canadian introducer used a few Danish signs. One of the Americans remarked to him, "Oh, you know International Sign Language! (b) A European teacher of the deaf, who is deaf himself, spent a year as a graduate student at Gallaudet. An American student asked him if he planned to take American Sign Language back to his country. The teacher looked surprised and said, "No, what for? We have our own sign language in my country." The student was astonished. Prior to his departure for the U.S., the same teacher had announced to his class of ten-year-old deaf pupils that he was going to America for a year of study. The class erupted with expressions of dismay. When asked why they thought it was so terrible, the pupils answered, "Because you'll have to learn American Sign Language!" These European youngsters, who had seen many foreign deaf people come and go, had a clear idea of the separation of different sign languages; while the older American college students did not.

3. We have two other major kinds of evidence to show that people keep their sign languages "separated." The first involves people who move to a different country. By all reports they forget their own signs rapidly as they acquire the sign language of their new country. We can report only one exception to this, a Finnish woman who moved to Denmark. Other foreigners in Demmark were surprised that she retained her native Finnish Sign Language.

4. It is also interesting to note what happens when one of these expatriates has visitors from his native country. All of them report that they have difficulty readjusting to their first language and that it takes several days of interaction with their guests before they begin to feel normal. They also report that they can understand but not express themselves very well in these situations.

5. Another type of evidence which shows that signers are capable of keeping their languages separate is what happens when a multilingual person mistakenly substitutes one language for another. We can illustrate this with an event which occurred two separate times: Two Finns, a Dane, and an American were travelling in a car. The two Finns were father and daughter and were having a conversation in Finnish Sign Language. The Dane was multilingual and attempted to interpret from Finnish to American signs for the benefit of the American. However, in the confusion he started signing to the American in Danish signs, and went on like that for a minute before the American stopped him and asked him to interpret into a language he could understand!

Attitudes. Finally let us consider attitudes toward language and language users. Since much of our material on language attitudes is from European signers collected during a three-week period in the United States, these generalizations are not without limitations.

Europe consists of many small countries whose deaf people interact extensively through travel and emigration. The United States is large, relatively homogeneous, and linguistically isolated from the rest of the deaf world. Possibly because of this isolation, deaf Americans seem to mirror the language attitudes of the American hearing majority culture. This involves ethnocentrism, language chauvinism, and linguistic naïveté.

Europeans claim that Americans are rigid and inflexible in their language and hard to understand. One deaf couple from Europe had to resort to pencil and paper to communicate with deaf people when they first arrived in the U.S.. They could make themselves understood, but could not understand the Americans when they signed, because they claimed, the Americans did not modify their language or slow down at all.

There were several reports of American students being surprised that foreigners had different sign languages, and also that deaf people needed interpreters to go from one sign language to another. When asked how foreigners communicate with each other Americans would describe their communication with labels like "home signs", "all pictures", "basic gestures", "mime", and "poor sign language". Europeans who knew about these American attitudes suggested that the Americans were not judging them on their own national sign languages but on the gestures and mime that they used when communicating with foreigners.

To illustrate how language-related attitudes can affect cross-cultural interaction, we offer the following story of two foreign deaf students at Gallaudet College. Although they came from two separate countries, they had very similar backgrounds. Both were profoundly deaf, had deaf parents, and were native signers of their own national sign language. They learned English before arriving in the United States, and they had an excellent command of written and spoken English. Possibly because of this prior knowledge, and possibly because they first were exposed to American signs in a classroom, they used American signs with English syntax, just as most hearing people do. As a result, the other students

thought they were either hearing or orally-oriented, awkward signers. The American students were not willing to believe that they had deaf parents, because they did not sign like the children of deaf parents should. Because of this "suspicious" behavior, one of these foreign students was falsely labelled as a narcotics agent and briefly ostracized.

Mistaken identity worked the other way, too. In spite of the fact that they had been signing all their lives, several foreign students said they could not distinguish deaf Americans from hearing Americans on the basis of their signing, for the first six months or so. To them, "Everyone signs the same."

For the European visitors during the W.F.D. Congress, America was full of pleasant surprises also. Most of them were awed by the fact that people from California could really understand people from the East Coast without any problems, and that the U.S. had a truly national Sign Language. Many people from the European drama troupes, all of whom perform in mime, dance, and gesture, were astonished at the National Theater of The Deaf's performance in American Sign Language. Several of them had previously commented that a play in real sign language would be impossible to stage. And finally, many Europeans commented on how well sign language was accepted here in the United States—it was used in the schools; hearing people learned it; and deaf people could sign on the street and not feel ashamed. These people were surprised, since these contrasted with their own experiences in their own countries.

Conclusions. We have established and examined a number of questions relating to sign language communication between deaf people from different countries. From personal interviews and observations we can suggest partial answers to some of them.

From examining some of the many sign language dictionaries available and from our records of communication with deaf foreigners, we do know that signs vary considerably from country to country. This much is certainly not in dispute.

From the personal reports of travellers and immigrants alike, we know that sign languages are not understood by signers who are not familiar with them—certainly not as easily understood as some stories would have us believe. Comprehension of a second language exceeds correct expression in that language; receptive skills exceed expressive skills.

The fact that deaf signers can and do communicate despite not sharing the same sign language is interesting, and it bears more investigation. While being skilled in sign language may prepare one for dealing with mime and for communicating in difficult cross-cultural situations, the two should not be confused. Signers consider them separate tasks.

The data we have gathered gives us little reason to believe that sign languages are much different from spoken languages as regards cross-cultural communication. To the extent that sign languages are separate entities, communication is hindered between groups. We need more information about the limitations and potentials in communication between foreign signers. We also feel there is a need for intensive linguistic investigation of national sign languages everywhere.

References

Baker, Charlotte (1975) Regulators and Turn-Taking in American Sign Language. Paper presented at the 50th Annual Meeting of the LSA.

Battison, Robbin (1974) Phonological Deletion in American Sign Language, *Sign Language Studies* 5, 1-19.

Bellugi, Ursula, & E. Klima (1975) Aspects of Sign Language & its Structure, in *The Role of Speech in Language,* Kavanagh & Cutting eds. (Cambridge, MIT Press), 171-205.

Berthier, Ferdinand (1854) Observation sur la mimique considérée dans ses rapports avec l'enseignement des sourds-muets. A M. le President et a MM. les Membres de l'Academie Imperiale de Médecine. Paris, L. Martinet.

Bjurgate, Anne-Marie, & M. Nilsson (1968) Tekenspràk för döva. Stockholm, Sö-Förlaget;Skolövers-tyrelsen.

Bornstein, Harry, & Lillian Hamilton (1972) Recent National Dictionaries of Signs, *Sign Language Studies* 1,42-63.

British Deaf & Dumb Association (1960) *The Language of the Silent World* (Paisley, Scotland).

Frishberg, Nancy (1975) Arbitrariness and Iconicity: Historical Change in American Sign Language, *Language* 51, 696-719.

Gallaudet, E. M. (1880) (Personal diary for the year 1880) Archives of the Gallaudet College Library, Washington, D.C.

Jeanes, D., R. Deanes, C. Murkin, & B. Reynolds (n.d.) *Aid to Communication with the Deaf* (Melbourne, Victorian School for Deaf Children).

Jordan, I. King, & R. Battison (1976) A Referential Communication Experiment with Foreign Sign Languages, *Sign Language Studies* 10, 69-80.

Klima, Edward (1975) Sound and Its Absence in the Linguistic Symbol, in *The Role of Speech in Language,* eds. Kavanagh & Cutting (Cambridge, MIT Press), 249-270.

Liddell, Scott (1975) Restrictive Relative Clauses in American Sign Language. Working paper, the Salk Institute, LaJolla, California.

Long, J. Schuyler (1918) *The Sign Language: A Manual of Signs.* (Reprinted 1962, Washington, D.C., the Gallaudet College Library).

Magarotto, Ceasare, & D. Vukotic (1959) First Contribution to the International Dictionary of Sign Language—Conference Terminology (Rome, World Federation of the Deaf).

Mallery, Garrick (1881) [1972] Sign Language Among North American Indians (Washington, D.C., Government Printing Office [The Hague, Mouton], (=Approaches to Semiotics 15, ed. T. A. Sebeok).

Michaels, J. W. (1923) *A Handbook of the Sign Language of the Deaf.* (Atlanta, Southern Baptist Convention).

Oléron, Pierre (1952) Études sur le langage mimique des sourds-muets, *L'Année Psychologigue* 52, 47-81.

_____ (1974) *Elements de Repertoire du Langage Gestuel des Sourds-Muets* (Paris, Centre National de la Récherche Scientifique).

Padden, Carol, & H. Markowicz (1975) Crossing Cultural Group Boundaries into the Deaf Community. Paper presented at the Conference on Culture and Communication, Temple University, Philadelphia.

Stokoe, William (1960) Sign Language Structure: An Outline of the Visual Communication Systems of the American Deaf, *Studies in Linguistics:* Occasional Papers, 8 (Repr. Linstok Press).

_____ (1970) Sign Language Diglossia, *Studies in Linguistics* 21, 27-41.

_ _ _ _ _, & Robbin Battison (1975) Sign Language, Mental Health, & Satisfying Interaction, Proceedings of 1st National Symposium on Mental Health Needs of Deaf Adults and Youth, eds. Mindel & Stein (New York, Grune & Stratton, to appear).

_ _ _ _ _, D. Casterline, & C. Croneberg (1965) [1976] *A Dictionary of American Sign Language on Linguistic Principles* (Washington, Gallaudet College Press [Silver Spring, MD, Linstok Press, 2ed]).

Woodward, James C. (1973) *Implicational Lects on the Deaf Diglossic Continuum*. Ph. D. dissertation, Georgetown University.

(1976) Signs of ASL and FSL, *Sign Language Studies* 11, in press.

World Federation of the Deaf (1975) *Gestuno*.

CHAPTER 5

Deaf Culture

Hearing people, who have never met a deaf person, may wonder why a "Deaf Culture" exists. Why would people whose only difference seems to be their inability to hear, develop a separate culture? The answer to this question lies in understanding the experience of deafness.

Imagine you are attending a large family gathering. The event is taking place at a park. It is a beautiful sunny day. Everyone is catching up with long lost cousins and feasting on barbecue and potato salad. Now, imagine that you are deaf. Your mother is the only one who knows how to sign to you, but she is busy talking with her sisters. You are a good lipreader, but many of your relatives look away or cover their mouths when they speak. Perhaps everyone starts to talk at once. Your favorite Uncle Charlie is sporting a new, bushy moustache that conceals his lips. Your speech is good but not perfect and the family frequently asks you to repeat yourself. As the day wears on it becomes increasingly difficult to participate effectively in any conversation. If you can picture this situation, you should begin to appreciate what it is like to be deaf in a hearing world. You may also understand why deaf people seek out each other's company and prefer situations where sign language is used and communication is fluent.

Culture is based on shared experiences, values, and beliefs that are expressed through literature, art, humor, dance, film and language. American Sign Language provides a bond of communication that is the heart and soul of the Deaf Community. This solidarity has been further reinforced by residential schools in which deaf children, from a wide geographic area, are brought together to be educated away from their families.

Deaf Culture in America is vibrant and dynamic. An example of this is The National Theater of the Deaf (NTD), established in 1967. It is an organization of deaf professional writers and actors who perform classic plays and original works in American Sign Language. Their productions are inspiring. The talent of the company can be appreciated whether one is deaf or hearing. This chapter explores other aspects of Deaf Culture such as name signs, poetry, art and women's issues. The final article by M. J. Bienvenu discusses deaf humor as a reflection of American Deaf Culture. Her illustrations of deaf jokes will leave you laughing!

Inside the Deaf Community

Barbara Kannapell

"When I think of communication," the first thing that comes to my mind is the free flow of communication in the Deaf Community. Deaf people feel so comfortable in communicating with each other at deaf clubs, church services for the deaf, or any event for deaf people given by deaf people, as opposed to the discomfort that they feel outside of the Deaf Community.

Then what is communication? Eileen Paul wrote an article, "Some Notes On Communication . . .," in which she defines the meaning of communication which is most relevant to that in the Deaf Community.

This last statement is the theme throughout this paper. I will show how it is relevant to the communication in the Deaf Community.

Now, let's look inside the Deaf Community. The question I'd like to ask is: "What makes deaf people feel at ease in communicating with each other?" I will offer three explanations.

The First Explanation

Deaf people can understand each other 100 percent of the time, whereas outside of the Deaf Community they get *fragmentary information* or *one-way communication*. Fragmentary information means that the deaf person may get 50, 60, or 70 percent of the information communicated through a not-so-skilled interpreter, or through a hearing person who uses speech or who has just learned Sign Language.

One-way communication can mean an interpreter who can express from voice to sign, but can't interpret from sign to voice. It can also mean a hearing person who can express him/herself in

Sign Language, but cannot read the signs of a deaf person. Deaf people experience this kind of one-way communication very often when they are with hearing people.

The Second Explanation

Deaf people share a common language—American Sign Language (ASL). ASL seems to be the primary communication mode we use among ourselves. Everything else—English in different forms—is the secondary communication mode for some deaf people. It does not necessarily mean that all deaf people are fluent in ASL. It can mean that those who are not fluent in ASL are skilled in English, or it can mean that they have no skills in English. It is possible that there are deaf people who are bilingual in varying degrees. I'd like to show some variations in communication styles in the Deaf Community:

ASL monolinguals - Deaf people who are comfortable expressing themselves only in ASL, and in understanding only ASL. They have no skills in English.

ASL dominant bilinguals - Deaf people who are more comfortable expressing themselves in ASL than English, and are able to understand ASL better than English (either printed or signed English).

Balanced bilinguals - Deaf people who are comfortable expressing themselves in both ASL and English, and who are able to understand both equally well.

English dominant bilinguals - Deaf people who are more comfortable expressing themselves in English, and who are able to understand English (in printed English or signed English) better than ASL.

English monolinguals - Deaf people who are comfortable expressing themselves only in English (oral or signed English) and in understanding English (in printed or oral or signed English). They have no skills in ASL.

Semi-linguals - Deaf people who do have some skills in both English and ASL, but are not able to master either language fully.

Based on these variations, I would like to raise several questions: 1) Who is really in the core of the Deaf Community, and who is on the fringe of the Deaf Community? 2) Are English-dominant bilinguals and English monolinguals in the core of the Deaf Community, or are they on the fringe? 3) Are there deaf people who use only ASL and understand only ASL (ASL monolinguals)? In other words, are there deaf people who know absolutely no English?

Within the Deaf Community, deaf people have a complex system of evaluating who should be in the core or on the fringe of the Deaf Community. It is important to mention here that the degree of hearing loss is not the most important requirement for being in the core of the Deaf Community. Deaf people just identify themselves as deaf or hard of hearing, no matter what their degree of loss is. They do not need to show their audiogram to enter the Deaf Community. Sharing a common language seems, however, not to be enough to be admitted to the Deaf Community.

The Third Explanation.

"Communication is the process of sharing what things mean to us with ourselves and with other people." I think this is the most important explanation of all. Deaf people share what things mean to each other, i.e., the word "deaf" means different things to deaf and to hearing people. Also, the word "hearing" has a different meaning for deaf people. Deaf people communicate those meanings through ASL. Such meanings extend to the following:

The bond of communication and strong relationships - Deaf people experience a strong bond of communication because they have common topics to share which are based on common experiences, such as the history of deaf people, school experiences, family experiences, sports, movies, stories and jokes. They develop strong relations based on these common experiences with other deaf people. Many deaf people develop strong relationships during school years and maintain these relationships throughout their lives. This feeling may be carried over from residential schools, where they developed a strong bond of communication for the purpose of survival skills.

Cultural beliefs and values - Carol Padden offers a good explanation of cultural beliefs and values in her essay in *Sign Language in the Deaf Community*. These beliefs and values are also related to the complex system of evaluating who should be in the core of the Deaf Community and who should be on the fringe. For example, deaf people have a way of evaluating who behaves like a deaf person and who behaves like a hearing person.

If a deaf person behaves like a hearing person, other deaf people will sign "hearing" on the forehead to show "he thinks like a hearing person." Thus, he is on the fringe of the Deaf Community, depending on his/her attitudes. Conversely, if a deaf person behaves like a deaf person, other deaf people may sign "strong deaf" or "fluent ASL," which means that the person is culturally deaf. Thus, he or she is admitted to the core of the Deaf Community.

If a hearing person wants to meet a deaf person, the rules of the Deaf Community dictate that he/she must be introduced as a "hearing" person in the Deaf Community. Then, the deaf person being introduced will ask questions such as "you from Gallaudet?" or "from deaf family?" or "teach deaf children?" If the hearing person has something to do with working with deaf people, or comes from a deaf family, a deaf person would be satisfied, since this would meet his/her expectations of a hearing person. But, if the hearing person is just interested in learning ASL as a foreign language and has nothing to do with deafness, deaf people will become suspicious and on guard. It is true that a few hearing people who have nothing to do with the education of deaf children or who do not come from a deaf family may eventually be admitted to this Community. These are just two examples relating to cultural beliefs and values in the Deaf Community.

Feeling equal - The bond of communication and strong relationships and similar cultural beliefs and values are equated with feelings of equality among deaf people. Within the Deaf Community is the only place that deaf people experience equality with others. Usually, deaf people do not feel equal with hearing people outside of the Deaf Community.

Thus, ASL is a powerful tool for identity in the Deaf Community, along with the cultural beliefs and values that are expressed through ASL. This suggests that ASL is the cultural language of the Deaf Community.

However, I want to emphasize that the knowledge of ASL alone seems not to be enough to qualify a person to be in the core of the Deaf Community. Everything else—shared common experiences, and cultural beliefs and values which are attached to ASL also seem to be important requirements for admittance to the core of the Deaf Community. A deaf person who is in the core of the Deaf Community is considered to be "culturally deaf."

The more culturally deaf a person becomes, the further he or she moves into the core of the Deaf Community. I suggest that the Deaf Community can be compared to the majority community of hearing people in terms of language supremacy. Deaf people experience ASL supremacy in the Deaf Community similar to hearing people's English supremacy in the majority community.

In relation to deaf people's experience of ASL supremacy, we also need to look into the functions of ASL in the Deaf Community. Language can serve many functions, i.e., Pidgin Sign English functions as a way for deaf people to communicate with hearing people. ASL serves as a way for deaf people to communicate with each other, but there is much more to it than just a function of language. There is a symbolic function in relation to identity and power, and we often keep our use of ASL limited to ourselves to preserve these factors of identity and power.

As a protection of our own identities, deaf people keep thinking that hearing people cannot learn ASL, but really deaf people exert their power in using ASL. For example, we can talk about anything we want—right in the middle of a crowd of hearing people. They are not supposed to understand us. In a classroom, for example, deaf students often talk about the hearing teacher right in front of him or her. They may say "understand zero" or "it went over my head" in ASL. The hearing teacher is not supposed to understand ASL.

If hearing people understand ASL, then deaf people are no longer in power using ASL. Here is what happened to me several years ago: I realized that a deaf friend of mine and I were no longer in power using ASL in front of two hearing friends. One of them knew no Sign Language, but the other one knew ASL fairly well. As my deaf friend and I began a deep personal discussion, the hearing person who knew ASL was able to understand us and felt awkward intepreting to the other hearing person what we were talking about.

I did not expect her to understand our discussion in ASL or to interpret to the hearing person because hearing people are not supposed to understand the conversation of deaf people in ASL. That's how deaf people experience ASL supremacy. ASL is the only creation which grows out of the Deaf Community. It is our language in every sense of the word. We create it, we keep it alive and it keeps us and our traditions alive.

I suggest another reason why deaf people do not use ASL with hearing people: *Language choice reflects identity choice.* Somehow, deaf people learn not to use ASL with hearing people in their school years. Deaf persons choose ASL or English depending on the identity the system wants for them. When they are with hearing people, they try to communicate in English—trying to use voice or sign in English—or both at the same time. When they are with other deaf people, they feel more like themselves and use ASL, and experience a strong sense of group identity.

I also suggest that in relation to the theme of this paper again, these words, "hearing person," "speech," and "English," are equivalent. When a deaf person meets a hearing person, the word "English" is strongly attached to that hearing person, so a deaf person tries to communicate on a hearing person's terms—using voice or signing in English order or both.

All those explanations of why deaf people do not share ASL with hearing people support this statement:

"Communication is a process of sharing what things mean to us with ourselves and with other persons." This statement can be rephrased as follows: *Deaf people share what things mean to them with themselves and with other deaf people.* They do not usually share their own special meanings with hearing people probably because 1) Hearing people will never understand what it is like to be deaf; 2) Deaf people do not have a chance to share what things mean to them with hearing people; and/or 3) Deaf people think hearing people are not interested in hearing what we would like to share with them.

I can tell you from my experiences of sharing what the deaf experience or world means to me with deaf and hearing people. I needed to develop trust in myself before I could share my world with deaf and hearing people. The more I share with them, the more they share with me. In other words, we need to respect ourselves as deaf persons and respect our language first before we can share what the deaf world means to us with other deaf and hearing people.

In conclusion, I see this paper as only a beginning in the understanding of the meaning of communication in the Deaf Community.

Name Signs as Identity Symbols in the Deaf Community

Kathryn P. Meadow

In every culture, great importance is attached to the naming of children. There is a whole complex of legal as well as cultural norms attached to the assignment of first names and the changing of surnames. There are special customs, sanctions, rituals, and ceremonies attending the naming of children in particular religious and ethnic groups that symbolize the entrance, acceptance, and welcome of a new group member, and that reflect the importance of group cohesion. Names are a key symbol and summary of personal identity, the first identifying marker used for specifying an individual. The form of address that is used, the use of a title plus surname, the first name, the nickname, diminutive, or pejorative form of the formal name very quickly captures the symbolic essence of the relationship between two persons. The study of names and naming can often provide interesting and revealing insights about a particular subgroup within a larger culture. It was this general formulation that led to my interest in examining the assignment and use of name signs in the deaf community.

A *name sign,* in the context of the American Sign Language used by approximately three-fourths of deaf adults in the United States, is a formalized gesture, referring to an individual's proper name. A *sign,* i.e. a morpheme of this language, has three components: One is the shape and presentation of the hand (or hands); the second is the placement of the hand in relation to the body; the third is the action of the hand. The shape of the hand for a name sign is very often identical to the handshape of the American Manual Alphabet letter used in spelling out the initial letter of the individual's first or last name. The placement and movement used in name signs show more variation.

I had been casually interested in the characteristics of name signs for several years, and often asked deaf friends about the circumstances of the assignment of their name signs, their meaning, and usage. In a paper on sociolinguistics and deaf subculture, delivered at Western Maryland College in 1971, I mentioned this interest and suggested that it might be a productive area for study as a means of learning about the development of individual identity and as a reflection of the process of identification within the deaf community in a more general sense (Meadow 1972). This brief and casual reference aroused great interest and much excited comment from the audience, many of whom were deaf, and it became the stimulus for the collection of name sign data that are now being analyzed. This report is a brief and preliminary discussion of early examination of these data.

Source of Data

Sporadically, over a period of two years, name sign data have been collected, primarily by two persons, native deaf signers themselves, with complete access to the deaf community network in California. No attempt was made to obtain a random sample, and no pretensions are made that the data are representative of the deaf community as a whole. I will be unable to say anything, therefore, about the proportion of deaf children or adults who have name signs, but I can say something about the patterns of name sign assignment and usage within the possibly special group of persons reported on. Contacts were made with deaf people at social gatherings, at deaf clubs, at meetings of state and national deaf organizations, at meetings of professionals working within the deaf community, and at state residential schools for the deaf. Every person reporting was asked to describe his name sign (or signs if he had more than one). He was asked to describe the circumstances of its assignment, the identity of the person who created his name sign, its meaning if it had any, and whether or not it was used generally or was situation or person specific. In addition, data were collected about the age, sex, marital status, occupation, and education of each of the primary informants. Name signs were also collected for informants' immediate and extended family members. Finally, each informant was asked to report name signs for friends or acquaintances that seemed to the informant to be particularly interesting or memorable. A total of approximately 450 individual name signs were collected and recorded. About one-fifth of these were anecdotal, "third-person" reports.

Characteristics of the deaf community

The deaf community that formed the base of persons questioned about their name signs can be defined in a number of different ways. Those deaf individuals who choose to consider themselves members of the cohesive subgroup can be said to form a linguistic community, based on their knowledge and everyday use of American Sign Language (Meadow 1972: 19). Linguistic communities may consist of small groups bound together by face-to-face contact or may cover large regions. There appear to be a number of times in his life when an individual can enter the deaf community. The assignment of a name sign can be seen as a kind of rite of passage, defining this entrance to the community through the bestowing of a name that is signed in the language of the subculture. Of the 280 persons for whom we have

available this information, name signs were given as follows: 42% given their name signs at the age of five or before; 25% given signs between the ages of six through ten; 15% at ages eleven through fifteen; and 18% at sixteen years or older.

Let us look next at the identity of the person who conferred the name signs—in Western cultures it is parents who choose the names for their children. We have data for 371 deaf persons on name assignment. In only 30% of the cases was the name sign conferred by a parent or by some member of the extended family. Residential school counselors or teachers assigned 13% of the name signs; peers accounted for 43% of the signs; work associates conferred 10% (on adults obviously); and 4% were assigned by other, miscellaneous categories of persons.

I have speculated elsewhere (Meadow 1972) that, in general, there are three periods in the life of a deaf individual that may mark his entrance into the deaf community: (1) infancy (for deaf children of deaf parents); (2) at the time of enrollment in a residential school for the deaf (generally between the ages of five and thirteen); and (3) at the time of graduation from high school. It would seem that name signs are assigned at one of these general periods, in these general places, and by persons who are representative of the institutions that mark the various avenues to the deaf community.

There are several striking and quite unusual features about the identity of the persons bestowing name signs on deaf children: First, parents serve this function only rarely; second, teachers and counselors sometimes serve *in loco parentis* in naming deaf children; third, deaf children themselves often serve as name bestowers on their peers, as is evident from the fact that almost half of the name signs in this group of 371 persons were conferred by age-mates. I am sure that when these data are examined more closely, the proportion of persons receiving their name signs from parents will be seen to be artificially inflated because of the ways the data were collected. In other words, there are actually far fewer deaf children who actually receive their name signs from parents. Only those children whose parents are deaf (between eight and ten percent of the total) are likely to get their name signs in this way. In view of this, it is perhaps surprising that as many as 16% of the name signs collected have some kind of family meaning or significance. By this I mean that some deaf families may use the same hand position for each child's name sign, varying the hand shape to conform to the manual alphabet initial of the first name; e.g. the placement of the name sign for each family member may be at the temple, or beside the cheek. One family in the study used first name initial hand plus GIRL for all female children and first name initial plus BOY for all male children; i.e. the signs GIRL and BOY were made with normal placement and motion but with an initial hand substituted for the thumb up hand of GIRL and the thumb-opposed bent hand of BOY.

In one study of naming in middle class (hearing) families, it was reported that 62% of the children were named for a particular relative (Rossi 1965: 503); only 16% of the families did not name any of the children for a specific relative, and in 48% of the families, all the children had kin names. I must hasten to point out that the given names of the 450 deaf persons for whom I have name sign information may be kin names; thus they too would have the same symbolic name heritage as the group cited in the Rossi study—the name sign of a deaf child could be a means of positive identification and a source of prideful deaf self identity that is but seldom utilized.

The absence of parental involvement in many cases of bestowing name signs is the first important feature noted. The second is the frequent involvement of teachers and counselors in giving name signs to their pupils and clients. The way in which this most often happens is that the counselor takes the child's first name initial and randomly places some movement with it. This is done with little thought, quite casually. Thus, if there are several children in a single class whose names begin with the same letter, the major consideration for a new name sign is that it not duplicate one of a classmate. This impersonality, of course, is still several steps above the impersonality reflected in the early days of the Lexington School for the Deaf, when students "name signs" were simply their locker numbers. Apparently these students were known for years to each other by their locker numbers.

Although parents and school personnel bestow some name signs, the most likely person for name sign assignment is a member of the child's peer group. Forty-three percent of the name signs reported by our informants were assigned by peer-group members. Generally speaking, the sign language of the deaf community is acquired within the peer group rather than from parents. This is one of the most significant aspects of socialization within or into the deaf community, and is a feature that probably makes the acquisition of sign language unique in the universe of linguistic socialization practices. There are any number of consequences for parents as well as children stemming from this one feature. That hearing parents are quite unlikely to be fluent or even familiar with the language in which the deaf child may be most comfortable is a phenomenon with far-reaching consequences for child rearing, for family cohesion, for language proficiency, and for the self image of both children and adults.

I am speculating that this child-to-child socialization has another significant relationship to the character of many of the name signs that were reported. There were 86 name signs reported that reflected some aspect of the individual's personal appearance or behavior. Seventeen percent of these referred to a positive aspect of the self; 37% seemed to have a neutral referent; but fully 45% had a negative connotation. Very often the name sign in these cases referred to some visible secondary handicap; e.g. the name sign for someone who limps might be CRIPPLE. The name sign for a child with poor vision might be the iconic representation for "thick glasses". "Fatso" is a fairly frequent name sign (expressed in several different ways). Facial scars or freckles are also visible marks that become the basis for name signs.

This negative aspect of so many name signs seemed to me a particularly cruel and unhappy feature, and one that I felt might differ among deaf and hearing children. However, literature on the culture of childhood pertaining specifically to children's usage of names and to teasing around names and naming made it apparent that deaf children are carrying out a universal childhood custom. The Opies remark that "children attach an almost primitive significance to people's names," and that they are not respecters of names once they have learned them; children like names that fall into patterns, and "for more than one hundred years they have been fitting people's names into peculiar spell-like mocking chants such as Maggy, my baggy; Jenny, my benny; Joan, the roan; Shirley-wirley" (Opie & Opie 1976: 156-158).

One anthropologist investigating children's use of nicknames suggests that the motives for the use of derogatory epithets and names by children "may have deeper roots than the folklorist has been aware and that the results may be harmful if not downright devastating to the victim's personality" (Winslow 1969:255). Mary Ellen Goodman suggests that "the popular belief that 'of course he doesn't know what he's saying' is a piece of adult naivete or wishful thinking" (Goodman 1964: 232). Winslow categorized children's epithets into four: (1) those based on physical peculiarities (e. g. braces on the teeth, eyeglasses, racial characteristics); (2) peculiarities based on mental traits, real or imagined (e.g. Stupid, Dumbo, Bubblehead); (3) those based on social relationships; and (4) those based on the play on or parody of a child's name. Winslow observes further:

> Mockery of peers, especially those whose appearance or other traits appear different, had it's origin in group consciousness and esteem of the values traditionally held by the group. Ridicule is a form of expression that may be a symptom

of a wide range of attitudes and feelings. When one's group is placed in jeopardy, ridicule may be used as a weapon of self-assertion (1969: 257).

Wolfenstein's analysis of children's humor includes some interesting comments on the use and abuse of names. She points out that "one's name is a peculiarly valuable possession, the mark of one's sexual and personal identity" and that the focus of children's word play is to begin with the proper name, which is used jokingly long before play on common names is mastered; also that word play often has a sexual or aggressive focus. To distort another's meaning is to transform him radically, since what he means and what he is are the same (Wolfenstein 1954: 64-69, 90).

Examples of all the practices noted by these authors about children's general uses of epithets and play on names were found among the name signs that were collected. In some ways, name signs are used in the same ways as nicknames. In a number of cases, however, informants reported two, or even several different, name signs used in different situations or used at differing periods in their lives. For instance, a change in name sign can sometimes mark a change in status. A number of women reported that their name sign took on a different characteristic that was related to their husband's name sign. Sometimes a name sign changed when occupational status changed. Thus, when the principal in a residential school became the superintendent, some feature of his name sign changed to signify his increased status.

It has also been noted (Wolfenstein 1964) that children are fond of expressing aggression against adult authority figures by a teasing use or change in name. This was reported frequently by deaf informants, who gave any number of examples of the expression of hostility, particularly toward hearing teachers, through the secret use of a scatological or hostile play on their names. This was particularly enjoyed when the meaning of the sign was not understood by the hearing person to whom the sign was attached. Wolfenstein comments: "The discovery of a phrase which can be understood as both respectable and indecent makes it possible to express rebellion against forbidding authorities by a mocking compliance" (1954:160).

Finally, it is interesting to note the variation in the assignment or non-assignment of name signs to the hearing children and/or grandchildren of deaf parents. Some deaf parents reported with pride and pleasure the assignment of name signs to all their children, deaf and hearing, soon after birth. Other deaf parents seemed surprised and taken aback that the question would even be raised or that it might be a possibility. Again, these differing attitudes would seem to reflect a positive or a negative approach to identification with the deaf community.

Summary and conclusion

A number of examples have been given of the ways in which the usage of name signs reflects either a positive or a negative sense of identity, both personally and in the group. In this day of new awakening of feeling for and support of the notion of deaf pride, and positive identification with deafness, it seems appropriate to wonder if leaders in the deaf world might want to consider capitalizing on the positive possibilities for building identity and group identification through the encouragement and support of the notion of formal, ritualized assignment of name signs, which could reflect personal, family, and community identification and pride. The interest that the topic of name signs seems to elicit among deaf persons would indicate that it would not be difficult to propagate such an idea.

References

Goodman, Mary Ellen (1964) *The Culture of Childhood: Child's-Eye Views of Society and Culture* (N.Y., TCP, Columbia Univ.).

Meadow, Kathryn P. (1972) Sociolinguistics, Sign Language, and the Deaf Subculture, in *Psycholinguistics and Total Communication*, ed. O'Rourke (Washington, Amer. Annals).

Opie, Iona, & Peter Opie (1959) *The Lore and Language of Schoolchildren* (London, Oxford University Press; paperback ed., 1967).

Rossi, Alice S. (1965) Naming Children in Middle-Class Families, *American Sociological Review* 30, 499-513.

Winslow, D. J. (1969) Children's Derogatory Epithets, *Journal of American Folklore* 82, 255-236.

Wolfenstein, M. (1954) *Children's Humor, A Psychological Analyis* (Glencoe, Illinois, The Free Press).

Deaf Women: We Were There Too!

Roslyn Rosen

Looking over the history of deaf people, one may wonder, "Where were the deaf women?" Well, I can assure you *we were there, too!* In this paper I'm going to share with you the many contributions of deaf women towards making today's world a better one for all people. In the interest of space, I will focus on only those deaf women who were truly "firsts"; that is, they were the first deaf person, male or female, to do something.

First of all, let me tell you that most of the facts here were stolen from Jack Gannon's magnificent book, *The Deaf Heritage* (1981), published by the National Association of the Deaf. Jack will be the first to tell you that the production of that book was pure hard work. A lot of sweat, blood and tears went into it. Jack will also tell you that without the help of his teammate and wife, Rosalyn, he could never have done it. So you see, whether we deaf women were working up front or behind scenes, we sure were there, too! We were, and are, blazing trails in every aspect of life: Education, Sports, Arts, Communication, Advocacy and Organizational Development.

Education

A little girl, Alice Cogswell, started in motion the wheels of American education of the deaf when her path crossed that of Thomas H. Gallaudet. The influence of deaf women continued to mold the thinking of T. H. Gallaudet, in the person of his deaf wife, Sophia Fowler. T. H. Gallaudet founded the first school for the deaf in Hartford, Conn. and his son, Edward Miner Gallaudet, established Gallaudet College.

Did you know that 24 schools for the deaf in the United States were founded by deaf persons? However, in only one instance are both husband and wife credited for the founding of a school. They were Mr. and Mrs. Ellsworth Long, who established the Oklahoma School for the Deaf in 1898. Since the probability that most of the deaf founders were married is high, it makes one stop and wonder how many unsung heroines there were who worked with their husbands in starting programs. These women probably hid behind their husbands' trousers in conformance with social dictates that a wife's place was in the home.

Other Alice Cogswells have resulted in schools for the deaf, such as Jeanne Lippitt, who was the deaf daughter of the Governor of Rhode Island. Of course, there were probably some male "Alice Cogswells", too. Also, Mabel Bell, the wife of Alexander Graham Bell, and Jeanne Lippitt were accomplished speakers and lipreaders, and may have indirectly fostered an oralism movement in this country.

Deaf people have also pioneered in religious education. Bridget Highes became Sister Patricia in 1880, one of the first deaf nuns. She convinced Archbishop Ryan to establish a Catholic School for deaf children in Pennsylvania, later named the Archbishop Ryan Memorial Institute for the Deaf.

For the first time in 1887, three deaf black people were hired to teach children, at the Texas School for the Deaf. One of them was Mrs. Amanda Johnson, a product of the North Carolina School for the Deaf.

The perennial struggle to teach deaf children English was very much a concern of deaf educators in those days. When talking about language structure systems, the names Fitzgerald and Wing come to mind. Both educators were deaf; George Wing's Symbols were used in some schools such as the Minnesota and Illinois School for the Deaf, but Edith Fitzgerald's Key, also known as "Straight Language for the Deaf", was used in as many as 75 percent of American schools at one time. She was the principal of the Virginia School for the Deaf when the first edition was published in 1926.

The first deaf woman to earn a Ph.D. may be Nansie Sharpless, from Wayne State University in 1970. Her major was biochemistry. A number of women have since received doctoral degrees, but of primary interest is Judith Pachizarz, who got her Ph.D. in biochemistry in 1971 from St. Louis University. However, she decided the Ph.D. was not good enough, and obtained her M.D. in Kentucky. Dr. Pachizarz may be the first and only deaf person to hold both a Ph.D. and M.D.

Rehabilitation/Services for Deaf Adults

Petra F. Howard was probably the first deaf person to pioneer in labor and vocational rehabilitation. In 1915, she served as the chief of the newly established Minnesota Labor Bureau of the Deaf, first of its kind in the U.S.—a forerunner of Vocational Rehabilitation Bureaus. In 1930, the Labor Bureau was assimilated by the State Department of Vocational Rehabilitation. Dr. Howard worked as a counselor until 1956 and then as a specialist for the deaf until 1959. She was granted an honorary doctoral degree by Gallaudet College in 1960 as well as several citations, one of which was from President Eisenhower. A residential therapeutical center for the deaf in St. Paul bears her name.

Edna P. Adler worked in a federal project in Lansing, Michigan for severely disabled deaf adults. At that time little was being done for this special population, and she became a pioneer in the special field of program development for severely handicapped deaf adults. Today, Dr. Adler is known as the first and only deaf woman in a significant federal position of nationwide influence. She serves as the assistant chief of the Deafness and Communicative Disorders Branch of the Rehabilitation Services Administration in Washington, DC, where she has worked for the past 16 years. In the course of her work, she has facilitated the development and expansion of mental health services, interpreting, manual communication, training and research across the nation.

Sports

Even in sports, deaf women have had their share of "firsts." The first deaf pilot in the U.S. and probably in the world was a woman, Nellie Zabel Willhite, in 1928. Charles Lindberg had flown the *Spirit of St. Louis* across the Atlantic Ocean just the year before. Female pilots were a rarity in these days. Ms. Willhite became a folk heroine in her home state, South Dakota, and her plane is on permanent display in the Taylor Museum at Hill City, SD.

A woman, Gertrude Ederle, became the first hearing impaired person honored, in 1953, with a place in the Helms Foundation Hall of Fame, which was established in 1936 to honor those who promoted amateur athletics. Ms. Ederle, the first woman to swim across the English Channel in 1926, became deaf from this ordeal. Two deaf men were finally admitted to the Helms Halls of Fame 20 years later, in 1973.

When the American Athletic Association for the Deaf initiated its annual Athlete of the Year award in 1955, the first recipient was, Helen Thomas, from California, for her achievement as the Women's North American Skeet Shooting Champion.

Another star in the sports arena is Kitty O'Neil, who is known as the "deaf daredevil," in Hollywood circles. In her stunt work, she has jumped off a 10-story building, crashed cars, been set afire, plunged over a 100-foot waterfall, and leaped off a 105-foot cliff, the highest jump ever filmed of a woman. She has broken speed records in her rocket-powered cars and earned the title "Fastest Woman on Earth."

The World Games for the Deaf provide opportunities for athletes to prove their physical prowess. Two American super water athletes emerged from the 1976 WFD games, with 10 medals each and victory for the U.S. team: Laurie Barber from Pennsylvania and Jeff Float from California. What also makes Ms. Barber remarkable was that she was 14 years old at the time.

Journalism

Many deaf women have pioneered and contributed to the field of journalism, creative poetry and publishing. To highlight a few here is a difficult task and is not intended to diminish the achievement of many other deaf women.

Laura Searling, starting in the 1920's, was an accomplished newspaper reporter and poet. She wrote under the pseudonym Howard Glyndon. Her "Belle Missouri" became the battle song of the Missouri Union Army. Her name is one of very few deaf persons included in the *Dictionary of American Biography*. Her work was published in the *St. Louis Republican, the New York Times, New York Sun, Galaxy, Harper's* and other newspapers and journals.

Annually, several awards are presented to deaf youth for leadership and excellence. One is the Helen Muse Award for Fiction. Ms. Muse, author of *Green Pavilions* (1961), is a deaf faculty member of the Georgia School for the Deaf.

Communications

Bill Stokoe has earned the well-deserved honor of being the one to establish the American Sign Language as a valid language in and of its own right. However, did you know that he had two deaf colleagues, Dot Casterline and Carl Croneberg, working with him in his early days, and both of them also coauthored with Dr. Stokoe the first book on ASL, *Dictionary of American Sign Language on Linguistic Principles,* in 1965? Carol Padden has been intensely involved in research of ASL, has coauthored "A Basic Course in American Sign Language" (1980), and is now working on her dissertation for a Ph.D. in Linguistics. When she completes it she will be the first deaf person with a doctorate in this quickly mushrooming field of study of so much significance to us all.

In the area of signed communication there has also been a phenomenal growth in manually coded sign systems, which started in the early 1970's with a small group of educators and parents who believed that deaf children learn by seeing, rather than by stimulated versions of "hearing." Thus, they worked on ways to manually code English, that is, they devised signs that would make English completely visual and represented on the hands. Of the three manually coded English systems that developed, only "Signing Exact English" (SEE 11), has had nationwide impact in education of deaf children. The driving force behind SEE 11 was Dr. Gerilee Gustason, who has been deaf since childhood and who has taught deaf students in schools and colleges.

There are many characters involved in the continuing controversy relative to use of Signs, however, one person stands out as a pioneer in bilingual theory as applies to deafness. This is Barbara Kannapell, who has published articles and is currently working on a doctoral dissertation in Sociolinguistics on the subject of bilingualism and deafness. Both Ms. Padden and Ms. Kannapell have stressed the importance of the deaf culture and the deaf community in relations to research, education, or services relative to deafness.

Of great importance in spreading on an international basis the merits of sign language is a woman, Frances (Peggy) Parsons, who has earned the nickname of the "Total Communication Ambassador of the World." She has almost single-handedly developed significant contacts and growing acceptance of deafness and sign language in many nations where she has, on a voluntary basis, visited, worked and shared with natives. She has also opened doors for young deaf people in the Peace Corps, when she served as the first deaf participant in 1974 in the Philippines. Ms. Parsons, as a role model, opened the eyes and hearts of parents and teachers in other nations to the fact their deaf children, too, could develop skills, self-esteem and independence.

Television

A major break-through for deaf television viewers came in 1972, when Jane Wilk and Peter Wechsberg pioneered a daily live news program called NEWSIGN 4 in San Francisco. Although the first signed TV news occured in 1959 with John Tubergen, the 1959 program was a weekly, interpreted news program lasting 39 weeks. The success of the Wilk-Wechsberg NEWSIGN 4 resulted in a ripple of signed and interpreted news programs across the nation. Those were in the days before captioned television began, and probably helped to strengthen justification for more special programming and captions for deaf viewers.

Performing Arts

You undoubtedly know of the National Theatre of the Deaf, started in 1965. The NTD has been instrumental in educating the public about deafness and the beauty of sign language. The NTD has served as a much-needed approach for fostering positive social attitudes toward deaf people. Subsequently, NTD performers have become well-known personalities in their own right, and have appeared on national television and theatre: Audree Norton (e.g. *Mannix, Streets of San Francisco*), Linda Bove (e.g. *Sesame Street*) and Phyllis Frelich, who won the 1980 Tony Award for her leading role in *Children of a Lesser God*, a

Broadway play based on her relationship with her husband. This is the first time any deaf performer has won the Tony Award. Special shows for the deaf have also appeared on TV, such as the *Rainbow's End*, featuring Freda Norman as the Supersign Woman.

The Gallaudet College Dancers, who have amazed and entertained audiences with their skills for more than 20 years, also bear mention here. Albeit the fact that the director was a male, Dr. Wisher, the program would be nowhere without the dancers themselves, who are, for the most part, if not all, deaf females.

Art

Art and museums have long been a fascination for Debbie Sonnenstrahl, who had countless meetings, wrote countless letters, and walked countless miles to drive home the point that museums had to be communicatively accessible to deaf people. Her efforts paid off in spades: interpreters for deaf people, written texts, and the establishment of a special education unit within the regular education department mandated by large American museums everywhere. Currently enrolled in a doctoral program at New York University, Ms. Sonnenstrahl is the only deaf person acting as a liaison with museums, serving on an advisory board, conducting presentations and workshops nationwide, and developing publications so that museums can better respond to the special needs of deaf people and also that deaf people can better appreciate their visual world in terms of the arts.

Regina Olson Highes worked 33 years as a scientific illustrator in botany for the Agricultural Research Division. Retirement in 1969 did not still her pen; she went to work for the Smithsonian Institute. Her work has won her wide acclaim and honors: the Superior Service Award from the Department of Agriculture, the honorary degree of Doctor of Humane Letters from Gallaudet College, and the naming of a new species of Bromeliad, *Billbergia Regina* in her honor by the Smithsonian Museum. She may soon go "international" since her services have been requested in England.

Betty Miller may be the first deaf artist to portray in her art work the methodoligical war that has been ravaging the field of education of the deaf, i.e. Oralism vs Signs. Her paintings are to the point, playing up deaf students as pleasant and passive, wearing various auditory gadgets, with exagerated hands that, although restricted, plead to be freed and used. Dr. Miller is also the first Gallaudet female graduate to have earned a Ph.D., in 1976 from Pennsylvania State University, in art education. Dr. Miller was one of the founders and co-directors of Spectrum, which brought national focus to deaf artists and the deaf culture.

Library

When one talks about public libraries, the name that leaps to mind is that of Alice Hagemeyer. She wasn't the first librarian by any means, but she was a primary moving force behind creative accessibility for deaf people to public libraries nationwide. She initiated the observation of Deaf Awareness (Deaf Action) week in the DC Public Library in December, 1974, a program which has spread to libraries in other cities. Her reason for this observation in December, rather than May, the traditional Better Hearing Month, is linked to the fact that many pioneers in deafness share a December birthday: T. H. Gallaudet, Laurent Clerc, Ludwig Van Beethoven, and Laura Dewey Bridgeman, who was the first educated deaf-blind American and served as a model for Helen Keller. Thus, a week in December would strengthen acceptance of deafness and appreciation of the rich deaf culture. (Note: Deaf Awareness Week first took place in Colorado in November, 1972, spearheaded by Mr. & Mrs. Jerry Moers. Betty Moers appeared in television public spot announcements proclaiming deaf awareness week.) Mrs. Hagemeyer's *Red Notebook*, a resource book for

libraries on deafness, services and accessibility, became the first and only official book on library services for deaf people, endorsed at the White House Conference on Libraries and Information Services, and approved by the American Library Association and the National Association of the Deaf. In 1980 she was selected for the National Association of the Deaf President's Award for her pioneering efforts to spread deaf awareness in the library world and library awareness in the deaf community.

Litagation

It may be of interest to know that pioneering efforts to secure rights through the judicial channel were made by women. Frances Davis is a deaf woman who went all the way to the Supreme Court in 1979 to challenge the decision of a nursing college in North Carolina to deny her admission on the basis of her deafness. Although the Supreme Court ruled in favor of the nursing college, Ms. Davis may be the first deaf person to reach the Supreme Court. Through this courageous woman, it became clear that attitudes cannot be legislated and that we need to intensify awareness and understanding about deafness in our communities and states.

On the other hand, Ruth Ann Schornstein filed a suit against the New Jersey Vocational Rehabilitation Agency to secure interpreters for her education at Kean college, and got the federal district court to rule favorably, in 1980. Amy Rowley is a deaf daughter of deaf parents who successfully sued a New York public school for interpreters services.

Jr. NAD

The name "Jr. NAD" brings to mind notables such as Dr. Garretson and Frank Turk. Did you know that the Jr. NAD concept was first proposed at the 1960 NAD Convention in Dallas, Texas by a woman, Mrs. Caroline H. Burnes, the wife of NAD President Burnes? She encouraged the establishment of Jr. NAD with affiliates in schools for the deaf to develop leadership among deaf youths. Mrs. Burnes can well be considered the modern-day version of Juliette Gordon Low, who established the Girl Scouts, a great international Association, in 1912. Incidentally, Juliette Gordon Low, became deaf in one ear after dislodging wedding rice from her ear. Today, the Jr. NAD with its motto "Promoting the Tomorrow of All the Deaf by Working With the Deaf Youth of Today" has more than 100 chapters and a membership of over 3,000.

Melinda Chapel Padden, as a school student, chaired the first Youth Leadership Conference at the Indiana School for the Deaf in 1968, with the guidance of Gary Olsen. Mrs. Padden later became the National Director of Jr. NAD.

NAD

For the first time, the NAD has a woman in its presidential office. The NAD President for the 1980-1982 term is a woman with dynamic leadership capacity. She is Gertie Galloway, who works as the principal of the Maryland School for the Deaf at Columbia. She first coined the expression, "The deaf child has the right to be deaf."

The present NAD Board has five female board members. Fifteen of our 50 State Associations are now led by a female President. Muriel Horton-Strassler, the current editor of NAD publications, the *Deaf American* and The *Broadcaster* wields a mighty pen.

Summary

Deaf women of America have and are continuing to play vital roles in the making of the history and the future of deaf people everywhere. It is only relatively recent that deaf women started to view themselves as main actors, along with deaf men. Young deaf women do need to see female role models in action in order that they, too, may contribute to the weaving of the tapestry of deaf awareness and deaf rights. Behind each successful person is a score of women and men, past and present, providing support and inspiration.

Poetry Without Sound

Edward Klima and Ursula Bellugi

The Greek poet Simonides once called poetry "painting with the gift of speech." We have discovered a different kind of poetry, one that lacks the gift of speech but possesses in its place the gift of gesture. For some years we have been studying the structure of American Sign Language (ASL), a manual-visual language used by most of the deaf people in this country to communicate with one another. Among those who have aided us in our research have been member's of the National Theater of the Deaf, a remarkably talented group of actors who are either deaf or the hearing offspring of deaf parents. These creative artists are developing before our very eyes a poetic tradition unlike any other—a tradition based on the very special characteristics of "signing."

In order to appreciate the uniqueness of signed poetry, one must know something about the language in which it is composed. Hearing people, who have only limited contact with the deaf, sometimes confuse sign language with finger spelling, which is not a distinct language at all. Finger spelling is a derivative system based on written English, which, in turn, is a derivative system based on spoken English. One simply uses the fingers to form, in the air, symbols that represent the letters of the alphabet. Fluent ASL signers use finger spelling primarily for names and for borrowing English words. Some sign systems are also connected with spoken language. For example, Signing Essential English uses signs to match English word order in a virtual sign-for-word translation of English, down to the last if, and, and but, including sign markers invented to match English affixes. Such English-based systems are often used in educational settings.

American Sign Language, on the other hand, is passed on from deaf parents to deaf children, and is a language in its own right, a full-fledged linguistic system. ASL signs are not based on English words, and a sign may or may not have an exact single-word English equivalent, just as a word in Russian or German may or may not have an exact English equivalent. Furthermore, ASL has its own methods for modifying the meanings of signs—for changing a sign from a verb to a noun, for indicating plural or temporal aspects, for extending the meaning of a sign from the purely literal to the metaphorical, for coining new terms, and so forth. Just as in a spoken language, ASL signs are not situation bound; signers can refer to other times, other places. And, as with spoken languages, individual signs may be combined into an unlimited number of statements. The syntax of ASL, the rules that determine what is and is not grammatical, is not based on any spoken language, but makes full use of mechanisms available to a visual-gestural language, including the elaborate use of spatial constructs.

The radical differences between signs and words are apparent from the way they are organized. A spoken word consists of a sequence of contrasting acoustical segments called phonemes, arranged sequentially. For instance, the word "feeling" breaks down into the phonemes f, i, l, i, and n. A sign, on the other hand, is essentially the *simultaneous* occurrence of particular values of a limited set of formational parameters. Every sign is composed of a hand configuration

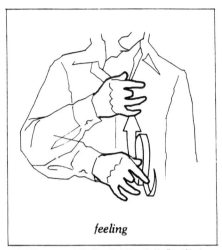

feeling

© Klima and Bellugi, The Salk Institute

(or sometimes two, if both hands are used), a relationship between the two hands, a particular orientation of the hands, a place of articulation with respect to the rest of the body, and movements of the hands. To make the sign that translates as "feeling" in English, a signer uses one hand with the palm facing the body (orientation). The hand is flat and spread, with the middle finger bent in (configuration). It contacts the middle of the chest (place of articulation), making repeated upward strokes (movement).

Contrary to common belief, signs in American Sign Language are not merely pantomimic gestures. Just as the particular sounds of a word have no logical connection to its meaning, the way a sign is formed in ASL does not necessarily have anything to do with the meaning of that sign. It is true that many signs originate in pantomime, and certainly the mimetic aspects of the language are still very much alive. However, as a new sign comes into widespread use, it tends to lose some iconic aspects and become stylized and conventionalized. Usually a nonsigner will not be able to guess the meaning of a sign simply from the way it is made—and neither, for that matter, will a deaf person who knows only British Sign Language or Chinese Sign Language, which are quite different from ASL.

We became interested in the study of signed poetry not only for its own sake but also because we felt that by analyzing the heightened uses of ASL—poetry, wit, plays on signs—we could learn quite a bit about the linguistic features of the language. In a poem, linguistic features are more than just fleeting vehicles for the expression of meaning. A person who wishes either to write poetry or to appreciate it must be sensitive to the form of the language as well as to meaning: to grammatical categories as grammatical categories, and, in spoken poems, to sound as sound. Thus, as far as meaning is concerned, it matters little that "June," "moon," "croon," and "swoon" have the same vowel and final consonant sounds—that they rhyme. But when the words are embedded in sentences patterned in a certain way, the sentences become verse, even though they may express inanities and the result is doggerel. We suspected that in signed poetry, too, we would find the manipulation of language for language's sake—the essence of the poetic function.

In spoken poetry, one finds various types of internal poetic structure, by which we mean structure that is formed by elements internal to the linguistic system proper: words, sounds, and so forth. At one level, there is a "conventional" structure determined by cultural tradition. In the English literary tradition, conventional structures make use of various metrical schemes, such as iambic pentameter, as well as end-rhyme schemes that dictate the recurrence of sounds in a predictable pattern. The Elizabethan sonnet is a conventional structure, as is the haiku form, borrowed from the Japanese poetic tradition. In structurally complex poetry, the conventional structure is overlaid by and interwoven with more innovative "individual" structures that involve the subtle patterning of sounds, words, grammatical forms, and meanings unique to the particular poem.

We have found that in signed poetry, the patterning of a poem is by-and-large individual rather than conventional. There is not yet anything analogous to the rigid, invariant structure of

Conventional ASL

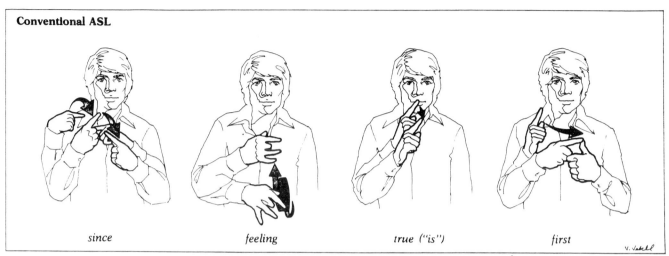

since   *feeling*   *true ("is")*   *first*

© Klima and Bellugi, The Salk Institute

there are at least two types of structure that are special to signed poetry and that greatly enhance its poetic effect. We call one of these the "external poetic structure"; it is produced by creating a balance between the two hands, or maintaining a flow of movement between signs. The other is a unique external structure that we call "imposed superstructure": a design in space, or a rhythmic and temporal pattern that is superimposed on the signs. In order to get at the distinctions between everyday signing and poetic signing, we asked Bernard Bragg, who is deaf and a master signer of the National Theater of the Deaf, to translate a poem by E. E. Cummings, "since feeling is first," into everyday sign and then into poetic form. The

Poetic sign

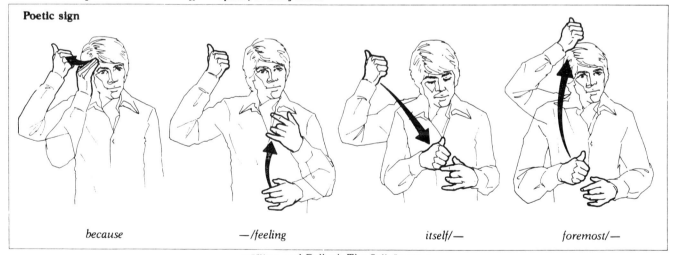

because   *—/feeling*   *itself/—*   *foremost/—*

© Klima and Bellugi, The Salk Institute
A dash and a slash before or after the name of a sign indicates that one hand from the preceding sign maintains the position and/or hand shape of that sign.

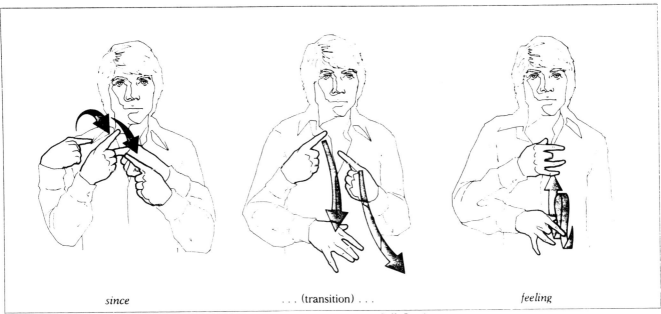

since   . . . (transition) . . .   *feeling*

© Klima and Bellugi, The Salk Institute

poem seemed peculiarly appropriate for linguists and artists to work on together:

    since feeling is first
    who pays any attention
    to the syntax of things
    will never wholly kiss you; . . .

We will discuss here only the first line. The drawings above show the signs that Bragg used to represent this line in conventional signing. In this version, each sign is a literal translation of the corresponding English word.

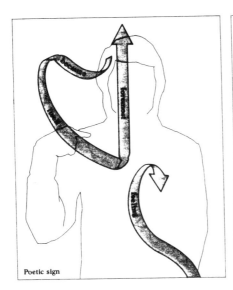

Poetic sign

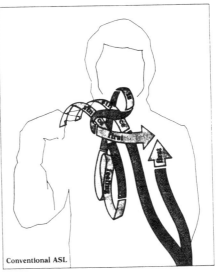

Conventional ASL

© Klima and Bellugi, The Salk Institute

"Summer" by Dorothy Miles (Miles rendition)

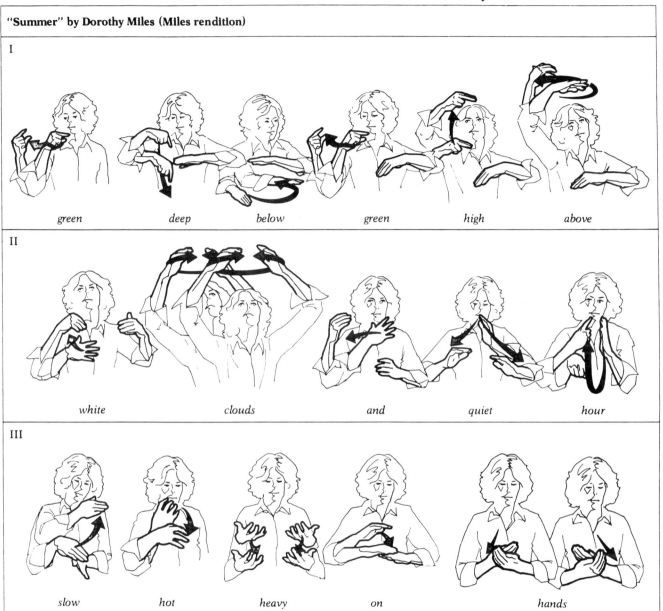

I

green   deep   below   green   high   above

II

white   clouds   and   quiet   hour

III

slow   hot   heavy   on   hands

Note that in the sign *since,* both hands are active, and they operate symmetrically. *Feeling* and *true* are one-handed signs. In *first*, one active hand operates on the other as a base. Since Bragg is right-handed, he makes the one-handed signs with his right hand and leaves his left hand lax,

by his side. As Bragg shifts from one sign to another, there are several changes in hand shape. The right hand starts with an "index" hand, changes to a "mid-finger" hand, and then changes back again to an index hand for the last two signs. The left hand starts with an index hand, drops

Five-finger hand

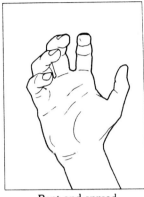 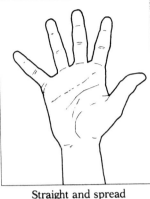 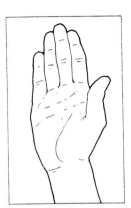

| Bent and spread | Straight and spread | Straight and compact |

© Klima and Bellugi, The Salk Institute

down toward the side of the body, and returns with a "fist" hand. There are various hand movements in the signs, and, although the illustration does not show them, there are also movements back and forth and up and down during transitions between signs. For example, at the end of *since*, the left hand relaxes and drops to the side, and the right hand moves down to the initial position of *feeling*.

Now consider the transformation of the poem into poetic style, in Bragg's capable hands. First of all, Bragg replaces all of the signs except *feeling*. The first sign of the original version, *since* is a literal translation of the English word, but it is not really semantically appropriate since in ASL it would ordinarily convey only the tem-

poral sense of the word. The form of the new sign, *because*, is very different froom that of *since*. Its final hand configuration is a fist with the thumb extended, and it moves from contact with the forehead to a final position off to the side of the head. The choice of *because* is related to the other choices in the line, because the other new signs share the same hand shape. Instead of *true*, Bragg uses *itself*, and instead of *first*, he creates a sign using a one-handed rendition of *most* (which is normally a two-handed sign), combined with a marker for the superlative, *-est*. Bragg translated the new sign as "mostest," and, we have called it "foremost." A deaf viewer would have no trouble interpreting it. The resulting line of poetry, then, has four signs made with one hand active, and the three made with the right hand share the same hand shape. We feel that this feature of hand shape similarity is probably analogous to the alliterative repetition of vowels or consonants in spoken poetry.

The choice of signs in a poem is part of its internal poetic structure. Bragg's translation also reveals an external poetic structure defined not by the choice of signs but by the pattern of their presentation. One aspect of this structure is balance. In ordinary conversation, a signer usually uses his or her dominant hand to make one-handed signs and as the active hand in signs requiring one hand to act on another. Since only about a third of all ASL signs involve the use of

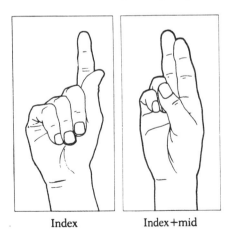

| Index | Index+mid |

© Klima and Bellugi, The Salk Institute

"Summer" by Dorothy Miles (Fant rendition)

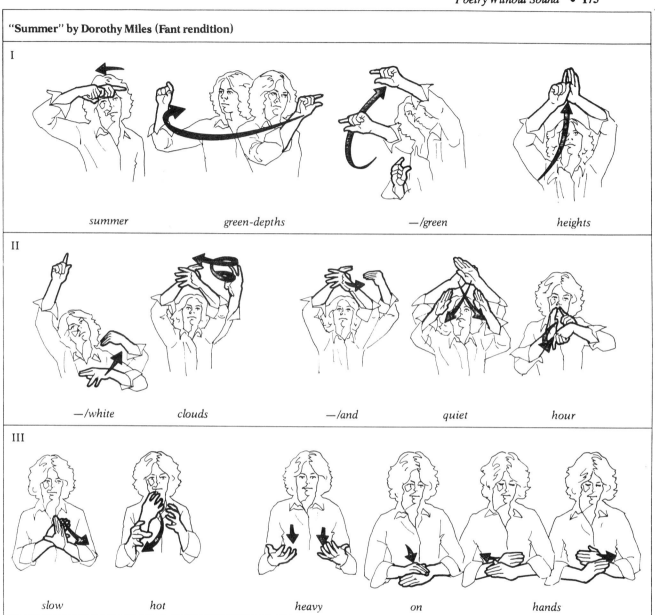

I

summer · green-depths · —/green · heights

II

—/white · clouds · —/and · quiet · hour

III

slow · hot · heavy · on · hands

© Klima and Bellugi, The Salk Institute

two active hands, most of the time there is an imbalance in the use of the hands. In the poetry being created by the National Theater of the Deaf, however, the signer may maintain balance by imposing a pattern of hand alternation that keeps both hands more equally in use. One method is to change hands with consecutive signs. Note that after signing *because* with his right hand, Bragg does not sign *feeling* with his right hand, as he ordinarily would, but with his left. He leaves *because* hanging in the air, as it were.

Another way to achieve balance is to overlap two distinct signs. After making the first sign, Bragg uses both hands at all times. While he signs

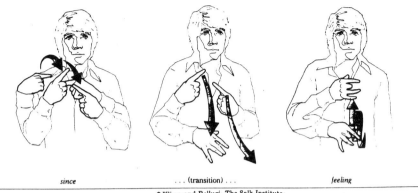

since   . . . (transition) . . .   *feeling*

© Klima and Bellugi, The Salk Institute

feeling he holds the sign *because* in its final position. Then he holds *feeling* (made with the left hand), and, in a way that would never occur in colloquial signing, he directs toward it the one-handed sign *itself* (made with the right hand). This emphasizes the fact that *itself* refers to *feeling*. Then Bragg continues to hold the hand configuration and final position of *feeling*, still with the left hand, while he makes *foremost* with his right hand.

Besides achieving a balance between the hands, Bragg also creates a continuous flow of movement of signs, another aspect of external poetic structure. We have found that to create this sort of continuity a poet may distort the form of the signs themselves, going beyond the grammatical code of the language, and may also manipulate the transitions between signs, as if to avoid any wasted movement.

The picture above shows the signs *since* and *feeling* in nonpoetic signing. The center drawing shows the transition between the signs. Notice that after *since* Bragg drops his left hand to his side, because it is not used in the sign that follows. During the transition, he moves his right hand from the final location of *since* to the initial location of *feeling,* at the same time changing hand shapes. In the poetic version of the line, however, Bragg manipulates the form of the signs so that effectively there is no transition: The final position of the hand after making each sign is

precisely the starting position of the next. The final position of *because,* which as we noted before is held during the signing of *feeling,* becomes the starting position of *itself,* and the final position of *itself* becomes the starting position of *foremost.* This continuity of movement would not exist in conversational signing of the same sequence of signs.

Finally, Bragg creates an imposed superstructure; it results partly from some of the distortions we have discussed, but is a separate level of structure. In this case a pattern of movement is superimposed on the signs of the line much as a melody is superimposed on the words of a song. We made flow charts of Bragg's hand movements in the nonpoetic and poetic versions of the Cummings line. You can see that in the poetic version there is a definite design in space, characterized by large, open, nonintersecting movements.

There are many problems in translating a poem from one language to another, and Bragg's task was even more challenging, since he was translating from one mode, the auditory, to another, the visual. In our laboratory we have also had the opportunity to study some original signed poetry. One of the poems we have analyzed, "The Seasons," by Dorothy Miles, is special in that the poet composed it simultaneously in American Sign Language and in English. (Miles, who has been profoundly deaf since the age of eight, has a brilliant command of both languages.) "The Seasons" consists of four verses; in the English version each verse is in the standard haiku form: three lines, with five syllables in the first and last lines and seven in the middle line. The compression and rich imagery of poems in the haiku style seem especially suited to sign language.

Here is the English text of the verse entitled "Summer":

Green depths, green heights, clouds
And quiet hours, slow, hot,
Heavy on the hands.

In addition to the conventional haiku structure, there is an individual structure that involves, among other things, repeated patterns of similar sounds. Here, though, we are more interested in the signed version. Miles's rendition suggests division into three "lines" as shown in the accompanying illustration (which we made by tracing images on a video tape of Miles performing her poem).

One of the most striking things about this verse is that it uses only a few of the possible hand configurations in ASL, variously estimated at between 19 and 40. Of the 16 signs in the verse, 13 use a "five-finger" hand in their citation form, either as the active hand or as a base, and sometimes both. The fingers may be bent and spread, straight and spread, or straight and compact, but in all 13 signs the five fingers are extended. Furthermore, through a distortion that is part of the external poetic structure, the five-finger hand becomes part of every sign in the verse after the first *green*. *High* and *green* are normally one-handed signs that do not use this hand shape, but Miles keeps the left hand in five-finger position as a kind of reference base or surface indicator throughout the signing of *deep below, green high above*. This modification provides a consistency to the forms of the signs in the first line.

In poetry, patterning is more important than mere frequency, and so we need to look at the patterning of hand shapes. The first line of the verse consists of two parallel halves, each beginning with an index hand (the first and second

appearance of *green*). Each half ends with an active five-finger hand operating below or above a base five-finger hand (the signs *below* and *above*), in similar arcs. The second sign of the first half, *deep*, uses an index hand as the active hand; the second sign of the second half, *high*, uses what we call an index+mid hand shape, which is only slightly different from the index hand. The first line is semantically patterned as well. The first signs of each half are the same (*green* and *green*). The second signs in each half are opposites (*deep* and *high*), and so are the third signs in each half (*below* and *above*).

The second line, *white clouds and quiet hour*, also reveals internal poetic structure. Notice that *white* and *and* are each one-handed signs with a five-finger hand closing to a tapered *O*. Both *white* and *and* are followed by a two-handed, five-finger sign (*clouds* and *quiet*, respectively). It is clear that the pattern forms an intentional individual structure, especially since the sign *white*, the first sign in the pattern, is not represented by a word in the English version of the poem. Finally, the last sign in the line, *hour*, echoes in its active right hand the index-hand motif of the first line, and combines it with the five-finger motif that dominates the second line and, in fact, the entire verse.

The third and final line of the stanza, *slow, hot, heavy on hands,* consists exclusively of five-finger hands in signs made in front of the chest with the hands touching or close together. There is variation in movement, orientation, and intensity of the signs.

So far we have been discussing only the internal poetic structure of the poem. The patterns of external poetic structure that we found in Bernard Bragg's translation of "since feeling is first" are for the most part absent in Miles's rendition of "Summer." When we talked to Miles about her poem, we learned that she intended to keep the signs as close to their normal form as possible. In this rendition, she does not alternate hands in order to create a sense of balance; she uses her right hand in all one-handed signs and as the

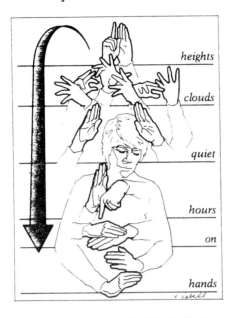

heights

clouds

quiet

hours

on

hands

© Klima and Bellugi, The Salk Institute

active hand in signs where one hand acts on another, just as she would in conversation. Nor does she make a special effort to overlap signs. During one-handed signs she leaves her left hand either by her side, as in *hot,* or off to the side and without a specific shape, as in *white* and *and.* She does make some minor variations in the forms of signs in order to produce certain effects, but she clearly does not make the major distortions necessary to create a design in space. Where Bragg displaced signs spatially to produce a kinetic superstructure, Miles makes all her signs within the normal signing space, not only in this verse but in her other ones as well.

However, a careful examination of "Summer" reveals a type of imposed super-structure that we did not find in the Cummings poem. It is not spatial, but temporal and rhythmic. Each of the three lines in the verse takes about 7.5 seconds to perform, although the individual signs vary in length. The first and second halves of the first line and the second half of the last line have a similar rhythm, with four accents. The other three half-lines of the verse have fewer accents. We can represent this rhythmic-temporal superstructure

in musical notation, and we are tempted to compare its effect with that of an operatic recitative, in which there is something of a cross between speaking and singing.

Different signers may favor different styles of poetic signing. Therefore we asked Lou Fant, who like Miles has been with the National Theater of the Deaf, to perform his own rendition of "Summer," working from the English text alone. First of all, Fant made the title a part of the first line of the poem. His other sign choices were not radically different from those of Miles, but neither were they identical. For example, he expresses the word "depths" from the English version not by a separate sign but by extending the sign *green* in a wide sweep of the arm, which gives the impression of *green* moving into the distance away from him. His rendition differs from Miles's in the direction of more structural regularity. All four signs in the first line use an index hand as active, and this motif has an echo in the last sign of the second line, *hour.*

But the most significant distinction between Fant's version and Miles's is in external poetic structure. Fant, like Bragg, modifies the form of the signs or aspects of their presentation to create an external structure. If you examine the accompanying pictures, you will see that he uses patterned alternation of the hands throughout the poem: *green-depths* is with the right hand, the second *green* with the left; *heights* with the right hand, *white* with the left, and so on. He also uses the technique of overlapping signs. By alternating the hands he can overlap even one-handed signs that occur in sequence: he holds the form of a just-executed sign with one hand, while he makes the next sign with the other. For example, the final position and shape of the right hand for *heights* remain through the signing of *white* with the left hand. In this way Fant can present two signs simultaneously to the eye of the viewer

When Bragg translated the Cummings poem, he controlled the flow of movement for poetic effect. Fant does the same in "Summer." Signs do not begin and end in the same positions as in ordinary signing. Fant also manipulates the transitions so that the final position of one sign becomes the starting position of the next. This eliminates superfluous movement, and one sign simply flows into another. There is also an obvious design in space that is consistent with the theme of the verse: heaviness. Fant makes the signs of the first two lines much higher than they would otherwise be. Beginning with the second line, the signs slowly descend from far above the signer's head—a location not used in everyday signing—to below the waist. At the end of the verse, the body is bent over, the shoulders are hunched, and the hands are low in the signing space.

This rendition of "Summer" exhibits one other feature that is quite prominent in signed poetry: In some of the signs, Fant exaggerates the representational or pantomimic aspects. Consider the title sign, *summer,* which Fant incorporates into the body of the poem. The usual form of this sign involves a bent index finger that brushes across the central part of the forehead. When we asked Shanny Mow, a deaf signer, to review our video tapes of the poem, he noticed that Fant elaborates *summer* by "increasing its length . . . thus producing a more pantomime-like action." He uses an outstretched index finger that gradually bends to form the conventional hand shape, and he "wipes" the entire length of his forehead—as if to wipe away the sweat caused by the summer's heat.

Mow also pointed out that in signing *clouds,* the hands rotate slowly across the space overhead, to portray the drifting of the clouds. The sign *heavy,* Mow observed, "certainly looks heavy, so heavy that the bottom drops. . . . One begins to feel the oppressive claustrophobic heat and time standing still as the long summer drags on." The sign *slow,* in Miles's rendition as well as in Fant's, is longer than usual in terms of both time and space. Ordinarily the finger-tips of the active, flat, five-finger hand brush once over the back of the base hand from the fingertips to the wrist. In Miles's version, the active hand, as it

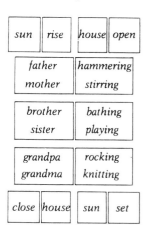

sun	rise	house	open
father mother		hammering stirring	
brother sister		bathing playing	
grandpa grandma		rocking knitting	
close	house	sun	set

This poem for four hands has great symmetry, even though — except for the opening and closing lines — the actors are portraying different words.

brushes over the base hand, continues well up toward the shoulder.

Poetry in sign language is still actively evolving and new poetic forms continually emerge. Joe Castronovo and Ella Lentz, two deaf signers who have worked with us, experimented with the signed equivalent of a duet. They were inspired by a well-known children's game called Double Personality. One person stands with his arms at rest and allows them to be replaced by the arms of a second person standing behind him. The effect is reminiscent of the many-armed Hindu god, Shiva. In the culture of the deaf, the game often involves signing. Castronovo and Lentz noticed that when both people signed, it seemed as if the person in front was talking to himself and was answered by his "other voice." They decided to compose a poem for four hands.

At the beginning of the poem, a male stands behind a female, and both sign. The resulting blend describes the sun rising on the horizon, where there is a house. As we approach the house, the door opens. At this point the two signers split apart, the male going to the right and the female to the left. Now each begins to sign a separate message. The male signs *father,* and then *hammering* (a very iconic sign that mimics the motions of hammering). At the same time the female signs *mother* and *stirring* (also iconic). The male signs *big* and *brother* while the female signs *little* and *sister.* The male signs *bathing* and the female signs *playing.* The male signs *grandpa* and *rocking* while the female signs *grandma* and *knitting.* The signs are made with strong, rhythmic beats, in clusters of three beats at the end of each line. Then, in the final section of the poem, the signers blend once again to describe the door of the house closing, the house receding into the distance, and the sun setting on the horizon.

An interesting feature of this poem is that the signs in the middle section form minimal pairs. The signs *father, brother,* and *grandpa* are exactly like their matched pairs *mother, sister,* and *grandma,* except that the male signs are made on the forehead while the female signs are made near the lower cheek. *Big* and *little* are identical except for location. *Bathing* and *playing* differ in location and handshape, but they are made here with similar up and down movements. *Rocking* and *knitting* have different hand shapes, but both are made with the same strikingly similar to-and-fro rhythmic movements. These similarities give the poem a very symmetrical internal structure.

Studies like these have taught us much about this soundless language. Many years ago, when we first began to study ASL, we read that sign language was "a collection of vague and loosely defined pictorial gestures"; that it was characterized by "grammatical disorder, illogical systems, and linguistic confusion"; that it was "a pidgin form of English on the hands with no structure of its own." Although these views have been dispelled, most people are not aware of the poetic tradition developing in the language. This tradition shows how human beings, deprived of spoken language, devise ways to express the poetic imagination.

For further information:

Bellugi, Ursula. "Formal Devices for Creating New Signs in ASL " *Proceedings of the National Symposium on Sign Language Research and Teaching,* ed. by William Stokoe. Cambridge University Press, 1978.

Bellugi, Ursula, Edward S. Klima, and Patricia Siple. "Remembering in Signs." *Cognition: International Journal of Cognitive Psychology,* Vol. 3, No. 2, 1975.

Klima, Edward S., and Ursula Bellugi. "Poetry and Song in a Language without Sound." *Cognition: International Journal of Cognitive Psychology.* Vol. 4, No. 1, 1976.

Klima, Edward S., and Ursula Bellugi. *The Signs of Language.* Harvard University Press, 1979 (in press).

Reflections of American Deaf Culture in Deaf Humor

MJ Bienvenu

Mainstream American culture teaches that "normal" people are born with five senses: hearing, sight, smell, taste, and touch. Of course, Deaf people can't hear, and this causes many people to view the Deaf as deficient and deprived. But nothing could be further from the truth—we have always had five senses: sight, smell, taste, touch, and a sense of humor.

Humor is one way that people share their perceptions of the world, express different levels of intimacy, and find comfort in knowing that others share their beliefs. I am going to focus specifically on four categories which reflect the values, norms, and belief systems of our American Deaf Culture.

Visual

As most of you know, Deaf people perceive most things through their eyes. We acquire language visually. It is worth noting that Sign Languages throughout the world adapt to meet the visual needs and comfort of the people who use them. We also acquire world knowledge visually. It should come as no surprise, then, that Deaf humor also has a strong visual base. To many Deaf people, the world is filled with comical sights. But the humor is not always apparent to the majority of hearing Americans.

An experience I had several years ago may illustrate this point: One night while I was coordinating an intensive ASL retreat for a group of non-Deaf people, we gathered together to watch the movie *King Kong* on TV. The volume was off, and for the first time, they realized what Deaf audiences have known all along: the actors' ex-

pressions are hysterically funny. As New Yorkers were running for their lives with the shadow of a monster ape looming over their heads, our group was laughing uncontrollably. I asked them what they found so funny. They replied, "Their faces!" The same people would have felt frightened if they had heard the actors screaming in terror or, with threatening music in the background. Instead, they got a glimpse of the movies from a Deaf perspective.

Deaf people find many visual things humorous which aurally dependent people may not. Often Deaf people are quite creative in their descriptions of people and events. This talent is fostered in residential schools where many children learn the art of storytelling, and most importantly, how to vividly re-create events and characters. When I was in school, no one was safe from our stories. Every identifying characteristic of a person would be imitated, right down to the way s/he walked. This intricate detail is a crucial part of the humor, because it reflects how acutely Deaf people perceive the world, and how adept a tool our language is for expressing our perceptions.

Often people who are not members of the culture will respond negatively to this form of humor. This is a common misunderstanding with outsiders. Deaf people are not insulting the individuals whom we describe; we are delighting in the precision of our language to accurately convey these details. Our culture is reinforced through the shared experience of how we, as a group, see the world and translate it into humor.

Can't Hear

As we all know, deafness is much more than the inability to hear. It is a complete culture, where one's decibel loss is far less important than one's allegiance to the Deaf Community. Yet, a significant amount of Deaf folklore contains jokes and stories which deal with the inability to hear.

There are many stories that have been handed down for generations in Deaf folklore which illustrate the convenience of deafness. The following popular tale shows how Deaf people can solve a problem creatively and humorously: *A Deaf couple arrives at a motel for their honeymoon. After unpacking, the nervous husband goes out to get a drink. When he returns to the motel, he realizes that he has forgotten the room number. It is dark outside and all the rooms look identical. He walks to his car, and leans on the horn. He then waits for the lights to come on in the rooms of the waking angry hearing guests. All the rooms are lit up except his, where his Deaf wife is waiting for him!*

Interestingly, in Ray Holcomb's book, *Hazards of Deafness,* the humor does not follow the culturally Deaf tradition, but rather focuses on stories in which Deaf people lament their "condition." This humor is typical of an "outsider's" view of deafness. Here is an example of one of the scenes in the book: *A deaf person is having a difficult time vacuuming the carpet. He goes over the same spot of dirt repeatedly, to no avail. In a fit of frustration, he turns around and notices that the machine is unplugged.*

This is a perfect example of humor that is *not* Deaf centered. Such a situation would never happen because a Deaf person would naturally feel that the motor was not running and immediately respond appropriately. What is most disturbing is the emphasis on hearing and the dependency on sound which the book portrays. Culturally Deaf people are quite articulate in defining the world in terms other than sound, and have adapted to technology as swiftly as non-Deaf people. The fact that the author does not address Deaf people's keenly developed sense of sight and touch is rather significant.

Linguistic

Another component of Deaf humor can be categorized as linguistic. Production and misproduction of signs is a common way to elicit laughs in ASL. One example, described in Bellugi and Klima's book, *The Signs of Language*, is how we can change the root sign, UNDERSTAND, to LITTLE UNDERSTAND by using the pinkie rather than the index finger.

Much of this linguistic humor is lexically based, and the punch lines to many ASL jokes are related to the production of the words. One of my favorites is the "giant" joke. It is funny both culturally and linguistically: *A huge giant is stalking through a small village of wee people, who are scattering through the streets, trying to escape the ugly creature, The Giant notices one particularly beautiful blonde woman scampering down the cobble-stoned street. He stretches out his clumsy arm and sweeps her up, then stares in wonder at the slight, shivering figure in his palm. "You are so beautiful," he exclaims. The young woman looks up in fear. "I would never hurt you," he signs, "I love you! We should get MARRIED." Producing the sign MARRY, he crushes her. The giant then laments, "See, oralism, is better."*

There are several components which make this joke successful in American Sign Language. First, it is visually active, because the expressions of the townspeople, the beautiful girl, and the giant can be dramatized to perfection. Secondly, it is linguistically funny because of the sign production MARRY which causes the girl of his affection to splat in his palm. Thirdly, it is humorous in its irony. Culturally Deaf people detest oralism; therefore, the irony in the giant's conclusion that oralism would have saved his beloved girl is funny.

Response to Oppression

It is no secret that Deaf people are an oppressed minority, and one way that minority cultures deal with oppression is through humor. Often this category of humor, sometimes called "zap" stories, features Deaf people getting even.

Often when Deaf people are naturally conversing in public, hearing people will stare at them in disbelief. When they finally gain the courage to initiate conversation with a Deaf person, they will inevitably ask, "Can you read my lips?" Well, of course, Deaf people are keenly aware of the configuration of this one sentence, and will always answer "No!" which is pretty funny, indeed.

Another way Deaf humor fights back at oppression is to show hearing people being outsmarted by a Deaf person. One famous example, which is a true story, provides the required ending: *A group of Deaf people was at a restaurant, chatting away when a group of non-Deaf people at the next table began to rudely mimic their signs. One of the Deaf women decided she'd had enough. She walked to the public telephone, inserted a coin, and making sure she was being observed by the hearing group, signed a complete conversation into the handset, including pauses for the person on the other end to respond. When the Deaf group left the restaurant, they were amused to see the hearing people run over to inspect the phone.*

Deaf people love this one, because we finally have the last laugh. These tales are rich with justice, and always the rude offender is put in her/his place.

In the same way that American Deaf Culture, as well as European Deaf Culture, is oppressed by the majority community, so our language is oppressed. From oralism to Signed English systems and other forms of English/sound coding, Deaf people have suffered under the thumb of hearing educators for many years. From the signs that these "experts" invent, it is obvious they have little knowledge of Deaf Culture or ASL. Often the invented signs already have an established meaning. Many of them look sexual, and are really inappropriate for young children to see, which is ironic, since school systems teach them. It's even worse when they are printed in "sign language" books. Deaf children leaf through these sign-code manuals with delight, snickering at all the "dirty" signs pictured in the textbook.

As one response to these oppressive attempts at linguistic isolation, Deaf people have chosen to incorporate into their discourse some of the artificial codes created from the oral/cued speech/Signed English systems. Coded signs for IS, AM, ARE, WERE, BE, -ING, -ED, etc. have all been reclaimed by Deaf speakers, and used with sarcasm directed toward those who created them. Of course, the humor is most pronounced when a contorted face accompanies the deviant signs—an editorial on the ineffectiveness of these codes.

In closing, let me say that humor is an essential part of our lives. I'm sure you've all heard the expression, "laughter is the best medicine." Well, there is much truth to that, particularly when you analyze minority cultures, and realize that they all incorporate fighting back at oppression into their humor. It is a common response to the frustration of our everyday lives, for in humor, the storyteller determines who will "win." Someone told me this joke the other day, and it seemed like a perfect way to end my presentation:

Three people are on a train—one is Russian, one is Cuban, and one is Deaf. The Russian is drinking from a bottle of vodka. She drinks about half the bottle, then throws it out the window. The Deaf person looks at her, surprised. "Why did you throw out a bottle that was only half-empty?" The Russian replies, "Oh, in my country we have plenty of vodka." Meanwhile, the Cuban is smoking a rich, aromatic cigar. He smokes about half the cigar, then throws it out the window. The Deaf person is again surprised, and asks, "Why did you throw out the cigar?" He replies, "Oh, in Cuba we have plenty of cigars!" The Deaf person nods with interest. A little while later a hearing person walks down the aisle. The Deafie picks him up and tosses him out the window. The Russian and Cuban look up in amazement. The Deaf Person shrugs, "Oh, we have plenty of hearing people in the world."

Chapter 6

Family Life

All families confront complex issues of communication. Bridging the generation gap, sibling rivalry and resolving differences among family members are examples of the dilemmas that frequently face families. Families with deaf and hearing members have the added challenge of finding a common language with which to communicate. Are hearing parents skilled in American Sign Language? Do deaf children have intelligible speech or an adequate command of English? Are deaf and hearing family members fluent in the same language? The answers to these questions affect the basic quality of family life.

A further complication is that experts in the field of deafness have differing opinions about how parents should communicate with a deaf child. The oral philosophy counsels parents to use spoken English in family communications. They believe sign language impedes the acquisition of speech and the mastery of English. Oral educators argue that good speech, efficient lipreading and competence in English are critical for deaf children to achieve success in "the hearing world." They discourage *any* form of signing with deaf children.

Other professionals believe that manual communication is the best and most efficient vehicle for deaf children to learn language. Within this school of thinking, however, there exists a further difference in opinion. One group believes Signed English enables deaf children to become competent in English. A second group suggests that parents and teachers communicate with deaf children primarily in American Sign Language. Par-

ents become caught in the middle of this controversy and the contradictory advice given them by professionals creates a Towel of Babel in the home. It affects the very core of family life.

As students read the articles in this chapter, the impact of deafness upon family life should become clear to them. Hearing parents struggle to master ASL and use it consistently. Deaf siblings may find speaking and lipreading frustrating. Deaf family members may be inadvertently excluded from a conversation when several people speak at the same time. If families do not use a common language, parents and children are isolated from each other in their own home. This predicament is described in the poignant story told by the hearing father of a deaf girl in the book Deaf Like Me (Spradley and Spradley, 1978).

The authors of the articles in this chapter have lived these dilemmas daily. They write eloquently about family life, their love of sign language and the painful struggle to communicate with loved ones.

The issue of family communication is especially critical when a deaf child needs foster care. In the urgency to place a deaf child, agencies may give little consideration to language-compatibility between parents and the child. Deaf children may be put in homes with well-meaning parents who are totally unfamiliar with the range and complexity of communication problems that arise between deaf and hearing individuals. This problem is discussed in the article by Acari and Bateman ("The Deaf Child in Foster Care"). Furthermore, these agencies may not have the resources to manage the challenges brought to them. Armed with knowledge and sensitivity, professionals can be responsive to the needs of deaf children for an effective means of communicating with members of a foster family.

The Jeach Family, From Dad with Love

Timothy Jeach

Dear Kids,

This letter is long overdue. I've often wanted to talk to you about communication in the family, especially when we have deaf and hearing people all living together under the same roof. Aunt Marilyn and I are the only deaf persons on both sides of my family as far back as we know, but your mother came from a family that has a strong history of deafness on both sides. It won't be long before some of you get married and have children. It's possible that you might have deaf children of your own someday, and I feel it is important that we discuss this business of communication.

Sometimes people think it is altogether a different proposition when deaf parents communicate with hearing children as compared to hearing parents with deaf children. I think this is true only when the children themselves are not given the means to convey information and needs as well as that of others in their environment. When a family truly shares with each other, I don't think it matters who is deaf or hearing.

Your grandmother was one of the best teachers I ever had. She had the ability to teach me things without making it "like school." Interested in developing my speech and speech reading, as well as my sister (Aunt) Marilyn's, "Gram" had a knack for making a game out of something we had to practice.

I can remember when she would make us leave a quarter orange peel in our mouths and ask us to talk to each other, trying to lip read what was said. Another "game" was when she'd tilt the lamp shade and have one of us stand between the lamp and the wall. That was great fun, because we learned you can lip read a shadow! Your grandmother never learned how to use Sign Language, but she shared all she had, and she communicated the fact that she loved me and wanted me to learn as much as possible. I hope I have conveyed this to you, also.

Before you start to wonder if it wasn't necessary for your grandmother to learn how to sign, let me assure you that I have been asked this question a hundred times by others. I'm convinced that if she had seen the advantages of using whatever means of communication (voice, signs, fingerspelling and hearing) that were available, she would have done so and we would have been even better off.

Today, they call this use of all available modes of communication "Total Communication." The term was coined by Roy Holcomb, a deaf educator, but more importantly, "Total Communication" (TC) has led to:

. . . . an unequivocal acceptance of deaf people as people, a belief that the language of signs is legitimate, that it belongs, that it is the cultural language of deaf people and the best possible tool that we have to become part of their existence and, as a consequence, to grow with them (Benderly, Dancing Without Music).

The above statement was made by a hearing person, and it is in direct opposition to the usual cliche that the deaf "must learn to live in a hearing world." While the latter is always true, it does me a world of good to see that people are beginning to recognize that a "deaf world" exists and has much to offer, just as Blacks, Hispanics, Orientals and other minorities have.

Did we use TC at home? Can we say we grew up during the last 20 years using a combination of voice, signs, fingerspelling and hearing? No, we didn't. We were content to use signs and fingerspelling because it was all we needed. We used voice, depending on who was talking with whom. You used voice with me, because I did with you. However, with your Mom you didn't, because she did not feel comfortable with her voice. Was that TC? Yes it was, because it was a situation where individuals in our family were accepted for what they were, not for how well they spoke or put together a sentence.

You may or may not remember how we were upset with you when you forgot to sign for us when you were talking among each other. We tried to explain that it was rude to leave people out of a conversation when they were in the room or right in the group. It was a while before you were able to show us that hearing kids don't always make it clear to their hearing parents what they are talking about either! The reasons why people don't always seem to acknowledge each other are not as conventional as we would like them to be.

Why was it that some of your friends felt ill at ease around us and yet others would feel perfectly at home with us? Was it ignorance? Was it a fear of the unknown? Was it personalities? Perhaps it was what some people call "vibes!" At any rate, you were able to communicate to us that it did not always have to do with the fact that we (the parents) were deaf, but that people are different, some more sophisticated and mature than others.

When you became older, you developed more meaningful relationships with certain friends. These people came over more often, stayed longer and had more reason to want to know your parents better. This was something we hadn't realized before.

I realized that the more I involved you in discussions regarding communication with the deaf, the more able you were to articulate the same ideas to your friends. Armed with knowledge, they gradually overcame their natural dis-

comfort and became more interested in knowing us as persons other than their friend's parents.

You see, this business of communication in the family has got to be a two-way street. I sometimes think there is too much emphasis on "if you sign it, say it, and if you say it, sign it." I don't mean to say it's not important, just that it's too shallow. As parents, we need to understand how a child with normal hearing thinks and develops, just as you need to learn about deaf people other than your parents.

Improving my style of communicating with you became a priority after your mother and I went out to dinner with good friends of ours. I had just finished ordering dinner for us when our friend proceeded to order for himself and his wife, using signs and speaking at the same time. After the waitress left, I asked him why he had signed to the waitress. His reply was, "But how would you know what I was saying to her?" Right then, I realized that I had been guilty of leaving deaf people out of what I thought was inane conversation.

The lesson in this is not so much deciding what or which conversation is important to be simultaneously signed and spoken, but rather, developing a conditioned reflex to signing and speaking simultaneously.

To tell the truth, I did this primarily for your mother's sake, so as to never leave her out of a conversation. Every time I forget to sign and speak in the presence of others "listening in," the restaurant scene manifests itself. However, after Mom passed away, I slipped to old habits and stopped signing when I talked with you. I'm sure it affected your signing skills, but at the time, I didn't think anything of it because we communicated pretty well as it was. What I did not realize until later was that it certainly affected your communication skills with my deaf friends and acquaintances.

I have noticed considerable improvement in your ability to sign, during recent months. I'm quite sure it has to do with my marriage to another deaf woman. Perhaps it is also the fact that Silvia is from Mexico City and has only recently become comfortable with American Sign Language that makes you more aware of the need to *communicate* effectively. Perhaps another factor is that the English language has to be explicit, due to the switch from Spanish. Boy! It's hard enough to have a deaf stepmother to adjust to, but to have one from another country truly adds a multi-cultural dimension.

As if this array of situations weren't enough, you've found there's an eight year old deaf girl named Rosangela in the package! On the day I took the plunge and proposed to Silvia, I can remember my thoughts: "Now I'll have a deaf child—a ready-made one, too—and all my beliefs on how to raise a deaf child are going to be put to the test!"

It has been nearly a year and a half now. I'm quite sure it would have been much easier making the adjustment had you been younger or Rosangela a baby. I know that the subject of stepmothers and stepchildren is a whole field of study by itself, but I want you to know that you've come a long way in making adjustments. Oh, we still yell, argue, cry and take pot-shots, but we can *talk*. Not just sign fluently, but communicate our feelings much better than before. I hope we all have learned that it's not only *how* but *what* we are able to get across.

There are some people who insist that TC means you sign and talk in the presence of the deaf person, no matter what that deaf person is doing, as long as he or she has the same opportunity to "overhear" or "pick up" snatches of conversation. The whole idea is to provide equal opportunity and respect human dignity. After all, who wants to be the poor deaf person in a room sitting like a bump on a log while everyone chatters away, oblivious to his or her presence?

I used to get pretty fired up about scenes like that and I still do. However, there are times when 100 percent compliance to a "rule" of TC can backfire. People are only human and don't always mean to be rude by leaving deaf persons out. It is important to teach children like Rosangela how to be assertive, rather than aggressive, so she can develop strategies for getting people to sign for her, rather than laying back and fading into the wallpaper because nobody had the presence of mind to acknowledge her.

People simply do not respond to being yelled at or ridiculed into doing something that needs to be done. At least, they aren't as willing as if they were *taught* what they need to do. The general public is basically ignorant of the needs of the deaf and only a good public relations gimmick is going to enlighten them. The "gimmick" is education of the general public *and* showing the deaf how to be diplomatic, if not assertive, regarding their rights as human beings.

I only hope that you have learned from me as much as I have learned from you. It is important that we realize that answers to questions can never be used for universal solutions and that solutions often depend on individual needs and aspirations. Because man is not a machine, diversity is the basis for a rich and creative life.

At the beginning of this letter, I said that you might someday have deaf children—and you might not. Whatever happens, I will be one happy father with the knowledge that you are part of a growing segment of the "hearing world" which recognizes that deaf people are a cultural entity and have a right to shape their own destiny.

With *much* love,

Dad

Nothing is Impossible—the Hughes Family

Patty Hughes

As the second child of deaf parents who have four deaf children, I would not want to replace our comminication method with any other. We have a very good communication line among each member of the family. All of us are profoundly deaf, and we all use American Sign Language. Each of us children acquired language when we were about nine months old.

My two sisters, my brother and I were all born in Missouri. My oldest sister, Bonnie, and I received most of our education from the Missouri School for the Deaf in Fulton, and some from the Virginia School for the Deaf and the Blind in Staunton. My younger sister, Mary, and my brother, Billy, attended both schools too, but stayed at the Virginia School longer. My parents both graduated from the Missouri School for the Deaf.

I don't recall if I ever felt that I was "deaf" when I was a child. My parents taught us to rely upon ourselves first, and being in a deaf family made it hard for me to realize that there was anything different about being deaf.

We shared a lot of things in growing up together. For example, we'd watch TV programs and guess together what was happening. We'd exchange our guesses with each other and usually agree on some conclusion. It didn't matter if our conclusion was right or wrong, since we had no way to find out what was actually occurring on the TV screen.

Before we owned a TDD, we used to ask one of our neighbors to make occasional phone calls. If our neighbors were not available, we'd have to ask a stranger to make it. That could be embarrassing at times. However, my parents always made the point to us that we could not help but to swallow some of our pride and approach strangers for help if a phone call was urgent.

Our family would go out to eat once or twice a week. During these dinners out, my parents set an example for us in writing down their orders and encouraging us to do the same. They emphasized to us that it made things much easier to write the order down, than trying to talk, as talking could lead to unnecessary misunderstandings and frustrations. We were also encouraged by my parents to write down a note for our doctor, before the actual appointment, to save time and to make sure the doctor got an accurate description of what the problem was.

The only time in my childhood years that I actually wished my parents were hearing was when I was introduced to some "bad" signs for the first time by friends at school. I knew I could not use them in front of my parents, because I'd be punished, whereas my deaf friends who had hearing parents could sign all the "bad" signs they wanted at home without their parents understanding a word!

In my family, it almost seemed as if my parents had two separate families to raise. Bonnie and I are less than two years apart, but Mary and I are five years apart. Thus, there were different things about Bonnie's and my upbringing, and Mary's and Billy's.

Bonnie and I grew up in Missouri whereas Mary and Billy grew up in Virginia. When we lived in Kansas City, Missouri, there were clubs for the deaf, a kindergarten for deaf children, and oral programs in the schools. My parents usually took Bonnie and me to the clubs for the deaf so we could play with the other kids there. They also sent us to a kindergarten with a program for deaf children, and Bonnie and I also attended the Troost School, which had an oral program.

The main reason we attended the Troost School was so that we could associate with the hearing kids. My parents thought this was very important for us. About the time that Billy and Mary would have entered school, we moved to a town up north in Missouri, and all of us attended the Missouri School for the Deaf.

We moved up north so that my Dad and his deaf partner could establish themselves in a dry-cleaning business in Moberly, Missouri. Then he and the partner decided to open up two more dry-cleaning businesses in Kirksville, Missouri. Bonnie and I spent our summers helping Dad by working at the counters (with customers coming in). We communicated by writing, and memorized most of our frequent customers' names. By watching Dad, we learned how to be comfortable with different communication modes, such as writing, with the customers.

When I was younger, I did not fully realize how frustrating it must have been for Dad when he opened up the businesses, as many of his deaf friends discouraged him from doing this just because he was deaf. Some people even stopped by the store and told Dad he was crazy. But these frustrations only made him more determined to prove to both deaf and hearing people that deaf people *can* do it!

Dad and his partner operated the businesses for eight years. Then Dad got a job offer to teach dry-cleaning at the Virginia School for the Deaf and the Blind. He grabbed the opportunity because he felt that he needed a change in his life and because he wanted to be able to spend more time with the family. He also felt we could get a better education at the Virginia School, and he wanted to go into the field of missionary work with deaf young people. Thus we moved to Virginia, and all of us girls have graduated from the Virginia school. Billy is still a student there.

In spite of the differences in ages the communication link in my family is very strong and powerful. We usually spend hours and hours talking together during and after supper. My parents believe strongly in encouraging us to share our thoughts and feelings with each other.

When my parents quarrel, all of us know what they are quarreling about, as they believe in open communication between them and us. There is a funny incident I remember well. When Billy was about four years old, my parents were quarreling one evening and Billy was trying hard to figure out what was going on. Finally, in the middle of a hot moment, he politely interrupted and asked them to slow down so he could understand better!

We rarely visit our relatives, because we don't enjoy feeling "left out of it" as we do when we visit them. All of our relatives except an uncle and a cousin are hearing, and most of them don't know Sign Language. I do wish sometimes that we had better communication because it would be nice to get to know them better.

When I was about 20 years old, it was the first time I really worked with hearing people, and my first experience in realizing that I am deaf and will experience some frustrations as a deaf person. The building where I worked was nearly full of people who had never met a deaf person before. When my boss and I were introduced to each other, he looked awed, and I was tempted to say, "Hey, I look normal, don't I?"

But we shook hands, and his first question to me was if I could lip read. I told him yes, but I'd rather write. Thus, all afternoon on that first day we spent hours writing back and forth to get acquainted.

The first week at work was very frustrating, since it was the first time I'd really had to deal with a communication barrier. As time passed, things became much better at work. I felt great working there for the summer as I felt I had won a battle in learning how to cope with communication barriers, and when I was asked to work there again, I felt good about it.

Sometimes I imagine that my family was hearing, and wonder if I would encounter this kind of frustration. But most of the time I am glad I have encountered it, and consider myself very lucky to be born into a family where my parents succeeded in teaching me to let nothing stop me just because I am deaf. That is the greatest lesson I have learned from them.

Bilingual Experiences of a Deaf Child

Judith Stein Williams

My husband and I had long expected that our children would have impaired hearing. Our genetic makeup showed this: Our parents, my uncle,and his four sons are deaf on my side, and four uncles on his side, and so are we. I was born deaf. My husband lost his hearing at the age of six months during an attack of whooping cough, which could be a sign that he was easily susceptible to deafness. When our son Todd was born, he showed so much alertness with his eyes and was so unresponsive to normal sounds that we knew he was like us.

My main concern was not his inability to hear (he is nearly five now and I still don't even give it a thought), but was instead how well he could live within the hearing world. His language acquisition was far more important, since this could open many channels for him including speech, lipreading, manual communication, and writing. The most important part was being able at an early age to express himself linguistically in the simplest forms. Lack of this ability can lead to personality and psychological problems. So I started talking to him like all mothers do, cooing, babbling, singing nursery rhymes and the like— but I added signs and fingerspelling while doing all this.

It was not until he was nine months old that he finally expressed himself clearly in sign language. He loved to throw his spoon on the floor from his highchair and yell for me to pick it up. I always asked him, signing and speaking, "Where is the spoon?" pointing to it before picking it up. This time he threw it again but asked me in signs, WHERE SPOON? and pointed at it. This led soon to his substituting in this frame other signs

(words) like ball, light, cat, dog, and book; and we went on to using the "Pictionary" and "First Objects" and other books I read to him from while he looked at the objects pictured. By the time he was one year old he was able to identify about fifteen different things in short sentences. His vocabulary increased, but it was not until after he was toilet trained (at about twenty months) that I introduced him to fingerspelling and put a lot of stress on this way of presenting words. He mastered this kind of communication of sentences on his level in a few months, and he associated the manual alphabet with the printed alphabet. At twenty-five months he started reading, and when he was turning three, he had five hundred words in his reading vocabulary and loved to read prep-rimers and beginning-to-read books. His language developed in the simultaneous sense, that is, through lipreading my speech, fingerspelling, printed matter, and signs. I see no conflict in his bilingual acquisition of English and Sign but believe that it greatly aided him. He loved nursery rhymes and was able to recite them himself. He eventually used his speech and sang some syllables out loud.

I enrolled him in the Gallaudet preschool when he was thirty months old, and its program gave him a lot of auditory training and speech work which I was not able to give him at home. His hearing aid did wonders (although he has an 85 decibel loss in both ears across the whole frequency range), and he responded more to speech and showed willingness to learn to say words accurately.

From this point everything else seemed to come naturally, and his curiosity brought him even further, until I would say that he is progressing just as normally hearing children do except that he is less vocal. He learned English very readily in expressive exercises, routines, monologues, and interpretations as well as in social responses and requests for information as the situation required. Simplification of grammatical structures was necessary in the early stages, but now at four years and ten months he simplifies them himself for his sister, Tiffany, two years younger, and elaborates them for his Daddy.

His bilingual experience is in some ways like and in others unlike that of the American-Japanese bilinguals studied by Susan Ervin-Tripp (1964). Todd has a more general knowledge of Sign, because that is the language more often used at home, and a specific knowledge of English from his education at home and in school. His is really a merger of the two languages, therefore, as in the case of the Japanese women who tend to use Japanese for social intercourse and as their base language when with other bilinguals but who do use English as the situation and the persons talked to require. Todd relies more on his Signs than on his English with his family and more on spoken English in the classroom.

As Ervin-Tripp says, ". . . bilinguals who speak only with other bilinguals may be on the road to merger of the two languages, unless there are strong pressures to insulate by topic or setting." Her hypothesis is that "as language shifts, content will shift." And she presents examples of the Japanese women's monologues in which *moon, moon-viewing, zebra-grass, full moon,* and *cloud* are in Japanese, and *skyrocket* and *cloud* are in English. This kind of difference needs more study in the case of Sign-English bilinguals. There may even be a trilingual situation—some words in signs, some spoken, and some in English spelled in the manual alphabet, depending on the who, where, and what of the communication.

Another observation Ervin-Tripp makes is that the Japanese women "were in an abnormal situation" when one was asked to speak English

with another Japanese woman. The effects on the style of English were clear when the two situations were compared. With the Japanese listener there was much more disruption of English syntax, more intrusion of Japanese words, and briefer speech.

This is also true in cases where two deaf children are forced to speak English to each other. I notice that Todd shortens his statements and tries to add signs between them. He uses more complex ideas, structures, and words in Sign than in spoken English.

In school Todd's English is more or less that of a four-year old in a preschool situation. But at home, when he was three years old, he asked me at the table (in signs), "Where does the meat go?" I asked him what he meant, and he replied: "Look, I swallow the meat, and where does it go?" I then explained to him in details he could understand, and he was pleased and satisfied with the answer. Another time, about six months later, he asked me where a sound he was listening to came from. I told him that I couldn't hear anything at all but that he and Tiffany and Daddy have a little hearing. He was very much hurt by this and offered me his hearing aid, hoping I would respond to sound. When he learned that it was of no help, he cried and was upset for a while. Later I told him he could help me by telling me to move the car over when he hears fire engines or ambulances passing by, because I must give them right of way. He now delights in telling me when he hears a siren, and he lets me know when he hears a sound and identifies it for me—the vacuum cleaner, someone knocking on the door, and the like. He doesn't have much hearing but uses his residual hearing well and intelligently.

Are there any deaf children this age without sign language who can express themselves this well, ask such questions, and make such distinctions? There are none that I know of. Knowing signs also helps Todd in learning English vocabulary. For example, Todd learned about a zebra in school but not the sign for it. When he came home, he told me about the characteristics of this new animal so I could easily identify what he was trying to find out—both of us using his "base" language of signs.

For young deaf children the most important contribution of sign language is to the child's expression of his needs, questions, and responses. With it he can also develop other channels of language and expression. Without it he may have some receptive competence, if he happens to be a very good lipreader, but he will be terribly hampered in his formative preschool years. Moreover, the spoken language the teachers are trying to instill in him becomes warped because he can't really use it expressively to ask questions and to make and try out corrections after being told of his grammatical mistakes.

Sign language has advantages for the hearing children of deaf parents as well. Their bilingual experience of serving their parents by making phone calls and receiving spoken messages can be very valuable. As they use both languages they translate from one to the other. The need to interpret for deaf parents makes them listen to adult conversation with more than normal childish attention. In return they get top grades in reading, spelling, grammar, and other subjects in school, as I found when I made a personal survey of my parents' deaf friends who have hearing children, about forty children in all.

These observations agree with the results of Meadow's study (1968). She notes that many professionals warn parents against sign language in case children are motivated not to learn speechreading and speech. Her study proves these fears false and shows that deaf children that are exposed to sign language in early childhood have better reading, speechreading, and written language scores. She concludes that "the deaf children of deaf parents [who use sign language] have a higher level of intellectual functioning, social functioning, maturity, independence, and communicative competence in written, spoken, expressive, and receptive language."

Sign language is not incompatible with English. In fact, with some care about its order and by spelling English function words, it can be made into a visual equivalent of English utterance. Unfortunately, there is not a school in the United States that uses it as a medium of communication between teacher and pupil, except in the advanced department. That is too late.

References

Ervin-Tripp, Susan (1964) An Analysis of the Interaction of Language, Topic, and Listener, *American Anthropologist*, 86-102.

Meadow, Kathryn P. (1968) Early Manual Communication in Relation to the Deaf Child's Intellectual, Social, and Communicative Functioning, *American Annals of the Deaf*, 113, 29-41.

The Empty Crib

Lou Ann Walker

Ever since she could remember, Shirlene Timmons had wanted to be a mother, so she was thrilled when she learned that she and her husband, Joey, were expecting their first child. Joey, Jr., was born on November 24, 1981. The Timmonses, ecstatic, brought him to their home, in rural Okeechobee, Florida, where they had readied a crib and an array of toys for the infant. But their happiness was short-lived.

Just three months later, Shirlene stood in the small, spotless home, sobbing in panic and frustration. She was living every mother's worst nightmare: Her baby had been taken from her, and she didn't know how to get him back. Shirlene picked up little Joey's teddy bear and hugged it—just as she ached to hug her son. She sobbed as she looked at her child's empty crib.

Joey, Jr., had been healthy but tiny at birth, weighing less than five pounds. Worried by his size and lack of appetite, the Timmonses took their son to a hospital in nearby Stuart. The doctor who examined the two-week-old infant said he had salmonella poisoning, and he characterized Joey, Jr., as a "failure to thrive" baby—a damning phrase that indicates parental neglect.

The diagnosis was later proved wrong. Joey, Jr., was suffering from an inherited allergy to milk, not from salmonella poisoning. But it was too late. The Timmonses had already been reported to a state agency that would take away their child and lead them through a bureaucratic labyrinth for the next four years.

How could a child be taken from loving, caring, concerned parents? Joey, Sr., explained the only way he could: in sign language. "It's because we're deaf," he signed to his distraught young wife.

But Florida's Department of Health and Rehabilitative Services had a somewhat different answer. Counselors in HRS's Okeechobee office said that the Timmonses lacked parenting skills and, because of their deafness, could not give their child enough verbal stimulation.

Tragically, however, the HRS workers reached that conclusion without consulting any experts on deafness.

Contrary to what the agency counselors believed, the vast majority of hearing children who grow up with deaf parents have normal childhoods. With the help of relatives, teachers and friends, some children find that having deaf parents can be an enriching experience.

I know this is true. My parents are deaf. Though I am hearing, I grew up signing and eventually became a sign-language interpreter and a writer and editor. My experience is similar to that of other hearing children of deaf parents: As I grew older, I interpreted for my mother and father and became their bridge to the hearing world.

A bridge is needed because, as Helen Keller once said, "Blindness cuts people off from things. Deafness cuts people off from people." This was particularly true for the Timmonses. The state never provided a fully certified sign-language interpreter for their conferences with the couple or for court proceedings, so the Timmonses had only a fragmentary understanding of what was happening. And they had difficulty making themselves understood as well. "Hearing people think we're stupid," Joey, Sr., signed to me as we talked about the tragic case.

Battling a bureaucracy

From the start of their ordeal, the Timmonses were faced with a series of obstacles that seemed almost impossible to overcome. Because there were no teletypewriters (used by the deaf to make phone calls) anywhere in the Okeechobee area the couple couldn't call HRS. Instead, Joey, Sr., and Shirlene had to go to the agency just to make an appointment to see a counselor. When they did get an appointment, they found that trying to communicate with the counselors was almost unbearably frustrating. Most disturbing of all, the Timmonses never understood that they were entitled to an attorney in their battle with HRS.

Despite these difficulties, Joey, Sr., and Shirlene were determined to get their baby back.

But in early 1982, just a few months after Joey, Jr., was born, the Timmonses' case looked bleak. After placing the infant with Joey, Sr.'s brother and sister-in-law for a few weeks, HRS put Joey, Jr., in a foster home in Okeechobee. There seemed little hope of his being reunited soon with his parents.

Baffled and fearful, Shirlene and Joey, Sr., went to the HRS office to find out when they could have their son back. The couple paced up and down the agency's halls, agitatedly stopping employees and begging to know when Joey, Jr., could come home. Finally one counselor took the time to write them a note. It read only: "I don't think you'll get the baby back."

That night, a distraught Shirlene signed to her husband: "I want to hold Joey." Feeling that he had no choice, Joey, Sr., drove the next day to the baby's foster home.

After he pulled into the driveway, Joey, Sr., walked into the house and straight to the baby's crib. "I want Joey," he signed, and he gently picked up the baby. The guardian ran to call the sheriff. Joey knew he wasn't welcome, but he had no way of hearing the telephone call. He stood chucking the baby under its chin, smiling, doing what every proud father does. As Joey, Sr., was leaving the house with his son, a police car pulled up, its lights flashing. A sheriff got out and pointed to Joey, Sr.'s car, telling him in the simplest possible terms to leave.

The father handed over his son and returned home. "I knew they would stop me," Joey, Sr., later signed to Shirlene, "but I had to try."

In order to get their baby back, the Timmonses did their best to comply with a list of court-approved conditions drawn up by just one of the many "alternative case plans" and "performance agreements" that are part of the agency's baffling vocabulary. HRS demanded that the Timmonses demonstrate their ability to budget their money and maintain a stable home. The agency also complained about the couple's dogs, even after Joey, Sr., told them, "They're hearing-ear dogs." In a further effort to placate the agency, Joey and Shirlene later agreed to take classes in "effective parenting" and "hygiene," although Shirlene was already a meticulous housekeeper.

Joy—and heartbreak

In December 1982, nearly a year after Joey, Jr., had been taken from the Timmonses, their prayers were finally answered. A judge ruled that he was satisfied with the couple's efforts to comply with the conditions specified by HRS. Shirlene and Joey, Sr., could have little Joey back.

It's going to be a wonderful Christmas after all, Shirlene thought. She wanted a tree with all the traditional decorations, candy canes, toys wrapped in red and green paper—a truly special Christmas, the first she would enjoy in peace with her son.

But HRS still exerted a great deal of control over the Timmonses' lives. Caseworkers were free to make unannounced visits for inspections. "They just walked in," Joey, Sr., recalled angrily. "And they even came when we weren't at home and snooped around."

Ironically, Shirlene's eagerness to follow HRS instructions led to the family's being criticized by a worker for the agency. Shirlene, seeing the employee arrive for an inspection and remembering that she had been told in hygiene class to put everything away, quickly gathered the baby's toys and stored them in the closet.

In the report on the visit, the inspector said the couple had failed to provide toys for their son!

The state seemed determined to view the Timmonses in the worst possible light. In April 1983 a clinical psychologist issued a report saying that Joey, Jr., "had notable deficiencies . . . in language and cognitive skills development . . . it is felt that he is definitely lacking in adequate stimulation . . . This is a direct consequence of the parental limitations and impairments." But at that point, Joey had lived most of his life in a *hearing* foster home.

Joey, Sr., refusing to be discouraged, vowed to keep his family together—and to provide for them. "I want to be responsible for my family," he told a friend.

The task was not an easy one. Okeechobee is a depressed area, with a high rate of unemployment. Most of the area's few jobs are on dairy farms. Joey had worked at odd jobs whenever any were available. He now took the only steady job he could find—at a dairy in a nearby town. But the hay aggravated his asthma, and an allergy to milk and cows caused him to break out in rashes and hives. Every evening after work, Joey, Sr., came home to his wife and son with a hacking cough. Every day Shirlene watched him grow weaker and weaker. Joey, Sr., finally had to quit the job after three months because of his ill health. It was a bleak time; the family barely made ends meet.

At the end of 1983, one year after Joey, Jr., had been reunited with them, the Timmonses decided to go to HRS and ask the agency for help in applying for financial aid.

But when the couple walked into the office of Chuck Coles, an HRS supervisor, for a scheduled meeting, they found that Shirlene's mother had been called in. (Shirlene's parents, John and Shirley Ledford, didn't get along with their son-in-law. The middle-class Ledfords seemed to feel that Joey, Sr., one of eleven children in an impoverished rural family, was not good enough for their daughter.)

Coles took Joey, Jr., from his mother's arms and gave him to Mrs. Ledford, according to the Reverend Quentin Hampton, a volunteer worker who had accompanied the Timmonses to the office.

"It's only for thirty days," Coles told the couple. "Just until you get settled."

"No, it's not!" Joey, Sr., signed furiously. He shook his fist in frustration. Shirlene burst into tears. Finally, an armed police officer escorted Mrs. Ledford and Joey, Jr., home.

Angry and disheartened, the parents at first refused to go to court again. "They keep tricking us," Joey, Sr., signed angrily.

HRS now demanded that the Timmonses put Joey, Jr., in day care for eight hours a day, five days a week, so he could get enough auditory stimulation. The cost: $2,000 per year. Until the couple proved they could pay, they could not have their son.

Hampton, who grew close to the Timmonses during their ordeal, spoke later of the "unfairness" of the HRS demand. HRS didn't explain where they could find the money, and they were ignoring the fact that they had a radio, a television set and hearing friends who came over."

"Besides," Shirlene added, "I wanted Joey home with me. I stay home so I can take care of him."

Advocates of the couple also point out that there are many poor people in the area whose children do not speak English. But these sons and daughters of migrant farm workers are not required to go to day-care centers in order to remain with their parents.

While the Timmonses were fighting to regain custody of their son, Shirlene gave birth to a second child, James, in June 1984. Once again, the parents were delighted; once again, their hopes were dashed. Within four months, HRS asked the court to take James away from his parents, saying that a neighbor reported the child cried "for an hour at a time"—something that is common among newborns.

Joey, Sr., promised that he and his wife would watch the baby even more closely. While a counselor stood on the Timmonses' doorstep, Joey, Sr., signed to his wife: "Watch the baby all the time, or they'll take him away, too!"

The first victory

Eventually, Sid Garcia, a young lawyer with Florida Rural Legal Services, heard about the case from another lawyer. Garcia says, "He told me he thought the rights of these people were getting trampled on." A native of Cuba, Garcia is bilingual and speaks passionately about human rights. He took the case immediately.

In January 1985, Garcia went before Judge Burton Conner, of the Circuit Court in Okeechobee, arguing that the Timmonses should be allowed to keep their younger child. He won. Conner turned down HRS's request to take James from his parents.

The Timmonses, elated by their first victory over the bureaucracy, shook Garcia's hand. "Now you get Joey back for us," they told him.

Garcia was angered by the inconsistencies in the case. "Here the court was allowing James to stay in the home, but they still weren't allowing Joey to go home! That's what I don't understand," he says heatedly. "How could they allow one child to stay in the house when conditions supposedly weren't right for the other?"

By mid-1985, Garcia's efforts had begun to pay off. Joey could stay with his parents for a few days each week.

Finally, in the fall of 1985, Joey, Jr., began living full-time with his parents. But the family faced one more court appearance, in February 1986.

In the courtroom, the interpreter used a form of sign language that was incomprehensible to the Timmonses, who use American Sign Language. As Shirlene looked anxiously at the faces of the people who would determine her family's future, she understood only a small part of what they were saying.

Suddenly the proceeding was over. "What happened?" Shirlene signed to another interpreter, who had come to testify. "Do I get to keep little Joey?"

"Oh, yes! Yes, you do!" the interpreter signed. "It's all over! Finished!"

Shirlene cried and bent down to hug her sons.

HRS officials said that the final hearing was not a victory for the Timmonses but merely a natural "winding down" of the case. "We never want to *keep* the children," says a supervisor. "Our goal is to reunite the families."

But the agency's conduct during the case angered deaf people and children of deaf people across the country. The National Center for Law and the Deaf, in Washington, D.C., received so many calls that it offered Sid Garcia legal materials from similar cases.

"It was an outrage in this day and age for such a thing to have happened," says the Center's Legal Director, Sy DuBow. "It was a stereotyped decision, based on wrong assumptions."

Looking back on the case, Garcia says "HRS was primarily motivated by the fact that Joey and Shirlene were deaf. They tend to be overzealous. The Timmonses may not have the nicest living area in the world. But they're good people. They love their children, and they are entitled to their children. I'm just glad it's over for them."

Together again

Today the Timmonses are a family once more, living in a neat, comfortable trailer just beyond the Okeechobee town limits. Joey, Jr., had been required by the court to continue in day-care classes for a time, and he now goes to a school that has agreed to take him free of charge.

Although HRS had insisted that there would not be enough auditory stimulation for a hearing child in the Timmonses' home, the trailer is not a silent place. Joey, Jr., and James talk to each other and to their parents. The boys' pet bird chirps in a cage. Two crowing roosters strut around the yard. The television set is often on. But it is the blond, blue-eyed youngsters who are the center of attention.

When I told the Timmonses that my own parents were deaf, both Joey, Sr., and Shirlene quickly and excitedly asked me, "Were you ever taken away from your parents?"

"No, never," I answered.

"Your parents are very lucky," Joey, Sr., signed gravely.

Shirlene and Joey, Sr., were so angered by their ordeal that they may bring a lawsuit against HRS workers.

The couple were robbed of most of their first-born's infancy, and the battle with HRS led Joey, Sr., to have a vasectomy, even though he and his wife would have liked to have a larger family. We don't want them to take any more children," he explained.

But the Timmonses are determined to make up for lost time. After their final court battle last year, the family was invited by a friend for a once-in-a-lifetime four-day spree at Disney World, in Orlando. Joey, Sr., loves showing visitors photos of the family's only vacation. As his father recalls the trip, Joey looks up from a coloring book. "I loved Mickey Mouse!" he says.

The Timmonses are also teaching their sons American Sign Language, molding the boys' tiny fingers into real words—words the children will use one day as interpreters between their parents and a world that has too often been insensitive and cold.

Joey, Sr., looks at his children proudly and tells me: "I taught them to sign 'Hello, Daddy. I love you.' "

The Deaf Child in Foster Care

M. Teresa Arcari and Beth Gwinn Betman

Although considerable emphasis has been placed on the issue of permanency planning for children in foster care, significant barriers must often be overcome in order to attain this goal. This is especially true when children who have special needs—in this instance, deaf children—are placed in homes ill prepared to meet their needs, and when workers responsible for planning for them do not have sufficient information about the disability or available resources. Although reference is made to foster care throughout this article, all points made are equally valid in the identification of appropriate adoptive homes.

Advocates for Hearing Impaired Youth, Inc., which was formed in 1982 for the specific purpose of assessing the needs of the estimated 4,000 to 5,000 children with hearing impairments placed under the care of social service agencies, is committed to providing child placement professionals with some awareness of and sensitivity to these special needs. The effort has grown out of the perception that in most cases, deaf children are inappropriately placed in substitute care. Increased knowledge of the issues specific to hearing impairment will help to ensure progress toward the goal of permanency planning for deaf children and avoid needless multiple moves.

A central area of concern involves the identification of foster families with communication skills that match the needs of individual deaf children. Those children with severe to profound hearing loss will most often use manual communication—sign language—in place of, or in addition to, speech. In seeking parents with sign language proficiency, the value of working with the child to attain as much speech as possible should not be overlooked. However, the use of total communication (both signing and speech) in order for deaf children to achieve early exposure to language is also important.[1] Whatever the final decision regarding the most appropriate communication style, it must be based on adequate knowledge about these issues.

Placement Concerns

Typically, social workers have had little, if any, exposure to deafness and have only a limited idea of what the "individual needs" of a deaf child are. Because of family crises, placements frequently occur without much time for planning. The deaf child is often placed with foster families who have boundless good will but no knowledge of the disability and no sign language skills.

In those rare cases where the social worker has some beginning knowledge of sign language, his or her skills most often fall short of the ability to explain to a child the events that are taking place. Frustration and disappointment for family and child usually result. The child faces two alternatives: quiet "adjustment" to a setting that affords very limited communication and often results in a sense of isolation that is extremely damaging,

---

1   E. Mindel and M. Vernon, "Oralism Only or Total Communication." in *They grow in silence,* Silver Spring. Md., NAD Press, 1971.

or acting out behavior that precipitates one move after another.

Angie's case illustrates the difficulties that may be encountered by the child, the foster family and the social worker.

Angie, an 11-year-old girl living in a large institution for dependent children, was one of the first children assigned to the social worker—who had had no previous contact with deaf individuals—for placement in a foster home. Prior to that, Angie had been placed in a residential center for severely disturbed children with the diagnosis—later to be found inaccurate—of "selective mutism" thought to result from Angie's experiences with her schizophrenic mother, whose bizarre behavior left her without any clear idea of normal, day-to-day life. (The children in this family often needed to beg meals from the neighbors or look for food in the trash. The mother performed strange religious rituals in the home and was often found wandering naked in the streets.) Based on this history, the original diagnosis was, in fact, a good guess, but wrong. The correct diagnosis of profound hearing loss was finally made when Angie was 10 years old and she was moved to the institution.

Although neither the worker nor the prospective foster parents had any sign language ability, they tried to prepare Angie for placement through drawings, gestures and carefully planned day trips. Despite their efforts, the final placement was quite traumatic. When she saw her suitcase, Angie knew that this was to be a big step and she was terrified. She threw a temper tantrum and attempted to get out of the car while it was moving on the highway.

After arriving at the new foster home, Angie sat on her suitcase for several hours. Through drawings and the kind, patient behavior of the new foster parents—and perhaps because she was too tired to fight anymore—Angie agreed to stay overnight. This began a long, uphill battle toward successful adjustment and growth.

Unlike Angie's foster family, most do not follow through to learn sign language—a process that takes a significant investment of time and energy—even after expressing an initial interest. While they are trying to help the child fit in with the new family, foster parents of a deaf child are simultaneously working cooperatively with special school placements, learning about the care and use of a hearing aid and taking the child for further audiological tests and perhaps additional speech therapy. Only the very committed succeed with so many demands.

In order to be fair to both the deaf child and foster family, foster parents must be identified who already possess basic communication skills and a knowledge of the disability.

Recruitment

Where would a child placement agency begin to recruit foster parents with the necessary knowledge and skills? If the agency has the good fortune to be located near a school for the deaf, this facility may have staff with sign language ability who would be interested in accepting a child into their home. Parents with a deaf child who have developed self-confidence from dealing successfully with their own child's disability may possess the needed communication skills and be willing to extend themselves to other children.

Individuals who grew up with a deaf sibling or whose parents were deaf often have fluent sign language skills and the needed sensitivity. Because these individuals frequently have regular contacts with hearing impaired adults in the deaf community, they can provide their deaf children with successful role models. The well-developed network of deaf clubs and deaf church congregations provides additional major meeting places for those with the skills necessary to raise deaf children, and these sources should not be overlooked in any serious effort to recruit appropriate foster homes.

This, of course, raises the question of active recruitment of deaf adults as foster parents. Why not tap this ready-made resource? The practical problem that must be confronted is the communication barrier between worker and prospective foster parents—a barrier that is not insurmountable.

A fundamental question that may need to be addressed first is whether agency administrators and workers view deaf indivduals as "handicapped." When deaf adults are seen in this light, they are perceived as those who *receive* services rather than as possible service *providers*. Often, child placement professionals do not see the deaf community as having capable adults who can impart valuable coping skills to deaf youngsters. Agencies do not seem to be aware of a responsibility to hire qualified sign language interpreters to facilitate the process of identification and matching of deaf children with deaf foster parents. These service gaps tend to be pervasive in spite of the provisions of Section 504 of the Rehabilitation Act of 1973 (P.L. 93-112). This Act states that any agency may not deny a handicapped person the opportunity to receive benefits or services that are equal to those offered non-handicapped persons, and may not provide them with benefits or services that are not as effective as the benefits or services provided to others.

Issues During Placement

With the arrival of a deaf child in the foster family, new demands are inevitable. Accommodation always requires a shift in attention and efforts to help the newcomer gain an equal footing with existing family members. Obviously, this does not happen overnight. Considerable adjustment is required for each person in the home. For example, any discussion in the presence of the hearing impaired child, whether directly related to the child or not, should be signed. Allowing conversations to be "overheard" enables the child to become privy to the thousands of incidental exchanges that normally occur in any

household. A considerable amount of information about relationships and day-to-day living is learned in this way.

If the family does not already have strong ties in the deaf community, special efforts may be required to find appropriate church congregations and social clubs. Visits with deaf peers from school, who often live some distance away, will need to be arranged. Such requirements must be identified and discussed with prospective foster parents ahead of time. They should also be encouraged to ask themselves two basic questions: Will I become tired of the extra effort? Will I wish these special needs would go away?

Frequently there is the subconscious hope, by both natural and foster parents, that if enough energy is invested, the deaf child will eventually become like a hearing person. Helping the child to maximize residual hearing through the use of hearing aids and fostering development of verbal skills through speech therapy are desirable steps to be taken. However, when the disability does not magically disappear, many parents become discouraged. The reality is that the deaf child does not become like them, a part of their hearing world. At this point parents often feel that they have failed and greatly curtail efforts on behalf of their child. Realistic recognition of the child's limitations from the beginning and encouragement of his or her strengths, interests and abilities can guard against their fantasy of "rescuing" the child from deafness.

Natural parents raising a deaf child need to know something about how hearing loss affects the stages of development.[2] Foster parents must consider this information, as well as additional factors related to the more complicated life experiences of children who come into foster care.

It may also be that the child's natural parents—overwhelmed with personal problems and unable to communicate effectively—abandoned

2 For a discussion of this issue, see H. Schlesinger and K. Meadows, *Sound and Sign, Childhood Deafness and Mental Health,* Berkeley, University of California Press, 1972.

any effort at consistent discipline. In addition, the child probably harbors deep anxieties about the meaning of the placement. Without clear and consistently available communication to ease these anxieties and set up behavioral guidelines, the child's activity level may be well beyond what is acceptable.

At the opposite extreme is the youngster who has deep-seated feelings of worthlessness related to the handicap. This child is convinced that the disability, which may have represented additional stress for the family, ultimately resulted in his or her rejection. In the new foster home the child pushes aside needs and worries in an effort to be found acceptable. If the child learns that it is desirable to express feelings and that people are sensitive to concerns, such groundwork will build a foundation for healthy interpersonal relationships.

The young deaf child who "adjusts" to a foster home and to the measure of security it provides in spite of very limited communication initially presents few difficulties for foster parents or the agency. This is not to say that the situation is problem-free for the child. Rather, issues tend to lie dormant, only to appear with the onset of adolescence.

For example, the concern has often been voiced that deaf individuals are slow to develop an appreciation for the feelings of others.[3] This should not be a surprise if the deaf child has not had continual help in sorting out the reactions of others to specific behaviors or in the comparison of feelings. Again, professionals working with deaf teenagers in foster care say that these youngsters seem to have missed out on internalizing the foster family's rules and values. The question to be answered is the same: Can one internalize values without continued exposure to them through family communication?

Yet another problem to be considered is that many children come into placement as the result

of physical and sexual abuse. Deaf children are particularly susceptible to both. Physical abuse may have occurred because of the added frustration the disability posed for the family. The incidence of sexual abuse is believed to be high because of the perception that deaf children cannot "tell" about these experiences. Because most deaf children do not receive help in sorting out these events, they are ill prepared to deal with such normal adolescent issues as developing self-esteem and sexual development.

Adolescent Concerns

Parents and workers who do not have a means of coping with significant issues early in placement face almost certain failure during adolescent years. This point is illustrated by Dana, a teenager who grew up in foster care.

During the early years Dana exhibited few difficulties and, in fact, was exceptionally compliant and not very outgoing, even among deaf peers. She had been sexually abused as a child but no one had helped her to work through these incidents. In an effort to protect her, her foster parents set up strict limits regarding her socialization outside the home, while communication at home remained on a superficial level.

Adolescent conflicts brought extreme rebellion from Dana, sexual acting out and an inability to discuss her feelings or to be helpful in making decisions regarding her future. She was finally admitted to an inpatient psychiatric unit, a placement which helped her to stabilize and then move on with her life. It seems clear that a crisis of this proportion could have been avoided 10 years earlier by more sensitive planning that included help with building on the understanding, self-esteem and communication necessary to cope with adolescent pressure.

While identity is an issue faced by all teenagers, it is further complicated for those in foster

---

3   Ibid.

care by the need to resolve conflicted feelings related to both birth and foster families. The issue of security vs. independence can also trigger heightened anxieties. Because the deaf adolescent in foster care deals with these issues and with identity as they relate to the disability, problems of wanting acceptance and not wanting to appear different become intensified. Often, there is a time of rejecting either the deaf or the hearing world in an effort to find a "fit" that is comfortable. The deaf adolescent is seeking answers to the questions of Who am I? and Can I negotiate both worlds?

Preparation for independence from the foster home presents a final area of concern. Do the foster parents have a sufficient grasp of career possibilities for their deaf youngster to encourage creativity in setting up employment goals? Or do they—through a lack of knowledge of these possibilities—demonstrate overprotectiveness and the expectation that deaf individuals will always have to depend on others? Deaf teenagers must possess the confidence that comes from knowing that they have been prepared for independence. Without this, the future is bleak, and serious depression can develop.

Worker-Agency Responsibilities

Helping foster parents to cope with so many issues on a daily basis underlines the role of the social worker and agency. The worker must be attuned to many factors that affect success in planning, including the implications of the degree of hearing loss; the pros and cons of various communication methods and educational placements; and the validity of psychological/I.Q. testing methods. In addition, the worker must be knowledgeable about the use of TDD'S, T.V. decoders, interpreters and signaling devices; Social Security benefits and other aspects of federal law as it relates to education and access to other public services; and career planning and vocational rehabilitation services.

Open communication with the deaf child is as important for the social worker as it is for foster parents. A social worker who can use sign language effectively is able to communicate directly with the child and can broach the many ongoing problems needing clarification. When social workers do not have this skill, they need to know how to identify qualified interpreters and how to use them appropriately. Workers demonstrate an understanding of the importance of maintaining confidentiality and impartiality by following these procedures and avoiding the use of family and friends as informal "interpreters."

It is important that agency policy backs these efforts fully. For example, agencies need to spell out clearly how a social worker is to obtain an interpreter for court appearances or for an individual interview with a deaf client. Who pays? Is there a special contract for hiring interpreters? Is the procedure clear and reasonably quick?

Traditionally, social service agencies have not made an effort to hire deaf social workers or workers with any specialized knowledge of deafness. As a result, cases involving deaf children are often randomly distributed among workers, a procedure that precludes the identification of special needs and the development of adequate services. Resources remain scattered. The recruitment of foster parents who already possess an awareness of deafness-related issues and communication skills is not generally recognized as necessary. Moreover, recruitment of deaf foster parents—ready-made role models for deaf children—has rarely been pursued as a solution.

It is imperative that child placement agencies begin to develop increased sensitivity to these issues. Until tangible changes occur, permanency planning for deaf children simply will not exist.

Chapter 7

Sign Language Interpretation

A sign language interpreter facilitates communication between people who use sign language and those who use spoken language. Interpreters perform several functions. One is to listen to spoken language and translate it into sign language. The other is to process sign language visually and render it accurately into spoken English. A competent interpreter will be able to perform these interpretations if a deaf person uses American Sign Language or Signed English.

The Registry of Interpreters for the Deaf (RID) is the professional organization that represents sign language interpreters. It currently issues two types of certification. A Certificate of Interpretation (CI) is awarded to individuals who demonstrate the ability to interpret between ASL and spoken English in sign-to-voice and voice-to-sign modalities. A Certificate of Transliteration (CT) is awarded to one who is able to translate literally between Signed English and spoken English in sign-to-voice and voice-to-sign modes.

The role of the sign language interpreter has evolved over time. Years ago it was not uncommon for interpreters to have close personal ties with the deaf person for whom they interpreted. Although these early interpreters were skilled signers, they encountered unforseen problems while interpreting. Remaining impartial when conveying certain information to a deaf friend or family member was difficult for them. At times, they left out offensive information, softened the message, or altered content to protect their deaf friend or relative.

Legislation passed in the 1960s required the government to pay for interpreting services for deaf people as part of the vocational rehabilitation process. The need for a forum to recruit and educate professional interpreters became urgent. In 1964, a workshop for vocational rehabilitation workers, interpreters and educators was held at Ball State College in Muncie, Indiana. At this meeting, the Registry of Interpreters for the Deaf (RID) was established. RID has become *the* national organization devoted to overseeing the profession of sign language interpretation and English transliteration in the United States. It advocates a strict code of ethics that protects both interpreters and deaf consumers of interpreting services.

Today, sign language interpreters are found routinely in hospitals, offices, classrooms and courtrooms. Interpreting is a complicated, demanding process. It takes hard work and perseverance to become proficient. Interpreters must be sensitive to the communication needs of others and adept at interpersonal relationships. Sign language interpretation is still a young profession and many issues in the field are unresolved. The articles in this chapter give an overview of the profession. Perhaps they will pique students' interest to pursue a career in this field.

Being Ignored Can Be Bliss: How to Use A Sign Language Interpreter

Barbara Fink

Much can be learned about an individual from the family, friends, and colleagues who are close to that person. Some understanding of deaf people and what it is like to be deaf and to live independently can be acquired from learning how Sign Language interpreters perform their work.

While an interpreter is a communication aid, he or she has a more extensive working relationship with a deaf person than a reader has with a blind person.

Nevertheless, this relationship is not as intimate as between a personal care attendant and a person with a severe mobility impairment. Most interpreters work with a deaf person for only three or four hours at a time. Rarely do they work repeatedly with the same individual, and when that does happen, it happens sporadically.

Deaf persons do not select interpreters from a group of interviewed candidates. Almost never does a hearing impaired person train an interpreter to the work. In fact, in many instances, interpreters, unlike attendants, are not working for a deaf person, but for the agency, school, or meeting in which deaf persons participate.

Finally, an attendant is involved with many aspects of a disabled person's life, from bathing to transportation. A sign interpreter is there for one specific purpose: Communication between the hearing world and deaf persons.

There is a poster at the bookstore at Gallaudet College, a post-secondary school for deaf persons in Washington, DC. A little elf smiles down saying, "I'm not deaf, I just ignore you." How well that describes my own situation!

Ironically, as a Sign Language interpreter, I am constantly in situations where I have to ignore people. I am most successful when I can get others to ignore me, too.

What's the big secret? Because I am certified by the Registry of Interpreters for the Deaf, I must follow the code of ethics they have established. Confidentiality is first and foremost. *Nothing* can be revealed about an interpreting assignment, including the fact that it even occurred.

So if you arrive late at a meeting or duck out for a cigarette, don't ask me what happened; I won't tell you. But all is not lost. Simply ask me to interpret while you ask one of the deaf people. That's why I am there.

Basically, it comes down to the fact that I wouldn't be there if it weren't for a communications problem between two parties. Deaf people have the same right to privacy as anyone else. It's not my right to take that away from them.

Suppressing just names and places doesn't work. The deaf community is so small, it is very easy to figure things out with a minimum of information. Suppose I tell you I'm going to traffic court on Wednesday morning, and later you meet a deaf person who has "some legal problems to take care of on Wednesday, but nothing serious." If that person also has a dented fender on his or her car, it's not hard for you to realize who else is going to court.

Other situations that can jeopardize confidentiality are more obvious. For instance, teachers ask me how deaf students are doing in school. Or employees want to know if their hearing impaired boss made the phone calls as promised. Also, many hearing people expect interpreters to be thoroughly familiar with the deaf individuals for whom we interpret.

Frequently, when I arrive at a new job, the teacher or the lawyer will question me about the deaf person's residence, employment, and other personal matters. It's hard for them to believe that, nine times out of ten, I have never met the deaf person before either. In all cases, my answer to questions about deaf individuals is the same: I will be happy to interpret when you ask the deaf person directly.

Another part of the code of ethics requires me to refrain from influencing in any way the communication I am facilitating. This means more than simple impartiality. Interpreters must in a real sense fade into the background. Sometimes, however, I can't help intruding.

Once while interpreting before a packed auditorium, I made the sign for "dream" and swung my arms wide. (Signs are made as large as possible on stage so that they are easily seen from a distance.) Somehow I knocked an entire pitcher of ice water off the podium and into the face of the speaker.

Another interpreter, also before an audience, once locked arms with a wildly gesticulating speaker. Needless to say, on such occasions, the interpreter unavoidably influences what happens next.

Actually, the code prohibits deliberately altering what someone says. I cannot add my own opinions, change that angry "damn" to a modest "heck," or leave anything out. Anything. If you say, "Ask her if she took any science in high school," I sign exactly that, including the "Ask her."

If the deaf person replies "Tell him just a year of biology," I vocally communicate every word to the hearing person. Usually, people soon realize how stiff they sound to each other and begin to speak more directly.

Sometimes, however, people are determined to involve me in the conversation. This is something I must resist. If you ask me a question or speak to me directly while I am interpreting, I will sign what you say, but I will avoid making any eye contact. Occasionally, people become aggressive, grabbing my arms in frustration and yelling, "You. You. I'm talking to you!"

Ideally, all parties will arrive early and give me a chance to explain my work. Sometimes this actually occurs, but most often people don't show up until the time for the class or the appointment, leaving me no opportunity to clarify my role.

This clarification is important for the hearing person unused to depending on a third party for communication. How unnatural this arrangement is became clear to me while learning Sign Language. Every night my classmates and I would come back from our practicum assignments and moan, "When, oh when, will people stop this 'tell him' and 'ask her' and talk directly to each other?"

Then one day we had a lecture on interpreting for deaf-blind people given by a person both visually and aurally impaired. This was the first time that many of us found ourselves having to communicate through an interpreter. The first question someone in the class asked began, "Ask him if . . ."

We all looked around in shock. If we, who supposedly knew better, found ourselves talking to the interpreter instead of to the lecturer, was it any wonder that the rest of the world was having the same problem?

American Sign Language (ASL) provides a means for deaf people to express themselves and to comprehend others as naturally as speech does for persons who hear and speak. But ASL does not simply *translate* spoken English. It *interprets* English into a different language with its own grammar, rules, and forms of expression. Like written characters in the Chinese language, many signs in ASL express concepts, not simply individual words.

Because eyes strain and get tired after even brief periods of concentration, ASL is very economical. What might take ten words to say in English is communicated in ASL by two signs and some facial expression. Even the position of the hands in relation to the body (and both the obvious and subtle movements of the hands) communicate meaning.

Still, as precisely as it has been developed, ASL has some limitations. It is very difficult to learn thoroughly and perfectly. Also, it sometimes requires more time to interpret spoken English into ASL than the interpreter has available. Consequently, we interpreters often mix interpreting in ASL along with "translating" into elemental signs some of what is spoken.

Sometimes signs and words just do not match. Nothing stops an interpreter faster than a joke like "What's black and white and red all over?" A newspaper, right? But when I sign the punch line for this type of joke, the deaf person usually wonders why everybody else is laughing. On the other hand, puns are possible in Sign Language that, when interpreted into English, mean nothing.

Fortunately, people need not worry themselves about the technical end of interpreting. That is my job. Nevertheless, if people understand the common sense limitations of interpreting, they can help me greatly. This goes for deaf people as well as hearing people. I've heard deaf people complain unjustly that their interpreter is lazy for failing to interpret conversations on the other side of a room.

While I am obligated to interpret everything I hear (including the dog barking outside or the airplane overhead), I can't hear what goes on outside in the hall or in a noisy crowd. Unfortunately, some people who always have been deaf just don't fully understand the limits on the sense of hearing.

Similarly, many hearing people do not understand the interpreter's basic need to be readily visible while working. On occasion, I have been positioned in out of the way spots, such as behind a post, or so far over to the side that deaf people couldn't possibly watch both the interpreter and the person actually speaking.

Another problem is fatigue. For a two- or three-hour class, a break after each hour gives my arms (and the deaf person's eyes) a needed rest. For a longer meeting, two interpreters should be hired to relieve each other periodically, usually every 30 minutes.

Interpreting is hard physical work. If you don't think so, try waving your arms constantly for 45 minutes. And I have the added stress of analyzing sentences to choose the correct signs and the dry throat from mouthing all the words while I interpret to aid deaf people who read lips. After fatigue sets in, it becomes harder to concentrate and I find myself thinking more about how tired I am than what is being said.

From experience, I have learned to dash for the door whenever a meeting calls a break. If I don't, invariably someone will decide they have to ask a deaf person some questions, and I spend my precious rest time interpreting. I'm only human, let me have my ten minutes.

Another thing. If you are running a meeting, look around and make sure I'm back before you resume business. I've returned to meetings before the end of the break time only to find business in full swing. The deaf people in attendance had no way of knowing the chairman, who appeared to be talking to someone across the room, had already called the meeting to order.

Another predicament can occur when a deaf person reads something while someone else gives verbal instructions, such as in many test situations. In one class I interpreted, the teacher would give out an exam, then talk constantly. For most students this was no problem, but the deaf student could not easily watch me and read at the same time. During one exam, the teacher started changing the questions verbally. To quickly get the deaf student's attention, I began flicking the light switch off and on.

The same teacher's love for slide shows also caused problems. At a moment's notice, the classroom would be plunged into darkness. My request for a little light during slide presentations was countered with the teacher's suggestion to wear day-glo gloves. But eventually he agreed to leave one light on during slide shows.

It is extremely difficult to interpret when more than one person speaks. (No, I can't sign one person on each hand.) Usually this happens when people are arguing, so it's even more difficult for me to follow along. Interpreters are divided on how to handle this. Some say it is alright to request people to slow down and stop interrupting each other.

Other interpreters feel you should just sign as much as possible, since the hearing people probably aren't getting it all either. Another difficulty: I usually point to whoever is speaking; and if people are cutting each other off, I spend more time pointing than signing.

A blind woman told me about a similar problem she had, but in reverse. At one meeting, the same interpreter vocalized what two different deaf people were signing. Since there was only one voice, the blind woman assumed only one deaf person had the floor and kept contradicting himself. When she finally realized the true situation, the blind woman asked the deaf participants to identify themselves each time one of them spoke. Some meetings avoid this problem altogether by hiring more than one interpreter.

This brings me to a sore topic. People hate to pay interpreters. Apparently, it is thought that this takes advantage of the deaf person's handicap. But then so do doctors, hearing aid dealers, and hospitals. No one denies that they should be paid for their services.

Look at the truth of the situation. First, we interpreters are professionals who have trained long and hard to perfect our skills. Secondly, if you are not willing to pay me, I have to take another job and not be available for the 10:00 a.m. conference or the 2:00 p.m. doctor's appointment.

Still, interpreters who volunteer do not necessarily act unethically. Occasionally, we donate services to worthy causes or to help out friends. Certainly, I am not going to send a bill for every joke I sign at a party. But generally, I have found that the people who are *always* willing to volunteer get into interpreting situations beyond their skills.

They also tend not to follow ethics because "after all, I wasn't really interpreting, I just went along to help out." That might be alright for a meeting or a chat at the water cooler. But it is a bad bargain for anything else. The money you pay an interpreter is well worth it.

Certification of interpreters is done by the Registry of Interpreters for the Deaf. Like other applicants, I was tested by a panel of both hearing and deaf interpreters. (Yes, there is such a thing as deaf interpreters. They work in special situations, usually with deaf people who have minimal English or minimal language skills.)

The panel questioned me about my background, my interest in Sign Language, and my reasons for wanting to be certified. Then came a series of ethical questions, mostly in the form of "What would you do if . . ."

A test of my expression skills involved my listening to two tapes and signing what I heard. The first was a story which lent itself very well to ASL: It was very descriptive with different characters and lots of action. The second tape was a lecture full of technical terms read by someone who spoke faster and faster as the tape progressed.

To demonstrate my receptive skills, I had to voice (in proper English and with appropriate word choices) what I saw being signed on a videotape. For the benefit of the deaf panelists, one of the hearing panelists sat behind me and signed to them everything I said. When he put his hands in his lap, they knew I was stumped.

Of course, certification is no guarantee of quality. It is only a guide. I know some excellent interpreters who, for various reasons, decline to take the test. On the other hand, some certified interpreters seem to memorize the code of ethics before the test and then immediately forget it. Still, unless you know the interpreter's skills personally, it is safer to hire a certified person.

When calling an interpreter to arrange a job, be specific about your needs. Realize that we are people and have different combinations of skills and expertise. Also, there are various types of certification. Interpreters are supposed to refuse any job for which they are not qualified, but we need to be able to make an informed decision.

Once, I arrived at a job which the referral center assured me was fine for my skill level. It turned out to be an interview between a person charged with a crime and an attorney. I turn down all legal assignments because I don't feel I have the proper skills. Also, I do not want the responsibility of a mistake that might cost someone their freedom or a great deal of money. I suggested to the persons involved that they hire someone certified for legal work.

Other situations are not as potentially dangerous, but the right interpreter can make an important difference. At a workshop or meeting where input from deaf people is needed, request someone with good skills in communicating vocally what deaf participants say in sign. Nothing inhibits a deaf person more than an interpreter who cannot communicate the deaf person's thoughts. In these situations, the interpreter's mistakes appear to be the deaf person's, and so the deaf person will tend to refrain from speaking.

A different, but related, problem once occurred at a medical school. A deaf student missed an entire lecture that accompanied an autopsy because the interpreter fainted at the sight of the corpse. Better advance information might have secured an interpreter who was a biology major, or, like one of my classmates at Gallaudet College, worked in a funeral home.

Another type of interpreter that is very new is the oral interpreter. Technically, they do not interpret, they mouth spoken English in a form that is more visible on the lips. This is more complicated than it seems. Skilled oral interpreters are familiar with how certain words and letter combinations appear on the lips and how to accentuate them. They will also use substitute words if they are more visible on the lips and have the same meaning.

Deaf people who hire oral interpreters choose not to use Sign Language and even find signing a distraction rather than a help. Most of the time, they prefer to rely on their own lipreading and speaking abilities and not on another person for communication. The oral versus Sign Language controversy in deaf education has been going on for hundreds of years and is still not settled.

The ideal interpreting experience happened to me about six months ago. I was interpreting at a meeting at which angry people were arguing with one another. My arms got progressively tired and my eyes more and more droopy. Then one of the deaf participants declared, "The interpreter needs a break."

That someone was so thoughtful was amazing. But what happened next was even more so. The hearing person who chaired the meeting turned to the deaf person who had spoken up and said, "Okay, tell the interpreter she can have a break."

I was shocked to the core. After all those months of having people talk at each other through me, these two were talking to me through each other! I had succeeded! I was being completely ignored while direct communication took place between these two people.

That may be the ideal interpreting experience. But in my mind it would be best if people took the time to communicate directly with each other through a medium they both understand. Deaf people and hearing persons have a lot to offer each other. If we all really took the time to find out what other people have to say, I wouldn't have to work so hard to be ignored. Then I'd become obsolete. And that would be terrific.

You're a What? Interpreter for the Deaf

Gallaudet University Public Service Programs

Imagine, for a moment, what it would be like to be deaf. You cannot hear what people say. Nor can you hear your own voice, and so you can learn to form words only with great difficulty. How would you make your ideas known? And how would you learn what others have to say?

This challenge confronts 14 million deaf and hearing-impaired Americans every day. Despite these obstacles, however, they do communicate effectively. Through methods such as sign language and finger spelling, they participate in schools, the workplace, and society generally. Some situations, however, call for a person equally skilled in speaking and signing to serve as a bridge between the world of silence and the world of sound. These people are known as sign language interpreters.

Bob Chandler is an interpreter who was introduced to sign language as a child. Both his parents are deaf, and he believes that he probably learned to sign before he learned to speak. After graduating from college with a degree in history, he did volunteer work with several organizations, including Alcoholics Anonymous. Work like this led to a position teaching sign language to mentally retarded deaf children. Eventually, Bob returned to school and earned a master's degree in rehabilitation/counseling of the hearing-impaired. Soon thereafter, he was recruited by Deafpride, Inc., an agency that provides interpreting services.

In the recent past, most sign interpreters were friends of deaf persons or members of a deaf person's family. But more and more people like Bob are earning their living as interpreters. Many, like Bob, graduated from training programs. Such programs are offered by colleges and universities in more than 30 States.

The trained interpreter is qualified in various manual communication systems, including American Sign Language and manually coded English.

Interpreters often differentiate between types of interpreting. Platform interpreting is performed near the speaker—on a platform or a stage—and in front of an audience. Such interpreters must use large, clear signs. In contrast, one-on-one interpreting is done face-to-face with the client. Janet Bailey, president of Sign Language Associates, Inc., an interpreting services firm, has experience with both types.

Janet became acquainted with sign language at an early age. Her mother, an instructor in a school for deaf children, taught her finger spelling. As an adult, her interest in signing was renewed when she helped a neighbor's child enroll in a sign language course at Gallaudet College in Washington, D.C. Janet decided to enroll, too. She completed several more courses and began to undertake some interpreting assignments. When *Good Vibrations,* a theatrical production, was staged at the college, she became part of the show, combining her interpreting skills and her acting talents. She has gone on to interpret for the Folger Shakespeare Theater, Arena Stage, Ford's Theater, and the John F. Kennedy Center for the Performing Arts, all in Washington.

Sign language interpretation places some unusual demands on its practitioners. Michael Jay Hartmann can attest to that. He's been interpreting for 12 years and has worked in a variety of situations, including owning and running his own interpreting services firm. He, too, began his career with voluntary work, interpreting for fellow students at the University of California and at religious services at the local temple. He now works as a program specialist for the handicapped for the U.S. Department of Health and Human Services, where his duties include being the official interpreter for the Secretary.

Bob, Michael, and Janet are among the 2,600 certified sign language interpreters in the United States. Certification is awarded by the Registry of Interpreters for the Deaf (RID), a nonprofit organization of professional interpreters. RID offers three different kinds of certification: comprehensive, performing arts, and legal.

Some of the principal customers of interpreters are schools, courts, and medical institutions. Most clients hire interpreters for one assismment at a time, so interpreters are usually freelancers. As a rule, they are paid by the hour, with rates starting at $10 and going up depending on the expertise of the interpreter and the complexity of the assignment.

Freelancing can be difficult. For Maureen Baglio, a freelancer affiliated with Sign Language Associates, the nature of the work is both a drawback and an advantage. "The uncertainty can be unnerving," she says, but adds that freelancing provides a freedom not found in salaried employment. Bob Chandler agrees. "You must be able to deal with an uncertain schedule and do without the fringe benefits that most people take for granted," he states. "But," he continues, "the thing I like is being in a different situation every day."

Bob's statement points toward one advantage of being a sign language interpreter. It's easy to move from job to job and place to place. Interpreters can find work all over the country. Michael Jay Hartmann says he was working 2 days after he arrived in Washington. "This is a good profession to be in if you've been properly trained," he says.

To be a good interpreter, you must possess certain talents. Sign language interpreters have excellent listening skills, clear mouth movements, and a good imagination. The best interpreters are excellent mimics. A shrug of the shoulders or a tilt of an eyebrow might be essential to impart not only the message but the nuances as well.

Sign language interpretation also demands fortitude. The energy and concentration necessary to listen to a speaker and provide a simultaneous translation to the client are considerable. For this reason, interpreters often work in teams when doing a particularly long session, alternating about every half hour.

According to Richard Dirst, former executive director of the Registry of Interpreters for the Deaf, there is a growing need for interpreters. He states, "Opportunities in interpreting for the deaf are increasing rapidly throughout the United States. The increased demand for interpreters in all facets of the deaf individual's life has created a shortage of qualified interpreters in almost every part of the country."

A career as an interpreter for the deaf can be challenging and rewarding. The ability to communicate in another language opens up a wide variety of opportunities and offers the chance to see the world from a wholly new perspective. To be an interpreter also provides the chance to be of service to those who can use your help.

On Gaurd!

Elaine Gardner

An interpreter who does not recognize the possible legal ramifications of interpreting is not a true professional. The interpreter who is familiar with the laws relating to interpreting not only does a great service to the deaf community and the profession, but also avoids many legal pitfalls.

Since the implementation of Title V of the Rehabilitation Act of 1973,[1] sign language and oral interpreters have been utilized to a greater extent and by a wider range of professionals and agencies than ever before. Hospitals, health clinics, mental health programs, courts, legal aid attorneys, public defenders and law enforcement agencies are now required to ensure effective communication for hearing impaired people by providing professional interpreters.

Like other professionals, interpreters must be aware of the legal implications of their behavior to avoid inappropriate, prejudicial or unethical conduct. Inadequate interpreter skills or lack of professionalism can have grave consequences for the deaf person and serious legal implications for the interpreter. Therefore, it is important for both the interpreting profession and the deaf community to understand interpreters' legal rights and obligations.

The Privileged Communication

Introduction to privilege

An issue of great concern to the deaf community and professional interpreters is whether an interpreter can be forced to testify about information obtained while interpreting. The fear that such information will be revealed by interpreters voluntarily, or involuntarily pursuant to court order, causes some deaf persons to withhold important information from professionals with whom they are meeting. It is important for all parties to such communication to understand which communications are protected by law and which communications the interpreter can be forced to reveal.

For public policy reasons, the law has chosen to protect certain communications from the court's power to compel disclosure. These communications, designated as "privileged," must meet the following criteria: 1) they must be confidential in nature; 2) this privacy must be essential to promote a successful and honest relationship between the parties; 3) the relationship must be one which society wishes to foster; and 4) the injury the disclosure of this type of communication would cause to the protected relationship must be greater than the benefit to the court of thereby gaining information.

Simply put, there are certain important relationships in which the parties need to be sure that what they say is private and cannot be disclosed

---

1   29 USC § 794, as amended.

by force of court order. Examples of some of these protected relationships are wife/husband, attorney/client, doctor/patient and clergy/parishioner. Additional privileges are sometimes also available, depending on the statutory law of the individual state. These can include psychologist/patient, therapist/patient and reporter/source.

Protection of interpreters from compelled disclosure of priveleged information

Not just any communication is protected as privileged communication. Even communication between two persons who share one of the relationships listed above must be made specifically in connection with this relationship, and without the presence of third parties.

Generally, the element of confidentiality essential to the establisliment of the privilege is missing when a third party is present during the communication. Therefore, the presence of most third parties destroys the privilege.

However, exceptions have been established to this third party rule. In an otherwise privileged situation, a third party's presence will not destroy the privilege if that third party is acting as the agent for the professional, the client, or both, and the presence of that agent is necessary for the conduct of the professional counseling. For deaf persons who rely on sign language to communicate, interpreters fit squarely into this third party exception. As agents of one or both of the individuals involved, they are unquestionably essential to furthering the relationship. As a result, an interpreter's indispensability in this area has been recognized by virtually every court reviewing this issue.[2]

When there is a need for a sign language interpreter, the presence of the interpreter should not dissolve the confidentiality of an otherwise privileged communication. However, circumstances do occur when deaf persons may desire the presence of family members, in addition to the interpreter, in situations which would otherwise be privileged. Especially when a deaf person is facing serious legal or medical problems, the presence of relatives can help provide background information and support to enhance free and accurate communication.

In a case before a Maryland court, an interpreter and close relatives were present during a jailhouse interview between an attorney and his deaf defendant charged with murder. An interpreter certified by the Registry of Interpreters for the Deaf (RID) was subpoenaed to testify before a grand jury as to the communication which took place at that time. The interpreter refused to testify, saying that she preferred to face jail than betray a confidence. In a major victory, the Maryland Circuit Court judge threw out the subpoena on the grounds that even in this situation a sign language interpreter is covered by the attorney/client privilege. The court stated: "When both attorney and client depend on the presence of an interpreter for communicating to one another, the interpreter serves the vital link in the bond of the attorney/client relationship."[3]

Moreover, the judge went a step further and found that the presence of close relatives during a deaf person's interview by an attorney does not necessarily destroy the attorney/client privilege. The judge, sensitized to the varying communication needs of the deaf individuals, stated:

---

2   *Hawes v. State*, 7 So. 302 (Sup. Ct. Ala., 1890); *Mileski v. Locker*, 178 NYS 2d 911 (1958); *DuBarre v. Linette*, Peake 108, 170 Eng. Rep. 96 (1791); *Parker v. Carter*, 18 Va. 273 (1814); *Foster v. Hall*, 29 Mass. 89 (1833); *State v. Laponia*, 85 NJL 357, 83A 1045 (1913); *Jackson ex dem Haverly v. French*, 3 Wend (N.Y.) 337 (Sup. Ct. 1829); *Hatton v. Robinson*, 31 Mass. (14 Pick) 416 (Sup. Jud. Ct. 1833); *Sibley v. Waffle*, 16 N.U. 180 (Ct. App. 1857); *Sample v. Frost*, 10 Iowa 266, 267 (Sup. Ct. Iowa 1859); *Tyler v. Hall*, 17 SW 319, 321 (Sup. Ct. Mo. 1891).

3   *Touhey v. Duckett*, 19 Crim. Law Rep. 2483, No. 23,331 Equity (Cir. Ct. Anne Arundel Co., November 30, 1976, slip op. at 3.)

It is readily apparent that the success of communicating through the use of Sign Language varies with the expertise of the deaf mute (sic). It would be to the advantage of any attorney who seeks to diligently represent his client, as in this case, to have members of the immediate family present to aid in the interpretation process.[4]

While an attorney, physician or member of the clergy must be duly licensed before a privileged communication with that professional can occur, there is no similar license or certification requirement for the interpreters they use. Because these interpreters are not professionals whose relationships are encouraged by law, it need merely be shown that the interpreter was an agent of either of the parties and was necessary to the communication.

The use of an interpreter should never destroy an otherwise privileged communication. Some states have taken the precaution of amending their interpreter statutes to ensure this privilege.[5] Such provisions, although often mistakenly called "interpreter privilege" legislation, do not create any new privilege; they simply ensure that existing privileges are not destroyed by an interpreter's presence.

Waiver of the privilege

Interpreters must understand that the privileges discussed above may be waived by a deaf person. In a privileged situation, the law clearly prohibits compelled disclosure of information. However, if the deaf client or patient consents to the disclosure of otherwise privileged information, a court may compel testimony by licensed professionals, or even by the interpreter who made communication possible between the professional and the deaf person. In some situations,

deaf persons themselves may subpoena interpreters to testify to otherwise privileged information. Interpreters have no legal basis for refusing to testify in these situations. The privilege belongs to the deaf person, not to the professional or the interpreter.

A waiver situation usually arises when the deaf person perceives that disclosure of the privileged communication will not prejudice—and may in fact enhance—his or her case. One example would be disclosure of an interpreted medical conference in a malpractice suit. Although an interpreter may have strong opinions about whether disclosure will help or harm the deaf person, it is not the interpreter's role to advise.

When the situation is not privileged

The majority of situations involving interpretation for deaf persons are not privileged. Employment and business situations, government benefit interviews, appointments with an accountant and public meetings are all examples of situations in which privilege does not apply. An interpreter can legally be compelled to testify about information obtained through such assignments.

Two common areas of confusion about the lack of privilege are police interrogations and private conversations between a deaf person and an interpreter. In either of these situations a privilege does not exist. However, in these circumstances, some deaf persons and interpreters mistakenly think that their communication can remain confidential.

The police interrogation situation clearly does not meet even the first criterion for privileged communications, as responses to the police are not confidential in nature. Indeed, the police are

---

4   This case was reversed on other grounds on appeal. 36 Maryland Appeals 238 (1977). *Touhey, supra,* slip op. at 4.
5   See the interpreter laws of Kentucky, 22 KRS 70 (1976), Tennessee, 123 TCA 24-108(j) (1977), New Hampshire § 521-A NHSA 11 (1977), Montana, 245 MCA 11 (1979), Florida, 19 FSA 6063 (7) (1980), Iowa, 622B ICA 6 (1980), North Carolina, 8A NCGS 5 (1981), Arkansas, 5 ASA 715.1(g) (1979), Texas, TCA Evidence Code, 3712a(c) (1979), Virginia, 37 VCA 8.01-400.1 (1979), and New Mexico, NMAS 38-9-1-1.

required to ensure that an arrested person understands the nonconfidential aspects of the communication by stating, prior to interrogation, that anything the arrested person says can and will be used against him or her in court.[6]

Many interpreters are surprised when called upon to testify regarding police interrogations which they interpreted. There is a general misconception that this critical communication is covered by a privilege of its own. But both professional interpreters and deaf persons should understand that interpreters may be legally required to repeat what is said at police interrogations.

Interpreters and deaf persons should also know that there is no legal protection for any conversation an interpreter and deaf person might have by themselves. Although they may assume that their communication is confidential, the relationship between an interpreter and a deaf person is not among those protected by privilege. Therefore, nothing communicated between an interpreter and a deaf person, in the absence of a professional carrying a privilege, can be assumed to be free from the threat of compelled disclosure.

To avoid confusion about when a privileged communication is occurring, an interpreter being used in an otherwise privileged situation may choose to step outside the room any time the professional does. This will ensure that no nonprivileged communication regarding confidential issues will occur.

Responding to a proper subpoena

There may be times when an interpreter will be subpoenaed to testify about nonprivileged communications. Many courts call upon interpreters to testify, instead of the hearing individual who used the interpreter. For example, a court may ask an interpreter to testify about a police interrogation, instead of calling the police officer who was there. This is because of the court's interpretations of the rule of evidence designated as the "hearsay rule." Under this evidentiary rule, testimony cannot generally be taken regarding communications which were not received firsthand by a testifying witness. Additionally, there may be times when the interpreter is called to testify as to information other than that communicated by the deaf person, such as which sign language mode the interpreter used.

In order to avoid subpoenas, some professional interpreters insist that nonprivileged, adversarial communications such as police interrogations be videotaped. This appears to be an excellent course, especially in serious felony cases. The videotaped communication can be played directly to another interpreter in court, thus assuring the court that accurate communication occurred, and it allows an interpreter's work to be reviewed by experts. Moreover, it relieves the original interpreter from a subpoena which may conflict with professional ethics or with that interpreter's standing in the deaf community. Many police stations are equipped with videotape equipment for recording drunk driving suspects. Therefore, it is a simple matter for them to videotape an interpreted interrogation.

The RID Code of Ethics, although compelling to many interpreters, is not legally binding in the face of a subpoena to testify. This code requires that "the interpreter/transliterator shall keep all assignment-related information strictly confidential." However, there may be circumstances in which an interpreter has no choice but to testify or risk a jail sentence for contempt of court. This is not to say, however, that the interpreter should not otherwise respect this canon to the highest degree possible. It may be advisable for the RID membership to consider the possibility of relaxing this canon to reflect the legal realities.

There are several means of alerting judges to the interpreter's quandary when subpoenaed.

---

6   *See* discussion of Miranda Warning.

Prior to testifying, or in open court, one can advise the judge of the conflict between the RID code and the compelled disclosure. The interpreter may also reduce the weight given this testimony by explaining that, as a simple conveyor of information, he or she experiences difficulties in recalling the processed information.

Liabilities of Professional Interpreting

The deaf person's recourses

Like all other professionals, interpreters are subject to complaints from those they serve, including, ultimately, malpractice lawsuits for money damages. It is critically important that deaf consumers and professional interpreters understand that there are recourses available to deaf people for the damages inflicted by poor interpreting.

Because of the need to protect deaf consumers from unscrupulous or unqualified interpreters, the RID has established a complaint procedure for the processing of complaints against member interpreters, with the ultimate penalty of decertification. Unfortunately, no professional complaint mechanism exists for interpreters who are not RID members.

Another recourse for the deaf individual is the malpractice lawsuit for money damages. Interpreters are not immune to this type of lawsuit. Realistically, they will most probably be included in a lawsuit against a professional, where both the interpreter and professional were guilty of negligence. It is important to note that even volunteer interpreters may be sued for malpractice.

Due to the growing national trend of suing professionals and the possibility of future malpractice suits against interpreters, the RID offers malpractice insurance to its members. However, the Chicago Insurance Company, which underwrites this plan, stated that it has never had a claim against an RID interpreter.

Due to the expense of a malpractice suit, a more practical means of removing a noncertified interpreter from practice may be to file an administrative complaint against the program using the interpreter, pursuant to Section 504. This is a lengthy procedure that will not recoup any losses for the deaf consumer, but its informality and low cost sometimes makes it the most viable solution.

There will be situations in which the agency or program that uses an unqualified interpreter is not covered by Section 504. In these circumstances, and prior to initiation of any Section 504 complaint, the program employing the interpreter should be contacted directly. If the reasonable concerns of the deaf person are made known, the program may voluntarily remove that individual's name from its list of available interpreters. In these situations qualified interpreters can greatly assist the deaf community in its protest over unqualified interpreters.

Avoiding malpractice claims

The best way to avoid complaints about one's interpreting skills or conduct are: self-evaluation of one's skills with respect to the individual deaf person in a given situation; complete understanding of one's role and responsibilities; and vigilant protection of oneself against attempts to misuse the interpreter's role.

The first step, self-evaluation, is perhaps the most important. Interpreters must understand that they are vouching for their own qualifications the instant they begin to participate in an assignment. It is crucial, therefore, that an interpreter honestly appraise his or her abilities to understand and be understood by the deaf person prior to initiation of the assignment. An expression of satisfaction by the deaf person should not alleviate this responsibility.

Similarly, interpreters must evaluate their qualifications to interpret in a given situation. Even if amply qualified to communicate with a deaf individual in some situations, an interpreter may not be able to communicate the terms and concepts of a specialized profession.

A second step in avoiding complaints about interpreting skills or conduct is the complete understanding by all participants of the interpreter's role. This role may vary with the needs of the deaf person involved. A well-educated deaf person may need only a translation into Signed English. However, the role of simple translator would not be sufficient for an interpreter involved in the investigation of a criminal defendant with low English-language skills. Although opinions, advice and editing are improper, in some situations it is necessary for interpreters to stress certain information to ensure the communication of important concepts. In a criminal situation, the police certainly understand the concepts and consequences of the situation; it is up to the interpreter to ensure that there is a mutual understanding of the full import of the situation.

The interpreter should be prepared in advance to educate all parties about his or her role—and to insist on doing so when necessary. For example, everyone involved should understand the neutrality of the interpreter. An agency that summons an interpreter might expect allegiance from the interpreter. Likewise, the deaf person may expect the same allegiance. Prior to initiation of an assignment, it must be made clear that the interpreter is no one's ally or advocate in an adversarial situation.

Interpreters should also discuss the best communication mode for the assignment with the parties involved. It may be necessary to explain an individual deaf consumer's need for more than simultaneous interpretation. To fulfill this responsibility, interpreters must have a knowledge of linguistics and the ability to communicate this in an understandable manner to persons who are not experts in this area.

Finally, interpreters must protect themselves at all times against the tendency of involved parties to misuse them. When an interpreter's services are not required, it is appropriate to remove oneself from the situation. Careful explanation of the interpreters role beforehand should dispel tendencies to ask an interpreter for an opinion. However, interpreters will encounter more subtle attempts to misuse them, and they must be on guard to protect themselves and their clients.

Emergency situations

The law of malpractice liability is eased somewhat in emergency situations. However, an interpreter who doubts his or her qualifications should express them so that a more qualified interpreter can be summoned. Moreover, the interpreter should question the summoning agency's designation of an "emergency." A criminal interrogation of a deaf defendant is usually not an emergency, nor is a medical procedure, short of emergency room treatment. Interpreters should not risk the serious consequences of inadequate interpreting and possible consumer complaints except in true emergencies.

Interpreting in a Legal Situation

The arrest situation

Interpreters and members of the deaf community must be familiar with deaf persons' rights in an arrest situation. The Department of Justice (DOJ) requires that law enforcement agencies receiving DOJ funding provide interpreters (certified, if possible) upon a deaf person's arrest.[7] The law enforcement agency is required to determine whether a deaf person uses American Sign Language (ASL) or Signed English, and to obtain an interpreter proficient in the preferred language.[8]

U.S. constitutional law requires that arrested persons understand certain rights and consequences at the time they are arrested. This requirement was affirmed by the Supreme Court in the case of *Miranda vs. Arizona*,[9] in which that

---

7   28 CFR Part 42, at 42.503(f).
8   45 Fed. Reg. 37630, Analysis of DOJ Regulation, (June 3, 1980).

Court set forth the Advice of Rights (the Miranda Warning) that law enforcement officials must present to arrested persons before interrogation.

The Miranda Warning is usually presented as follows:

1. You have the right to remain silent;
2. Anthing you say can and will be used against you in court;
3. You have a right to have an attorney present and consult with him before and while answering any questions; and
4. If you cannot afford an attorney, one will be provided for you without cost.

Most interpreters recognize that these warnings pose serious problems for many deaf persons. There are no commonly understood ASL signs that adequately convey terms and concepts in the Miranda Warning.[10] Because the warning is written at a sixth- to eighth-grade reading level,[11] it is meaningless to fingerspell these terms to deaf persons who read below that level.

Often, the only satisfactory means of interpreting these warnings is by rephrasing each one several different ways, and then asking the deaf person to explain what each warning means. If the police are unwilling to spend this amount of time with the Miranda Warning, the interpreter should resign from the assignment.

The exclusionary rule of evidence forbids the use of evidence procured in violation of one's constitutional rights. If an arrested person is not properly informed of these rights, statements made by that person may not be used in court. The exclusionary rule is often raised in trials involving deaf defendants. Interpreters who accept pretrial criminal assignments must be aware that interpretation of the Miranda Warning should be given a great deal of prior thought because their interpretation may be subject to scrutiny at the trial.

As noted above, interpreters can protect themselves by insisting that the procedure be videotaped. Interpreters who do not wish to subject themselves to the intensive critique that a videotape allows should not be interpreting in arrest situations.

Interpreting for deaf individuals can be a very rewarding and challenging profession. Interpreters who follow the guidelines here will avoid professional and ethical dilemmas while providing the best possible services to the deaf community.

Courtroom Hints

Prior to any court proceeding to which an interpreter is assigned, certain steps should be taken to ensure competent and professional interpreting. First, the interpreter should find out to whom he or she should report in the courtroom, and then do so. Second, the interpreter should meet with the deaf person involved to ascertain what the communication needs will be, whether simultaneous interpretation will be possible, and if a second interpreter, with a Reverse Skills Certificate (RSC), will be needed to ensure that the court will understand the deaf person.

Next, an interpreter should attempt to meet with the judge, or with both attorneys involved. Qualifications and information regarding an interpreter's professional role should be presented. The interpreter should also explain his or her physical needs, and the deaf person's communi-

---

9   *Miranda v. Arizona*, 384 US 436 (1966).
10 For example, there is no single ASL sign which is a satisfactory interpretation of the term "right." The signs commonly used are those for the concepts "all right," "can," or "correct." None of these adequately convey the total concept of a legal right. See McCay Vernon's excellent discussion of this issue for a more detailed analysis. Vernon, McCay, *Violation of Constitutional Rights: The Language Impaired Person and the Miranda Warnings*, Journ. Rehab. of the Deaf, Vol. 11, No. 4, pp. 1-8 (April,.1978).
11 Vernon, at 7.

cation needs. This is a good opportunity to ask the judge the proper means to make the interpreter's needs and limitations known during the proceeding.

The interpreter should be sworn in at the very outset of the trial. Interpretation should begin immediately and, in most cases, continue through the proceedings. An interpreter should interpret everything the deaf person says and not edit any testimony.

Physical positioning in a courtroom is important to competent interpreting. Exhibits should not block a deaf person's vision. The interpreter should be positioned within ten feet of, and in full view of, the deaf person.[12]

There is no impropriety in utilizing one interpreter to serve the needs of all deaf persons involved in a trial. Interpreters in this siuation are expected to remain totally neutral and must be very careful to protect themselves against future allegations of bias. One good solution is not to talk to any of the parties during breaks in the proceedings.

---

12 See the interpreter laws of Louisiana, 15 LRS 270B(1) (1968), Rhode Island, GLRI § 8-5-8 (1968), and Texas, TCA, Evidence Code § 3712a(b) (1979), for state statutes which mandate this positioning.

Code of Ethics

The Registry of Interpreters for the Deaf

1. Interpreters/transliterators shall keep all assignment-related information strictly confidential.

Guidelines: Interpreters/transliterators shall not reveal information about any assignment, including the fact that the service is being performed.

Even seemingly unimportant information could be damaging in the wrong hands. Therefore, to avoid this possibility, interpreters/transliterators must not say anything about any assignment. In cases where meetings or information become a matter of public record, the interpreter/transliterator should first discuss it with the person involved. If no solution can be reached, then both should agree on a third person who could advise them.

When training new trainees by the method of sharing actual experiences, the trainers shall not reveal any of the following information:

- name, sex, age, etc., of the consumer;
- day of the week, time of the day, time of the year the situation took place;
- location, including city, state or agency;
- other people involved;
- unnecessary specifics about the situation;

It takes only a minimum amount of information to identify the parties involved.

2. Interpreters/transliterators shall render the message faithfully, always conveying the content and spirit of the speaker using language most readily understood by the person(s) whom they serve.

Guidelines: Interpreters/transliterators are not editors and must transmit everything that is said in exactly the same way it was intended. This is especially difficult when the interpreter disagrees with what is being said or feels uncomfortable when profanity is being used. Interpreters/transliterators must remember that they are not at all responsible for what is said, only for conveying it accurately. If the interpreter's/transliterator's own feelings interfere with rendering the message accurately, he/she shall withdraw from the situation.

While working from spoken English to sign or non-audible spoken English, the interpreter/transliterator should communicate in the manner most easily understood or preferred by the deaf or hard-of-hearing person(s), be it American Sign Language, manually coded English, fingerspelling, paraphrasing in non-audible spoken English, gesturing, drawing, or writing. It is important for the interpreter/transliterator and deaf or hard-of-hearing person(s) to spend some time adjusting to each other's way of communicating prior to the actual assignment. When working from sign or non-audible spoken English, the interpreter/transliterator shall speak the language used by the hearing person in spoken form, be it English, Spanish, French, etc.

3. Interpreters/transliterators shall not counsel, advise or interject personal opinions.

Guidelines: Just as interpreters/transliterators may not omit anything that is said, they may not add anything that is said, they may not add anything to the situation, even when they are asked to do so by other parties involved.

An interpreter/transliterator is only present in a given situation because two or more people have difficulty communicating, and thus the interpreter's/transliterator's only function is to facilitate communication. He/she shall not become personally involved because in so doing, he/she accepts some responsibility for the outcome, which does not rightly belong to the interpreter/transliterator.

4. Interpreters/transliterators shall accept assignments using discretion with regard to skill, setting, and the consumers involved.

Guidelines: Interpreters/transliterators shall only accept assignments for which they are qualified. However, when an interpreter/transliterator shortage exists and the only available interpreter/transliterator does not possess the necessary skill for a particular assignment, this situation should be explained to the consumer. If the consumer agrees that services are needed regardless of skill level, then the available interpreter/transliterator will have to use his/her best judgment about accepting or rejecting the assignment.

Certain situations, due to content, consumer involvement, the setting or other reasons, may prove so uncomfortable for some interpreters/transliterators and/or consumers that the facilitating task is adversely affected. An interpreter/transliterator shall not accept assignments which he/she knows will be adversely affected.

Interpreters/transliterators shall generally refrain from providing services in situations where family members or close personal or professional relationships may affect impartiality, since it is difficult to mask inner feelings. Under these circumstances, especially in legal settings, the ability to prove oneself unbiased when challenged is lessened. In emergency situations, it is realized that the interpreter/transliterator may have to provide services for family members, friends, or close business associates. However, all parties should be informed that the interpreter/transliterator may not become personally involved in the proceedings.

5. Interpreters/transliterators shall request compensation for services in a professional and judicious manner.

Guidelines: Interpreters/transliterators shall be knowledgeable about fees that are appropriate to the profession, and be informed about the current suggested fee schedule of the national organization. A sliding scale of hourly and daily rates has been established for interpreters/transliterators in many areas. To determine the appropriate fee, interpreters/transliterators should know their own level of skill, level of certification, length of experience, nature of the assignment, and local cost of living index.

There are circumstances when it is appropriate for interpreters/transliterators to provide services without charge. This should be done with discretion, taking care to preserve the self-respect of the consumers. Consumers should not feel that they are recipients of charity. When providing gratis services, care should be taken so that the livelihood of other interpreters/transliterators will be protected. A freelance interpreter/transliterator may depend on this work for a living and therefore must charge for services rendered, while persons with other full-time work may perform the service as a favor without feeling a loss of income.

6. Interpreters/transliterators shall function in a manner appropriate to the situation.

Guidelines: Interpreters/transliterators shall conduct themselves in such a manner that brings respect to themselves, the consumers, and the national organization. The term "appropriate manner," refers to: (a) dressing in a manner that is appropriate for the skin tone and is not distracting, and (b) conducting oneself in all phases of an assignment in a manner befitting a professional.

7. Interpreters/transliterators shall strive to further knowledge and skills through participation in workshops, professional meetings,

interaction with professional colleagues, and reading of current literature in the field.

8. Interpreters/transliterators, by virtue of membership in or certification by the RID, Inc., shall strive to maintain high professional standards in compliance with the code of ethics.

Chapter 8

Resources

The mastery of any language is easier if extracurricular aids are available for students. The number of resources produced for students and teachers of American Sign Language is increasing annually. Unfortunately, there is no single source to which one can refer to find out about them. This chapter is a compilation of the principal resources available to anyone interested in the Deaf Community and American Sign Language.

Organizations, Agencies and Educational Institutions

Sign language students who live in or near the nation's capital are proximate to Gallaudet University. Gallaudet is a prominent liberal arts university for deaf people in the United States. The charter establishing it as an institution of higher education was signed by Abraham Lincoln in 1864. Since its founding, the University has been a cultural hub for Deaf Americans. The University has been active for over a century in educating deaf students, researching hearing loss and serving as an agency for disseminating information about deafness. Tours of the campus may be arranged through the Visitor's Center. Further information about Gallaudet may be obtained by writing the university at the address below.

Gallaudet University
Kendall Green
800 Florida Avenue NE
Washington, DC 20002-3695

Voice/TDD: (202) 651-5000

The National Technical Institute for the Deaf (NTID) is located at the Rochester Institute of Technology in New York State. NTID was established to provide post-secondary education for deaf students in technical and professional fields. Like Gallaudet University, it is an active research institution in the field of deafness. The Division of Public Affairs has additional information about the programs and mission of NTID.

National Technical Institute for the Deaf
Rochester Institute of Technology
Division of Public Affairs
Rochester, NY 14623-0887

Voice/TDD: (716) 475-6824

The National Information Center on Deafness (NICD), at Gallaudet University, is one of the leading sources of information on the language and culture of Deaf Americans in the United States. Staff at the Center network with professionals in governmental and educational agencies around the world. The staff will answer questions by phone or mail and make referrals of requests for information or services to organizations, agencies and experts across the nation.

NICD is well known for its publications on deafness and sign languages. Some titles are available free of charge. A maximum of five copies of each brochure are distributed per individual. Other publications may be purchased for a nominal fee. NICD will mail the brochure,

Publications from the National Information Center on Deafness, to any one who requests it.

The National Information Center on Deafness
Gallaudet University
800 Florida Avenue, NE
Washington, DC 20002-3695

Voice: (202) 651-5051
TDD: (202) 651-5052

The clearing house for information about legal issues affecting deaf persons is the National Center for Law and the Deaf (NCLD) on the campus of Gallaudet University. NCLD maintains a staff of competent attorneys who stay abreast of new developments in law which relate to the civil, rights of the deaf population. The staff provides legal representation as well as consultative and educational programs for interested parties in the Deaf Community.

The National Center for Law and the Deaf
Gallaudet University
800 Florida Avenue, NE
Washington, DC 20002-3695

Voice/TDD: (202) 651-5373

The National Association of the Deaf (NAD), founded in 1880, exists to advance the cause of deaf persons in America. NAD is the oldest consumer organization of disabled persons in the United States. Membership in NAD is not limited exclusively to deaf or disabled persons. All who share the philosophy and goals of the Association are welcome to join. Sign language students may consider joining NAD to support the organization and to become familiar with the major issues facing the Deaf Community in America today. *The NAD Broadcaster* is the leading publication of the National Association of the Deaf. It contains informative articles on the education, employment, history, communication and cultural status of Deaf Americans. *The NAD Broadcaster*

is provided free to members or may be obtained through an independent subscription.

The National Association of the Deaf publishes and sells a number of books, pamphlets and brochures on deafness and sign language. The Publishing Division of the NAD prints a catalog of the titles currently offered.

National Association of the Deaf
814 Thayer Avenue
Silver Spring, MD 20910-4500

Voice: (301) 587-1788
TDD: (301) 587-1789

When parents are informed that their child is deaf, they require the support and assistance of specialists in the fields of audiology, speech pathology, special education and rehabilitation psychology. These professionals assist parents in understanding the physical, educational and psychological needs of the deaf child. For years no resources were available for parents of deaf children. Fortunately, that has changed. The American Society for Deaf Children (ASDC) is a national organization founded to support the policies, programs and agencies that facilitate the development of all deaf children. Membership in ASDC entitles one to receive *The Endeavor,* a newsletter containing timely articles about raising a deaf child. Anyone interested in the mission or resources of ASDC may contact the association at the address below.

American Society for Deaf Children
814 Thayer Avenue
Silver Spring, MD 20910-4500

The organizations mentioned above are just a few of the many agencies in the United States whose mission is to increase public awareness of hearing loss, to advocate for persons with hearing, speech or language impairments and to disseminate information on deafness and American Sign Language to the public. Other agencies with similar goals are listed below.

American Deafness and Rehabilitation
Association
P.O. Box 21554
Little Rock, AR 72225-1554

Alexander Graham Bell Association for the
Deaf
3417 Volta Place, NW
Washington, DC 20007-2778

American Speech-Language-Hearing
Association
Consumer Division
10801 Rockville Pike
Rockville, MD 20852

Association of Late-Deafened Adults
P.O. Box 641763
Chicago, IL 60664

AT&T National Special Needs Center
2001 Route 46
Parsippany, NJ 07054-1315

Deafpride, Inc.
1350 Potomac Avenue SE
Washington, DC 20003-4412

Deafness Research Foundation
9 East 38th Street
New York, NY 10016-0003

National Captioning Institute
5203 Leesburg Pike
Falls Church, VA 22041

The National Theater of the Deaf
The Hazel E. Stark Center
5 West Main Street
Chester, CT 06412

World Federation of the Deaf
General Secretary
Ilkantie 4, P.O. Box 65
SF-00401 Helsinki, Finland

Professional Journals

Research on deafness began over a century ago. At that time two pioneers in the field, Edward Miner Gallaudet and Alexander Graham Bell, held diametrically opposite views on the methods of teaching deaf children. Gallaudet favored the use of sign language in the classroom. Bell was a passionate advocate of speechtraining and lipreading. Articles supporting each side of this debate began to be published. This literature gave rise to professional journals devoted exclusively to the study of deaf persons and their language. Some of those journals continue to exist today. The following list contains five prominent, contemporary journals on deafness and American Sign Language. Some of the articles in these journals may be too technical for introductory-level students; however, the list should serve to direct them to sources that are useful in writing term papers or conducting research for graduate and undergraduate courses.

American Annals of the Deaf
Donald Moores, Editor
KDES, PAS9
Gallaudet University
800 Florida Avenue, NE
Washington, DC 20002-3695

Journal of American Deafness and
Rehabilitation Association
Gerry Walter, Editor
P.O. Box 21554
Little Rock, AR 72225

SHHH Journal
Barbara Harris, Editor
Self Help for Hard of Hearing People, Inc.
7800 Wisconsin Avenue
Bethesda, MD 20814

Sign Language Studies
William Stokoe, Editor
Linstok Press, Inc.
4020 Blackburn Lane
Burtonsville, MD 20866-1167

The Volta Review
Richard Stoker, Ph.D., Editor
Alexander Graham Bell Association for the
Deaf
3417 Volta Place, NW
Washington, DC 20007-2778

General References on Deafness

Classic Titles

In every field books become classics because the authors contributed significantly to the field. All of the books below fall into that category. Although some may be out of print, the serious student of deafness should make every attempt to become familiar with them or obtain a copy for their personal library.

Crammatte, A. B. (1968). *Deaf persons in professional employment*. Springfield, IL: Charles C. Thomas.

Furth, H. G. (1966). *Thinking without language: Psychological implications of deafness*. New York: Free Press.

Furth, H. G. (1973). *Deafness and learning: A psychosocial approach*. Belmont, CA: Wadsworth Publishing Company.

Gannon, J. (1980). *Deaf heritage: A narrative history of Deaf America*. Silver Spring, MD: National Association of the Deaf.

Higgins, P. C. (1979). *Outsiders in a hearing world: A sociology of deafness*. Beverly Hills, CA: Sage Publications.

Jacobs, L. M. (1974). *A deaf adult speaks out*. Washington, DC: Gallaudet College Press.

Lane, H. (1984). *When the mind hears: A history of the deaf*. New York: Random House.

Levine, E. S. (1967). *The psychology of deafness: Techniques of appraisal for rehabilitation*. New York: Columbia University Press.

Meadow, K. P. (1980). *Deafness and child development*. Berkeley: University of California Press.

Mindel, E. D., & Vernon, M. (1971). *They grow in silence: The deaf child and his family*. Silver Spring, MD: National Association of the Deaf.

Schein, J. D. (1968). *The deaf community: Studies in the social psychology of deafness*. Washington, DC: Gallaudet College Press.

Schlesinger, H. S., & Meadow, K. P. (1972). *Sound and sign: Deafness and mental health*. Berkeley: University of California Press.

Stokoe, W. C. (1972). *Semiotics and human sign languages*. The Hague: Mouton.

Woodward, J. (1982). *How you gonna get to heaven if you can't talk with Jesus: On depathologizing deafness*. Silver Spring, MD: T.J. Publishers.

Current Books

In the last decade, the professional literature on deafness increased significantly. Gallaudet University Press, T.J. Publishers and the National Association of the Deaf are three major publishers in deafness. Scholars continue to study the medical, psychological, educational and sociological aspects of hearing loss. The following list is a sample of the kinds of books currently published in the field.

Bowe, F. (1991). *Approaching equality*. Silver Spring, MD: T.J. Publishers.

Garretson, M. (Ed.). (1991). *Perspectives on deafness*. Silver Spring, MD: National Association of the Deaf.

Holcomb, M., & Wood, S. (1988). *Deaf women: A parade through the decades*. Berkeley, CA: Dawn Sign Press.

Luterman, D. (1987). *Deafness in the family*. Boston: Little, Brown & Company.

Moores, D. F. (1987). *Educating the deaf: Psychology, principles, and practices* (3rd ed.). Boston: Houghton Mifflin Company.

Moores, D. F., & Meadow-Orlans, K. P. (Eds.). (1990). *Educational and developmental aspects of deafness.* Washington, DC: Gallaudet University Press.

Padden, C., & Humphries, T. (Eds.). (1988). *Deaf in America: Voices from a culture.* Cambridge, MA: Harvard University Press.

Schein, J. D. (1989). *At home among strangers: Exploring the Deaf Community in the United States.* Washington, DC: Gallaudet University Press.

Turk, F. R. (1990). *A Kaleidoscope of Deaf America.* Silver Spring, MD: National Association of the Deaf.

Vernon, M., & Andrews, J. F. (1990). *The Psychology of deafness: Understanding deaf and hard-of-hearing people.* White Plains, NY: Longman Publishing Group.

Wilcox, S. (Ed.). (1989). *American deaf culture: An anthology.* Silver Spring, MD: Linstok Press.

Autobiographies, Biographies and Novels

The period from 1970 to 1990 was a renaissance in literature on the language and culture of Deaf Americans. Novels, autobiographies and biographies by and about deaf persons captivated the attention of the nation at the time America was struggling to understand and accept the cultural differences among its people. These books are delightful to read. They tell intriguing stories about the triumph of the human spirit. Many are certain to appear on reference lists in sign language courses. They are excellent for leisure reading or for book reports.

Benderly, B. L. (1990). *Dancing without music: Deafness in America.* Washington, DC: Gallaudet University Press.

Bragg, B. (1989). *Lessons in laughter: The autobiography of a deaf actor.* Washington, DC: Gallaudet University Press.

Gannon, J. (1989). *The week the world heard Gallaudet.* Washington, DC: Gallaudet University Press.

Greenberg, J. (1970). *In this sign.* New York: Holt, Rinehart & Winston.

Harris, G. A. (1983). *Broken ears, wounded hearts.* Washington, DC: Gallaudet University Press.

Kisor, H. (1990). *What's that pig outdoors? A memoir of deafness.* New York: Hill and Wang.

Nieminen, R. (1990). *Voyage to the island.* Washington, DC: Gallaudet University Press.

Neisser, A. (1990). *The other side of silence: Sign language and the deaf community in America.* Washington, DC: Gallaudet University Press.

Parsons, F. M. (1989). *I didn't hear the dragon roar.* Washington, DC: Gallaudet University Press.

Sacks, O. (1989). *Seeing voices: A Journey into the world of the deaf.* Berkeley: University of California Press.

Schaller, S. (1991). *A man without words.* New York: Summit Books.

Sidransky, R. (1990). *In silence: Growing up hearing in a deaf world.* New York: St. Martin's Press.

Spradley, T. S., & Spradley, J. P. (1978). *Deaf like me.* New York: Random House.

Walker, L. A. (1986). *A loss for words.* New York: Harper and Row.

Sign Language Books

Selecting a book from which to study American Sign Language can be overwhelming. Fortunately, in formal coursework, the instructor usually will have made that decision for students. Nevertheless, if students wish to build a home library of sign language books, deciding which ones to purchase is difficult. Ironically, this difficulty did not exist prior to 1960 because then only a couple of sign dictionaries were published in America. One of them, *How to talk to the Deaf*, by Reverend Daniel D. Higgins, a Catholic priest, contained principally the signs used by Catholics in religious ceremonies.

Listing all of the books published on American Sign Language would be a volume in itself. While that is not the intent here, the following section should enable students to be informed when purchasing American Sign Language books.

Dictionaries of Signs

American Sign Language, like any other language, has a vocabulary and a grammar. Vocabularies of foreign languages are often found in dictionaries, whereas the formal rules governing usage of that language are in texts of grammar. This simple principle applies to sign language books. Dictionaries of signs are usually alphabetical listings of English words with an accompanying picture illustrating how the sign is produced. Most dictionaries use a sketch of a model producing the sign. Few ASL dictionaries use actual photographs of the signer. This technique reduces cost for the consumer. Because American Sign Language is a three-dimensional language, and the page of a book is two-dimensional, some sign dictionaries illustrate vocabulary with several sketches and arrows to show the direction and sequential motions essential in executing a sign. Learning vocabulary only from sign dictionaries is confusing for beginning students. To see the sign executed by a model in three-dimensional space is helpful.

Dictionaries of American Sign Language may be grouped as follows: (1) Comprehensive dictionaries; (2) Thematic dictionaries; and (3) Comparative dictionaries.

Comprehensive sign dictionaries include most of the vocabulary in use at the time the dictionary is printed, as does an unabridged dictionary for spoken languages. An example of a comprehensive dictionary of signs is listed be-

low. The hard-cover edition of this work contains a system of cross-referencing vocabularies from English to French, German, Italian, Japanese, Portuguese, Russian and Spanish.

Sternberg, M. L. (1981). *American Sign Language: A comprehensive dictionary.* New York: Harper and Row Publishers.

One of the most popular dictionaries of sign language was originally published in 1963 under the title *Talk to the deaf*. It's author, Dr. Lottie L. Riekehof, is a pioneer in sign language instruction and interpretation in Washington, DC. An appealing feature of this book is that the signs are grouped into classes (time, family relationships, animals) for easy reference. The most recent edition of this book contains approximately 1500 signs.

Riekehof, L. L. (1987). *The joy of signing* (2nd ed.). Springfield, MO: Gospel Publishing House.

Thematic sign language dictionaries are collections of sign vocabulary in specific content areas (e.g. signs for colors, animals or foods). These dictionaries are published in simple editions for children or in more esoteric themes. An example of each is found below.

Gillen, P. B. (1988). *My signing book of numbers.* Washington, DC: Gallaudet University Press.
Woodward, J. (1979). *Signs of sexual behavior.* Silver Spring, MD: T.J. Publishers.

Comparative dictionaries of sign language contrast the different ways a sign is made from one geographical region to another in the United States. An erroneous assumption often made about spoken languages is that single words or expressions are universally accepted in a culture to represent objects, persons or concepts. Daily experiences with English prove that is false. For example, a large sandwich might be called a "grinder," "sub," "dagwood," "club," or "hoagie" in different parts of the United States. A comparative dictionary of sign language alerts students to regional differences in signs across America. The following reference is an example of a comparative sign language dictionary:

Shroyer, E. H., & Shroyer, S. P. (1984). *Signs across America*. Washington, DC: Gallaudet University Press.

Texts of American Sign Language Grammar

Learning a new language involves mastering a new vocabulary and a new grammar. Grammar is the study of the rules which govern the relationship among the symbols of a language. American Sign Language is not English-on-the-hands. It has its own unique grammar, distinct from English grammar. Language scholars have discovered that some of the grammatical features of ASL are found in the facial expressions and body posture of the signer. Just as foreign language dictionaries usually do not contain explanations of the grammar of a language, sign language dictionaries do not contain descriptions of the grammatical rules governing the use of ASL. The following references are a sample of the many fine sign language grammars currently in print.

Baker, C., & Cokley, D. (1991). *American Sign Language: A teachers's resource text on grammar and culture*. Washington, DC: Gallaudet University Press.

Eastman, G. C. (1989). *From mime to sign*. Silver Spring, MD: T.J.Publishers.

Hoemann, H. W. (1986). *Introduction to American Sign Language*. Bowling Green, OH: Bowling Green Press.

Humphries, T., Padden, C., & O'Rourke, T. J. (1988). *A basic course in American Sign Language*. Silver Spring, MD: T.J.Publishers.

Madsen, W. J. (1982). *Intermediate conversational sign language: A bilingual text*. Washington, DC: Gallaudet University Press.

Linguistic Analyses of American sign Language

The professional student of linguistics may be interested in the growing body of research that is developing on American Sign Language. Professionals who study the manual languages of the world publish their findings in scholarly works. These linguistic treatises are written analyses of the syntactical and grammatical structures of sign languages. While some of these may be too technical for beginning students, intermediate and advanced students are certain to benefit from reading them. Those who further study sign languages should consider building a reference library of these technical works.

Baker, C., & Battison, R. (Eds.). (1980). *Sign language and the deaf community: Essays in honor of William Stokoe*. Silver Spring, MD: National Association of the Deaf.

Battison, R. (1978). *Lexical borrowing in American Sign Language*. Silver Spring, MD: Linstok Press.

Frishberg, N. (1990). *Interpreting: An introduction* (rev.ed.). Silver Spring, MD: Registry of Interpreters of the Deaf (RID) Publications.

Klima, E. S., & Bellugi, U. (1979). *The signs of language*. Cambridge, MA: Harvard University Press.

Lucas, C. (Ed.). (1990). *Sign language research: Theoretical issues*. Washington, DC: Gallaudet University Press.

O'Rourke, T. J. (Ed.). (1972). *Psycholinguistics and total communication: The state of the art*. Washington, DC: American Annals of the Deaf.

Schlesinger, I. M., & Namir, L. (1978). *Sign language of the deaf: Psychological, linguistic and sociological perspectives*. New York: Academic Press.

Siple, P. (Ed.). (1978). *Understanding language through sign language research*. New York: Academic Press.

Stokoe, W. C., Casterline, D., & Croneberg, D. (1976). *A dictionary of American Sign Language on linguistic principles.* Silver Spring, MD: Linstok Press.

Stokoe, W. C., & Kuschel, R. (1979). *A field guide for sign language research.* Silver Spring, MD: Linstok Press.

Wilbur, R. B. (1987). *American Sign Language: Linguistic and applied dimensions.* Boston, MA: Little, Brown and Company.

Books for children

Families with a deaf child need support, understanding and information to help them deal with the impact of deafness upon family life. Hearing parents of deaf children frequently ask if children's sign language books or storybooks on deafness are in print. These books are not only helpful to the deaf child but also to hearing siblings. Deaf parents often want their hearing children to share their language and culture and to understand hearing loss. Sign language primers and storybooks about deaf persons help hearing children understand their parents' deafness and master sign language.

More than a hundred children's books on sign language and deafness are presently in print. Deborah Oldman-Brown's annotated bibliography is a valuable resource. It lists books about Helen Keller, deafness and sign language and has a supplement that contains a directory of instructional resources for teachers. In 1989, Loraine DiPietro of Gallaudet University edited a supplement to this bibliography which is included with the original document when it is purchased from the National Information Center on Deafness.

Oldman-Brown, D. (1985). *Have you ever wondered about hearing loss and deafness? An annotated bibliography of children's books about hearing loss, deafness, and hearing-impaired people.* Washington, DC: Gallaudet University, National Information Center on Deafness.

Additional Aids for Sign Language Students

Videotapes

Sign language instructors differ about the value of videotapes as supplemental aids in learning the language. One side of the argument states that American Sign Language is a three-dimensional language and students will find learning signs from watching a television screen difficult. The opposing side of the argument suggests that contemporary students have been raised on television and are comfortable learning through that medium. Just as audiotapes supplement the teaching of a foreign language, videotapes are an excellent aid for teaching sign language. Regardless of this debate, the number of videotapes produced for sign language students and teachers is rapidly growing.

Two types of sign language videotapes are produced currently. One features models demonstrating the appropriate formation of the sign for a particular concept. The English word for that concept usually appears at the bottom of the screen. These videotapes are designed to build vocabulary skills outside the classroom. Also available are videotapes to teach the manual alphabet and fingerspelling.

A second type of ASL videotape presents dialogues among signers for students to use as translation exercises. In recent years, some leading Deaf Americans have filmed inspiring autobiographical tapes in American Sign Language. These videotapes are voice interpreted for the hearing audience. Through them, students not only get an exposure to ASL, but also gain an appreciation of the life journey of these prominent Deaf Americans. Videotapes on deafness and American Sign Language may be purchased from Gallaudet University Bookstore, T.J. Publishers, Harris Communications and Sign Media, Inc. The addresses for these companies are found in the summary at the end of this chapter.

Sign Language Flash Cards

Flash cards are popular aids to learning from preschool to college. Language flash cards, printed on 1 by 4 inch card stock, make mastering the vocabulary of a new language easy and efficient. The foreign word is usually printed on the front of the card. The back side of the card gives an English translation of the word as well as other relevant grammatical information.

Only a few sets of flash cards are published for sign language students. The most comprehensive set of these is the two volume edition by Harry and Shirley Hoemann. Each page is printed on 8 1/2 by 11 inch perforated stock which can be separated into nine 2 1/2 by 3 1/2 inch cards. The volumes contain a total of 1,000 signs, with an alphabetical index at the back of the book. The indexes for the respective volumes permit teachers and students to coordinate vocabulary learned with course content. Each card has a line drawing of the sign on one side. The reverse side has an English translation of the sign as well as additional linguistic information. The Hoemanns adroitly state in the Preface to Volume 1 that "learning signs is not the same thing as learning Sign Language." Sign language flash cards are a way of mastering vocabulary apart from class time which may be spent more productively on practicing sentence formation or studying the linguistic features of American Sign Language.

Hoemann, H. W., & Hoemann, S. A. (1988). *Sign language flash cards* (3rd ed. Vol. 1) . Bowling Green, OH: Bowling Green Press.

Hoemann, H. W., Hoemann, S. A., & Lucafo, R. (1983). *Sign language flash cards* (Vol. 2). Bowling Green, OH: Bowling Green Press.

Making a set of ASL flash cards can be fun. Using 3 by 5 inch index cards, students can print the English word on one side of the card in large bold letters. The opposite side of the card can be used for a simple sketch of the sign or a brief description of sign movement using homemade abbreviations such as LH for left hand, U for up, and MR for move hands to the right.

In American Sign Language, signs stand for concepts just as words represent concepts in English. Flash cards that help the student associate a sign with the concept it represents are the most helpful in mastering ASL vocabulary. One clever, inexpensive way to make ASL flash cards is with fellow students in a group project. Using a sheet of 8 1/2 by 11 inch white bond, students can divide the page into 6 or 9 equal parts with a ruler and pencil. A student with artistic ability makes a simple sketch of the signs like those found in ASL dictionaries. The master sheet is photocopied for each member of the group and cut on the lines to make 6 or 9 cards, respectively. The blank back of each card can be used to write the English translation of the sign or to paste a picture of what the sign represents. Master sheets may be passed along to other students in future semesters. This project sounds more complicated than it really is. Students who have tried this approach have found it a rewarding way to learn sign vocabulary.

Games

Not many sign language games are marketed for students today. *Keep Quiet* is a fingerspelling game like *Scrabble* for players ages seven to adult. The game comes with several cubes (like dice). On each facet of the cube is a printed letter of the manual alphabet. Players toss the cubes and try to construct as many words as possible in a minute's time from the manual letters which appear. The *Keep Quiet Reword Game* is a similar manual alphabet game.

Mystery of the Superintendent's House is a sign language videotape mystery game. It comes with a 100-minute videotape, clue cards, an instruction manual and other sundry pieces. All of these games are available from Gallaudet University Bookstore.

Because American Sign Language is an active language, gaming is a natural way to approach learning it. Mary Ann Royster and Susan Kirchner each published a collection of games for sign language students.

Kirchner, S. L. (1977). *Play it by sign: Games in sign language.* Acton, CA: Joyce Media.

Royster, M. A. (1974). *Games and activities for sign language classes.* Silver Spring, MD: National Association of the Deaf.

Students should not rule out the possibility of making their own ASL board or action game. Several of the authors' students have invented creative games that afforded them the opportunity to learn sign language in dynamic ways.

Computer Software

Software for computer-assisted instruction in American Sign Language is sparse, if contrasted to the other resources in the field. The quality of visual graphics on earlier models of the personal computer was extremely poor in comparison to the resolution of pictures on television, making the computer an inadequate visual medium for presenting signs to students. A few companies produced software for learning fingerspelling or recognizing sign vocabulary. *Talking Hands,* a fingerspelling program, is produced by EBSCO Curriculum Materials, P.O.Box 1943, Birmingham, AL 35201. Micro-Interpreter II, Computerized Animated Vocabulary of American Sign Language (CAV ASL), teaches sign language vocabulary through computer animation. The program was developed by A. Tolu-Honary, D.I.T. of Microtech Consulting Company, P.O. Box 521, Cedar Falls, Iowa 50613.

The future of this field should be promising. Computer specialists are working diligently on interactive learning programs that have excellent visual graphics. Interactive media allow the student to participate in the learning process by the selective study of pictures or videotapes in a content area. In the future, at student using this technology may sit at the keyboard of a personal computer and see on screen an ASL translation of the English text typed into the computer.

Telecommunication Devices for the Deaf (TDDs)

History and Explanation of the TDD

What does TDD mean? This question is frequently asked when one notices this three-letter code adjacent to the phone numbers of individuals and oganizations in the Deaf Community. TDD means telecommunication device for the dcaf. Telephones have been an integral part of the life of hearing Americans for decades. On the other hand, Deaf Americans have had the opportunity to communicate with each other over phone lines only since 1965. The original TDDs were teletypewriters (TTYs) used by news services to transmit printed copies of news reports around the globe. Two deaf scientists, Weitbrecht and Marsters, worked diligently to devise a way to connect the TTY to the telephone. They devised an electronic device called an acoustic coupler. This device consists of two foam cups, similar to headphones, positioned six inches apart from each other. Each "headphone" is wired to an electronic circuit that converts letters, numbers and characters (such as punctuation markers) into audible tones. One places the telephone receiver over the acoustic cups and dials another TTY number. When a connection is made with the distant TTY, anything typed on either machine appears as a printed message on the paper-roll of both TTYs.

The older, mechanical TTYs are rarely used today. The newer, solid-state telecommunication devices for the deaf (TDDs) have replaced them. TDDs are compact, portable, electronic devices with a keyboard configured like a typewriter. Just above the keyboard is a digital display upon which the alphanumeric characters typed by the operator appear. Some TDDs can be connected directly to phone lines; most, however, still use the acoustic coupling method of Weitbrecht and Marsters. Communications with a TDD are slower than voice conversations over the telephone. They proceed at the same speed as two persons typing messages to each other. For this reason, phone companies give special long-distance rates to deaf consumers.

With the revolution in microelectronics, the price of TDDs is dropping rapidly; however, deaf persons must invest several hundred dollars for a TDD and having a telephone and a phone line installed in their homes. Individuals or agencies who plan frequent contacts with the Deaf Community should purchase a TDD to insure that deaf persons have equal access to the programs and services. Many states mandate that emergency services and governmental agencies have a phone line dedicated to TDD access by deaf persons.

Telecommunications for Deaf, Inc. and Sign Media, Inc. have produced *Using Your TTY/TDD: An Educational Tape,* a twenty-minute instructional videotape on TDDs. A simpler, less expensive introduction to telecommunication devices for the deaf is the publication "What Are TDDs?" distributed by the National Information Center on Deafness.

Hearing persons consult the phone directory to locate telephone numbers. A TDD directory is printed for deaf (and hearing) consumers of TDD services. *The International Telephone Directory for TDD Users* may be purchased from Telecommunications for the Deaf, Inc., Silver Spring, Maryland. This directory is a comprehensive listing of TDD numbers of individuals, agencies, and other services for deaf consumers in the United States and Canada.

Telecommunications for the Deaf, Inc., a consumer-oriented organization, provides information and assistance to individuals about TDDs and other special electronic equipment for deaf persons. This group is an objective source of information about the range of products currently on the market. It publishes the newsletter, *GASK,* which addresses these topics.

Telecommunications for the Deaf, Inc.
8719 Colesville Road, Suite 300
Silver Spring, MD 20910-3919

Voice/TDD 301-589-3006

The Personal Computer as a TDD

The personal computer may be configured to become a TDD with the addition of a modem and special software. A modem is an electronic circuit which connects the computer to the telephone. A modem converts the electronic signals a computer generates into audible codes. Those codes are sent over telephone lines to another computer at the receiving site. Software (a set of instructions written to program the computer) for telecommunications is available from several commercial distributors. Having someone with experience in telecommunications to assist setting up a personal computer as a TDD is advisable.

Gallaudet University's Technology Assessment Program (TAP) developed "freeware" known as ASCII-TDD to facilitate telecommunications between deaf and hearing persons. Freeware is inexpensive software in the public domain. It is available from a programmer for the modest cost of the diskette and mailing. Norman Williams, author of ASCII-TDD, designed it to remove the technical hassles of going on-line. The operator provides the computer with some simple information and the computer "makes decisions" about setting up the call. It works with IBM-compatible computers and Hayes-compatible modems. The program may be purchased for a nominal fee from the Technology Assessment Program at the address below or it may be downloaded from the TAP bulletin board system (BBS).

Technology Assessment Program
Gallaudet University MSSD-200
800 Florida Avenue NE
Washington, DC 20002-3695

TAP BBS: (202) 544-3613

Electronic Signaling Devices

How do deaf persons "hear" the ring of the telephone or the whine of the smoke detector, "answer" the doorbell or "respond" to the wake-up alarm? They do so with the help of electronic devices, known as transducers. A transducer is an electronic circuit designed to change one form of energy into another form of energy. The speaker on a radio is a transducer. It changes the radio signal inside the receiver into sound. The homes of deaf people are equipped with special electronic components that convert sound into other forms of energy detectable by sight or touch (tactile sensations such as vibrations). While these devices are of little use to hearing students, to know they exist is important.

Some individuals enroll in sign language classes because they or an elderly family member are losing their hearing. In these cases, special electronic equipment and other assistive listening devices for deaf persons are extremely valuable aids to daily living. Gallaudet University distributes two publications, cited below, that summarize some of the more common electronic equipment for deaf persons. The devices described in those publications may be carried in the inventories of one or more of the companies listed at the end of this chapter.

Compton, C. L., & Brandt, F. D. (1985). *Assistive listening devices: A consumer-oriented summary.* Washington, DC: Gallaudet University.
DiPietro, L., Williams, P., & Kaplan, H. (1984). *Alerting and communication devices for hearing-impaired people: What's available now?* Washington, DC: Gallaudet University.

Continuing the Study of American Sign Language

Students often inquire about continuing the study of sign language if the institution from which they took an introductory class offers no further instruction in the language. Students can pursue many avenues in finding quality instruction in American Sign Language. Resources may even be found in one's own neighborhood.

Community colleges, colleges and universities are a good place to start the search for sign language classes. Some colleges offer both credit and non-credit (continuing education) courses. If the local college does not offer sign language instruction, students should not abandon the search there. Professors of special education, psychology, audiology, speech pathology or linguistics may know of other places the courses are offered. Deans and chairpersons of academic departments at local colleges also may know if a faculty member on staff can assist in the search.

Local Boards of Education sometimes offer a variety of courses in sign language for adult learners. These are most often taught in the evenings. Some Boards of Education mail catalogs or course schedules to taxpayers in their district. Carefully perusing these catalogs, students may discover a variety of courses that satisfy their needs.

Churches and synagogues in some regions of the country have special services for deaf persons. This fosters an interest in sign language among hearing members of the congregation. Usually deaf church members will respond to this interest and teach conversational sign language classes immediately before or after church services. Some religious groups offer extensive programs with beginning, intermediate and advanced courses, small class sizes, and much individual attention.

State and other public agencies, such as the Division of Vocational Rehabilitation, provide on site training for employees and other professionals in the community. Some of these programs are for building the sign language skills of employees. They may be open to the public or students majoring in a related field. A list of state agencies for deaf persons in the United States is published by the National Information Center on Deafness.

Private agencies that advocate for deaf persons now exist in many metropolitan areas across the Unites States. In some cases, sign language instruction is an integral part of the agencies' mandate.

In the Baltimore-Washington Metropolitan Area, The Bicultural Center, founded by M. J. Bienvenu and Betty Colonomos, two well-respected linguists in the field, offers classes, lectures, forums and public programs on American Sign Language. Anyone living in the local area has an outstanding resource within a reasonable traveling distance. The address of The Bicultural Center is provided below.

The Bicultural Center
5506 Kenilworth Avenue
Suite 105, Lower Level
Riverdale, MD 20737-3106

Individual tutoring from a deaf person, from an interpreter or from a sign language instructor is another option for continuing the study of American Sign Language. Students should be cautious when pursuing this avenue of instruction. Not everyone skilled in the use of American Sign Language is qualified to teach the language.

Private community agencies often welcome help from volunteers. Volunteer work may put students in contact with deaf people who come to the agency for assistance. These interactions could range from brief exchanges to more extensive outreach work. Any interaction with a deaf individual which taxes the language skills of an ASL student will be a valuable learning experience. It is likely to increase confidence, build vocabulary and promote fluency in the language.

The following story is an example of how community outreach can build fluency in ASL. In Annapolis, Maryland, Cynthia Abney Carter was appalled by the dearth of TDDs in public and private agencies. She realized that deaf people had little access, via telephone, to the range of services in the local county. Carter, on her own time and initiative, founded LINK, a private telecommunications relay service for deaf residents of Anne Arundel County. She worked tirelessly,

without personal compensation, to see her dream become a reality. At the start of the project, she had taken only a beginning sign language course. Several months later, after consulting with deaf citizens about improving LINK's services, she was fluent in ASL. Carter created her own "special classroom" within which to learn American Sign Language.

Professional sign lanauage interpreters sometimes teach courses in American Sign Language at local colleges, agencies or churches or know where the courses are taught. They are excellent sources of information about quality sign language instruction in the community.

Make friends with a deaf neighbor and start signing. It is a myth that one can only learn a language through formal instruction. People acquire their native language without classrooms, books, audiotapes and flash cards. They learn by listening, repeating and making mistakes. Students are encouraged to go to the places where American Sign Language is being used and meet the people who are using it. While this suggestion strikes fear in the hearts of beginning ASL students, sometimes it is the best way to continue to study the language.

Chapter Summary

This chapter contains a review of the many resources that are available to students of deafness and American Sign Language. Books, games, videotapes, flash cards and the like can take the drudgery out of learning and make it fun. Each person has a unique learning style. One student may benefit tremendously from using flash cards; another student may find them cumbersome and boring. Students should experiment with different techniques and not forget the instructor is a precious human resource in the mastery of course material.

No single distributor carries all of the items reviewed in this chapter. Some companies specialize in the sale of books, videotapes, assistive devices, or sign language novelties. The companies listed below provide literature on their line of products. The listing of a company does not constitute an endorsement of that company or the products it sells. Since errors occur in printing and proofreading, students may want to cross-reference all addresses with current literature from the company.

Gallaudet University Bookstore
Kendall Green
800 Florida Avenue, NE
Washington, DC 20002-3625

Harris Communications
6541 City West Parkway
Eden Prairie, MN 55344-3248

Modern Signs Press, Inc.
P.O. Box 1181
Los Alamitos, CA 90720
National Association of the Deaf
814 Thayer Avenue
Silver Spring, MD 20910-4500

Sign Media, Inc.
4020 Blackburn Lane
Burtonsville, MD 20866-1167

T.J. Publishers, Inc.
817 Silver Spring Avenue
Suite 206
Silver Spring, MD 20910-4617

Disclaimer

Errors inevitably occur when dealing with large databases. Every attempt has been made to record accurately the information about resources on hearing loss and American Sign Language presented in this chapter. The authors and publisher of this text will not be responsible for any inconvenience, expense, damages or harm which accrue to an individual as a result of using the material contained in this chapter or any other chapter of *Reflections on the Language and Culture of Deaf Americans*.

GLOSSARY

Some terms in this book may be unfamiliar to you. Be patient with yourself when you encounter them. You are learning the technical vocabulary of a new field. That takes time and effort. This glossary is provided as a convenient reference for you when studying. It does not include all the terms in the field of deafness.It has been developed to help you define some of the technical language found in the articles in this book.

Adventitious deafness - Acquired deafness. The loss of hearing due to accidental factors.

AMESLAN - An acronym for American Sign Language formed from the letters AME in American, S in Sign and LAN in Language.

Amplitude - The level of strength or intensity of a sound wave.

ASL sightline - An imaginary line between the signer and the receiver on which certain grammatical features are represented.

Audiogram - A graphic representation of the level of hearing loss at each frequency of sound within the range of human hearing.

Bilingualism - Equal competence in two different languages.

Certificate of Interpretation (CI) - The certificate, awarded by the Registry of Interpreters for the Deaf, verifying an individual is able to interpret from American Sign Language into spoken English and vice versa.

Certificate of Transliteration (CT) - The certificate, awarded by the Registry of Interpreters for the Deaf, verifying an individual is able to translate literally between signed and spoken English.

Cheremes - Those manual features essential to the production of signs in American Sign Language. This concept was developed by a linguist, William Stokoe, to analyze the components of signs. (Also see DESIGNATOR, SIGNATION and TABULATION).

Cherology - The study of the manual features (cheremes) of American Sign Language.

Classifier - A handshape in American Sign Language that resembles the concept it represents and is used to convey information about the action-status of that concept in a sentence.

Closed captioned decoder - An electronic device used with television receivers and VCRs to display on the bottom of the television screen written captions of the spoken dialogue or narrative in the television program.

Conductive hearing loss - A hearing impairment caused by congenital defects, an infection or an obstruction in the outer and/or middle ear.

Congenital deafness - Deafness present at birth due to genetic causes or non-hereditary factors such as maternal illness or birth trauma.

Cued Speech - A system, developed by R. Cornett, that uses a combination of hand cues and lip movements to facilitate speech reading in deaf youngsters. Cued Speech is not American Sign Language, and American Sign Language is not a form of Cued Speech.

Dactylology - A synonym for fingerspelling.

Decibel - The unit of measurement for the amount of energy required to produce sound. The scientific symbol for a decibel is dB.

Designator (DEZ) - The shape of the hands when making a sign in American Sign Language.

Directional verb - A verb in American Sign Language that specifies the nature of the subject-object relationship by the direction and manner in which it is executed.

Dominant hand - The hand most commonly used in daily activities, such as writing, eating and handling objects. In American Sign Language, the dominant hand is often the more active of the two hands in the production of signs.

Expressive language skills - The capacity to encode the contents of consciousness into the meaningful symbols of a conventional language.

Fingerspelling - Use of the manual alphabet to spell (on the hands) proper nouns as well as certain English and foreign words.

Fingerspelling space - The area just in front of the shoulder of the dominant side of the signer in which fingerspelling is most often produced.

Frequency of sound - The number of cycles or oscillations per unit of time a sound wave makes.

Gender marker - A manual prefix used in American Sign Language to designate masculine or feminine gender of the concept being represented by the sign.

Generativity - A principle of linguistics that the symbols of a language may be combined in an endless number of possible ways to form sentences.

Gestuno - An international sign language developed by the World Federation of the Deaf. Gestuno is rarely used.

Grammar - A system of rules in a language that specifies the agreement among the symbols of that language.

Homophony - A characteristic of the English language whereby different words or phrases look identical when formed on the lips. Homophony makes speech-reading extremely difficult for deaf persons.

Iconicity - The picture-like quality of some signs in American sign Language. A sign is iconic if it resembles the object it represents.

Idiom - A phrase in a language that makes no sense when literally translated into another language.

Incorporation - The simultaneous inclusion of several, distinct grammatical features in the production of a single sign.

Initialized sign - A sign made with the manual letter that correspond to the first letter of the English word the sign represents.

Interpretation - Transposing a passage as it is being spoken or signed into its equivalent meaning in another language.

Lanquage - A complex system of human communication using relatively arbitrary symbols and grammatical signals that change across time.

Lexical borrowing - The use of the symbols of one language in the vocabulary of another language. R.S.V.P. (please reply) in English is borrowed from the French *repondez s'il vous plait*.

Lexical item - A symbol in a language. In every language, the lexical item stands in place of or represents a concept.

Lexicon - All of the symbols in a language.

Linguist - A scholar who studies the structure and use of languages.

Linguistics - The scientific study of human languages.

Linguistics of Visual English - A system of manually coding English, developed by Dennis Wampler. The acronym for this manual code is LOVE.

Manual alphabet - Twenty-six specific handshapes used to represent each of the letters of the English alphabet. These manual letters are used in American Sign Language to spell proper nouns and English words.

Manually coded English (MCE) - A form of signing which preserves the word order and structure of English while using signs from American Sign Language. MCE has been referred to by some language scholars as "English-on-the-hands."

249

Mixed hearing loss - A loss of hearing caused by impairments in both the nervous system and the physical structure of the human ear.

Modulation - Change in the pitch and/or intensity of the voice for the purpose of emphasis in the language in which one is communicating.

Morpheme - Combinations of phonemes which form the smallest meaningful units of sound in a language.

National Association of the Deaf (NAD) - A national organization founded to represent and advance the cause of Deaf Americans.

Native language - The first language learned by a person.

Negative incorporation - Reversal of the direction of a sign's motion resulting in the negation of the sign's meaning.

Non-dominant hand - The hand used less often in daily activities. In American Sign Language, the non-dominant hand is usually less active in the production of signs.

Onset of hearing loss - The age at which a hearing impairment first occurs in the life cycle.

Oral Method - A philosophy of educating deaf children that relies exclusively upon speech training, lip-reading, and the use of residual hearing. The Oral Method, also known as "Oralism," does not allow deaf children to use any form of manual communication.

Phoneme - The smallest unit of sound in a language.

Phonology - The study of the sounds and changes in the patterns of speech in spoken languages.

Pidgin - A method of communicating between two cultures with different languages. A pidgin language shares some of the features of the respective languages from which it has come.

Pidgin Sign English (PSE) - A manual language which combines the grammatical features of American Sign Language and English.

Prelingual deafness - The loss of hearing before the stage in human development (18-48 months) during which the child acquires a language.

Postlingual deafness - The loss of hearing after the stage in human development (18-48 months) during which a child acquires a language.

Pronominalization - The process of representing pronouns in a language. A pronoun is the part of a language that stands in place of a noun.

Psycholinguistics - The branch of psychology devoted to the study of language as a complex symbol-behavior among human beings.

Receptive language skills - The capacity to decode the contents of spoken or signed languages into meaningful units of thought.

Reduplication - Repetition of a sign for a specific grammatical purpose.

Registry of Interpreters for the Deaf (RID) - A national organization, founded in 1964, to promote and represent the profession of the interpretation of American Sign Language.

Residential school - An educational institution that requires deaf children to live at the school during the academic year.

Residual hearing - The amount of hearing available to deaf persons to process sounds in the environment.

Rochester Method - A technique for teaching deaf children whereby the teacher fingerspells each word of the lesson being taught.

Second language - A language acquired after a person has mastered a native language.

Seeing Essential English - A system of manually coding English, developed by David Anthony. The acronym for this manual code is SEE 1.

Semantics - The branch of linguistics that studies the meanings of word and phrases.

Sensorineural hearing loss - A relatively permanent type of hearing impairment associated with a defect in the cochlea and/or auditory nerve. Hearing aids may be less effective with this type of loss.

Sign name - The unique sign used to name a person in the Deaf community. Name signs eliminate the necessity of fingerspelling of a person's name when it occurs in sign language dialogue.

Signation (SIG) - The distinct movement of one or both hands in forming signs in American Sign Language.

Signing Exact English - A system of manually coding English, developed by Gustason, Pfetzing and Zawolkow. The acronym for this manual code is SEE 2.

Signing space - The area in front of the body from the top of the head to the waist, and within the width of the elbows, in which the majority of signs are made in American Sign Language.

Simultaneous Method - The concurrent use of sign language and spoken English when communicating with a deaf person.

Syntax - The order of the symbols of a language as they appear in a sentence. Each language has a unique syntax. Without syntax, language is a meaningless sequence of symbols.

Tabulator (TAB) - The place on or near the body at which the sign American Sign Language.

Telecommunication Device for the Deaf (TDD) - An electronic device, with a typewriter keyboard, for sending alphanumeric characters across phone lines. TDDs are "telephones" for deaf persons.

Temporal signs - Those signs in American Sign Language that represent time concepts.

Total Communication - A philosophy of educating deaf children that advocates oral (speech/lip-reading) and manual (sign, finger-spelling, and pantomime) modalities and the use of residual hearing.

Translation - Transforming a passage from one language into another language. Translations are not made as languages are being uttered (Also see INTERPRETATION).

Transliteration - The process of rendering a passage from American Sign Language into its literal English equivalent.

Transparency - The recognizability of the meaning of a sign from the manner in which it is made.

World Federation of the Deaf (WFD) - An international organization of deaf people. WFD sponsors the World Congress of the Deaf where deaf leaders meet to discuss matters of interest to the Deaf Community throughout the world.

References

Abernathy, E. R. (1959). An historical sketch of the manual alphabets. *American Annals of the Deaf, 104*, 232-240.

Anthony, D. (1974-75, Winter). Seeing Essential English: SEE. *Gallaudet Today, 5*, 7-10.

Arcari, M. T., & Betman, B. G. (1986). The deaf child in foster care. *Children Today, 15*(4), 17-21.

Baker-Shenk, C. (1985). The facial behavior of deaf signers: Evidence of a complex language. *American Annals of the Deaf, 130*, 297-304.

Barnes, B. (1979, April 21). They finally listened. *The Washington Post*, p. 13.

Battison, R., & Jordan, I. K. (1976). Cross-cultural communication with foreign signers: Fact and fancy. *Sign Language Studies, 10*, 53-68.

Bellugi, U., & Klima, E. S. (1972, June). The roots of language in the sign talk of the deaf. *Psychology Today*, pp. 61-64, 76.

Berrigan, D. ASL and me. (1983). *The Reflector, 5*, 7-9.

Bienvenu, M. J. (1983). ASL: Adjective before noun or after noun. *The Deaf American, 36*(2), 27-30.

Bienvenu, M. J. (1989, September). Reflections of American Deaf Culture in deaf humor. *TBC News*, pp. 1-3.

Bornstein, H. (1974-75, Winter). New signs. . . the pros and the cons. *Gallaudet Today, 5*, 4-6.

Cokely, D. (1982). The interpreted medical interview: It loses something in the translation. *The Reflector, 3*, 5-10.

Cokley, D., & Gawlik, R. (1974). Options II: Childrenese as pidgin. *The Deaf American, 26*(8), 5-6.

Elliott, H. (1986, November/December). Acquired hearing loss shifting gears. *SHHH Journal*, p. 23.

Erting, C. J. (1985). Cultural conflict in a school for deaf children. *Anthropology and Education Quarterly, 16*, 225-243.

Fant, L. (1974-75 Winter). Ameslan. *Gallaudet Today, 5*, 1-3.

Fernandes, J. J. (1983). Thomas Hopkins Gallaudet on language and communication: A reassessment. *American Annals of the Deaf, 128*, 467-473.

Fink, B. (1982). Being ignored can be bliss: How to use a sign language interpreter. *The Deaf American, 34*(6), 5-9. (Reprinted from Disabled USA, Fall 1981).

Gallaudet, E. M. (1887). The value of the sign language to the deaf. *American Annals of the Deaf, 23*(3), 1887, 141-147.

Gallaudet College, Public Service Program. (1984). You're a what? Interpreter for the deaf. *Occupational Outlook Quarterly, 28*(3), 34-35.

Gardner, E. On guard! (1987, Special Issue). *Gallaudet Today, 17*, 31-38.

Geer, S. (1985, Spring). What are the legal issues in mental health? *Gallaudet Today, 15*, 3-5.

Golladay, L. (1980). Laurent Clerc: America's pioneer deaf teacher. *The Deaf American, 32*(7), 3-6.

Groce, N. (1980). Everyone here spoke sign language. *Natural History, 89*(6), 10-16.

Gustason, G. (1974-75, Winter). Signing Exact English. *Gallaudet Today, 5,* 11-12.

Higgins, F. C. (1983, Summer). William Mercer: Deaf artist of the Post-Revolutionary War Era. *Gallaudet Today, 13,* 28-32.

Hoemann, H. W. (1975). The transparency of meaning of sign language gestures. *Sign Language Studies, 7,* 151-161.

Hughes, P. (1981). Nothing is impossible: The Hughes family. *The Deaf American, 34*(3), 8-9.

Jaech, T. (1981). The Jaech family: From Dad with love . . . *The Deaf American, 34*(3), 5-7.

James, W. (1892). Thought before language: A deaf-mute's recollections. *The Philosophical Review, 1*(6), 613-624.

Jordan, I. K. (1988-89, Winter). Let us begin. . . . together. *Gallaudet Today, 19,* 14-15.

Kannapell, B. (1982). Inside the deaf community. *The Deaf American, 34*(4), 23-26.

Klima, E. S., & Bellugi, U. (1978). Poetry without sound. *Human Nature, 1*(10), 74-83.

Lane, H. (1977). Notes for a psycho-history of American Sign Language. *The Deaf American, 30*(1), 3-7.

Language is the key: An interview with Harlan Lane. (1985, Fall). *Gallaudet Today, 16,* 2-8.

LoCascio, E., Rubinstein, L., & Aymard, L. L., Jr. (1985). Deafness and dental health care. *Clinical Preventive Dentistry, 7*(4), 11-15.

Lowman, R. (1982, Fall). The Gallaudet poets 1930-1940. *Gallaudet Today, 13,* 6-9.

MacDonald, R. J. (1982). Communication: Our highest priority. *The Deaf American, 34*(4), 4-7.

McConnell, L. (1988, Spring). Dance fever. *Gallaudet Today, 18,* 29-31.

Meadow, K. P. (1977). Name signs as identity symbols in the deaf community. *Sign Language Studies, 16,* 237-246.

Mulrooney, J. (1972, October). *The newly deafened.* Paper presented at the National Conference on Program Development for and with Deaf Persons, Washington, DC.

Orlans, H. (1988). Confronting deafness in an unstilled world. *Society, 25*(4), 32-39.

Panara, R. (1983, Spring). Cultural arts among deaf people. *Gallaudet Today, 13,* 12-16.

Rosen, R. Deaf women: We were there, too! (1984). *The Deaf American, 36*(3), 4-9.

Sacks, O. (1988, June 2). Revolution of the deaf. *The New York Review,* pp. 23-28.

Stokoe, W. (1981). Signs and systems: What the student of sign language should know. *The Reflector, 1,* 5-8.

Vernon, M. (1987). Controversy within sign language. *The Deaf American, 38*(1), 22-25.

Walker, L. A. (1987, March). The empty crib. *Ladies Home Journal,* pp. 154-158.

Williams, J. S. (1976). Bilingual experiences of a deaf child. *Sign Language Studies, 10,* 37-41.

Wixtrom, C. (1988). Two views of deafness. *The Deaf American, 38*(1), 21.

Woodward, J. & Erting, C. (1975). Synchronic variation and historical change in ASL. *Language Sciences, 37,* 9-12.

ARTICLE EVALUATION SHEET

Student's name_____   Date_____

Title of the article_____

Major topic discussed in the article_____

List some of the KEY CONCEPTS discussed in the article and give a brief definition of each one. Use the glossary if necessary.

Concept   Definition

_____   _____

                                     _____

                                     _____

_____   _____

                                     _____

                                     _____

                                     _____

_____   _____

                                     _____

                                     _____

What is the principal idea proposed by the author in this article?

_____

_____

_____

_____

How does this article fit into the theme of the chapter in which it appears?

_____

_____

_____

_____

How does this article relate to the information presented in class or discussed in other readings?

_____

_____

_____

_____